ACE Group Fitness Instructor Manual:

A Guide for Fitness Professionals

Second Edition

Editors

Cedric X. Bryant, Ph.D.

Daniel J. Green

Christine J. Ekeroth

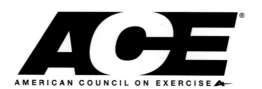

AMERICAN COUNCIL ON EXERCISE

Library of Congress Control Number: 2006909380

Second edition
ISBN 10: 1-890720-20-8
ISBN 13: 978-1-890720-20-9
Copyright © 2007 American Council on Exercise® (ACE®)
Printed in the United States of America.

C D E F G

Distributed by:
American Council on Exercise
P. O. Box 910449
San Diego, CA 92191-0449
(858) 279-8227
(858) 279-8064 (FAX)
www.acefitness.org

Editors: Daniel J. Green, Christine J. Ekeroth
Technical Editor: Cedric X. Bryant, Ph.D.
Associate Editor: Marion Webb
Design and Production: Karen McGuire
Production: Nancy Garcia
Index: Bonny McLaughlin

Acknowledgements:
Thanks to the entire American Council on Exercise staff for their support and guidance through the process of creating this manual.

NOTICE

The fitness industry is ever-changing. As new research and clinical experience broaden our knowledge, changes in programming and standards are required. The authors and the publisher of this work have checked with sources believed to be reliable in their efforts to provide information that is complete and generally in accord with the standards accepted at the time of publication. However, in view of the possibility of human error or changes in industry standards, neither the authors nor the publisher nor any other party who has been involved in the preparation or publication of this work warrants that the information contained herein is in every respect accurate or complete, and they are not responsible for any errors or omissions or the results obtained from the use of such information. Readers are encouraged to confirm the information contained herein with other sources.

Reviewers

Stephen A. Black, M.Ed., P.T., A.T.C., C.P.T., opened Sports Performance in 1991, a company providing testing, coaching, educational, and consulting services to multi-sport and endurance athletes, corporations, clubs, and organizations, with offices located in Boulder, Colo., Orlando, Fla., and Austin, Texas. With close to 25 years experience in the sports medicine field as a physical therapist, athletic trainer, and certified personal trainer, Black assists with research and development of new products, and conducts ongoing research and educational programs.

Sabra Bonelli, M.S., is the associate executive director for the Palomar Family YMCA in Escondido, Calif. Bonelli received her master's degree in exercise physiology from San Diego State University, and has been an ACE-certified Group Fitness Instructor since 1991. In addition to serving on the ACE Group Fitness Exam Development Committee, Bonelli is the author of three of ACE's fitness guides: *Aquatic Fitness, Stability Ball Training and Step Training.*

Karen J. Calfas, Ph.D., is the director of Health Promotion at Student Health Services, San Diego State University. Dr. Calfas is assistant clinical professor in the Department of Family and Preventive Medicine of the School of Medicine at the University of California, San Diego.

Richard Cotton, M.A., is the chief exercise physiologist for MyExercisePlan.com, a membership Web service that provides personalized exercise programs and support. Cotton is also the former chief exercise physiologist for the American Council on Exercise.

Ann Cowlin, M.A., C.S.M., C.C.E., is assistant clinical professor at the Yale University School of Nursing and the movement specialist for the Yale University Athletic Department. Cowlin is the founder of Dancing Thru Pregnancy, Inc. and the author of the *U.S. Army Pregnancy Fitness Train-the-Trainer Program.*

Denise Fandel, M.S., A.T.C., has served as executive director of the NATA Board of Certification (NATABOC) since 1997. Prior to becoming executive director, she served on the NATABOC Board for seven years and as president for four years. Previously, Fandel was the head athletic trainer at the University of Nebraska at Omaha as well as an instructor in the School of Health, Physical Education, and Recreation. She authored a chapter in the *ACE Personal Trainer Manual* and has been published in the *Journal of Athletic Training.*

Scott D. Flinn, M.D., is the director of the Sports Medicine Clinic at Marine Corps Recruit Depot, Parris Island, South Carolina. During his military career he worked with the U.S. Navy Seals for three years and in Italy as a family practice physician. He completed his Primary Care Sports Medicine Fellowship at San Diego Family and Sports Medicine Center affiliated with Stanford University. Dr. Flinn is board certified in family practice and has a Certificate of Added Qualification in Sports Medicine.

David L. Herbert, J.D., is senior partner of Herbert & Benson, Attorneys at Law, Canton, Ohio. He is the co-editor of the *Exercise Standards and Malpractice Reporter*, published by PRC Publishing, Inc. of Canton, Ohio. Herbert is a past presenter, consultant, or reviewer for ACSM, AFAA, ACE, NSCA, and a number of other organizations. He is the author or co-author of 10 books, a dozen book chapters, and more than 500 articles on a variety of topics dealing with the legal aspects of sport, sports medicine, negligence, exercise, and risk management.

Dale Huff, R.D., C.S.C.S., is co-owner of NutriFormance, a personal training and nutrition consulting company based in St. Louis, Missouri. Huff is a member of the *ACE FitnessMatters* Editorial Advisory Board and a frequent speaker and writer for IDEA and other professional organizations.

Irene Lewis McCormick, M.S., is an ACE, ACSM, and AFAA-certified group fitness instructor and personal trainer with more than 16 years experience. She is a master trainer, ACE faculty member, national fitness lecturer, presenter, and educator, and has contributed to *ACE Certified News, Better Homes & Gardens, ACE FitnessMatters*, and several specialty and instructional manuals. She is also the host of her own local cable fitness show. Lewis McCormick currently acts as the fitness program director at Ames Racquet & Fitness Center in Ames, Iowa, and is the spokesperson for the Better Homes & Gardens fitness Web site "The Personal Trainer" available on-line at www.bhglive.com.

Sabrena Newton-Merrill, M.S., has been actively involved in the fitness industry since 1987. Her focus has been teaching group exercise, owning and operating her own personal training business, managing fitness departments in commercial fitness facilities, and lecturing to university students and established fitness professionals. She has a bachelor's degree in exercise science as well as a master's degree in physical education from the University of Kansas, and has numerous certifications in exercise instruction.

John P. Porcari, Ph.D., is a professor in the Department of Exercise and Sports Science and executive director of the La Crosse Exercise and Health Program at the University of Wisconsin – La Crosse. He is a fellow of the American College of Sports Medicine and the American Association of Cardiovascular and Pulmonary Rehabilitation (AACVPR) and is a vice president on the Executive Board of AACVPR. Dr. Porcari's research interests have focused on the acute and training responses to exercising on a variety of exercise modalities, particularly new products on the market. He has more than 30 peer-reviewed publications and 60 national presentations.

Brad A. Roy, Ph.D., F.A.C.S.M., is the director of The Summit, Kalispell Regional Medical Center's facility for health promotion and fitness. He has more than 20 years experience in the field of clinical exercise physiology and serves as a reviewer for a number of journals.

Steve Sanchez, M.S.P.T., is the director of Physical Therapy at the Head, Neck, & Spine Center of San Diego in La Jolla, California. He is also a physical therapist at the University of California, San Diego Medical Center.

Larry S. Verity, Ph.D., F.A.C.S.M., is a professor of exercise physiology in the Department of Exercise and Nutritional Sciences at San Diego State University. He is a fellow of the American College of Sports Medicine and is a certified Exercise Specialist. He has served as an editorial consultant for ACE and has published refereed manuscripts and chapters on fitness assessment and screening.

Table of Contents

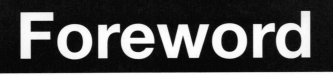

Foreword

The fitness industry is facing a unique and difficult time. While the expertise of fitness professionals has never been stronger, statistics still show that Americans are getting heavier and less active as each year passes. The American Council on Exercise has championed education and professionalism among its certified professionals for more than 20 years, and yet our mission of enriching quality of life through safe and effective physical activity remains as challenging as ever.

The benefits of eating right and exercising are almost universally known. Few Americans could honestly claim ignorance in this regard, as the benefits of physical activity are broadcast every day on magazine covers and television news programs. The difficult thing for many fitness professionals to understand is why the vast majority of individuals do not turn this common knowledge into practice. A sedentary lifestyle is as harmful to an individual's health as nearly any other risky behavior, so why is it so hard for people to get started and stick with an exercise program?

ACE has been working in recent years to reach directly to fitness consumers around the world. Instead of counting on our certified professionals to bring the ACE message to their clients, members, or participants, we've expanded our media presence and community outreach programs with a goal of directly communicating with potential exercisers. But the onus of this challenge still rests with the individual fitness professional, who is working with people on a daily basis that represent every shade on the exercise spectrum, from the completely sedentary to the elite athletes.

Group fitness instructors are in an advantageous position with regards to motivating potential exercisers, because the people attending their classes have already made the commitment to exercise, sought out a time and class type that suits them, and arrived at the session ready to work. Some of the major hurdles have already been cleared, but that does not mean that instructors are off the hook in terms of reaching out to potential exercisers. Aggressive and targeted marketing campaigns, volunteer opportunities, and well-considered networking are all means of acquiring new participants. ACE has been working with clubs and individual professionals to develop the tools that group fitness instructors and personal trainers need to expand their client bases and increase class attendance. It is important to remember that ACE is not simply a certifying agency, but is instead a partner and resource to be utilized throughout your career in the fitness industry.

National statistics and global trends can be a bit overwhelming at times, and they should be reviewed and understood by all members of the fitness community. But you should never lose sight of the fact that your goal, each and every day, is to positively influence people to have an enriching relationship with physical activity and acquire a lifelong fitness habit. If every ACE-certified Professional maintains that focus with every individual they work with, eventually these small successes will have a global impact.

Scott Goudeseune
President
American Council on Exercise

Introduction

The role of group fitness instructors is constantly evolving. Not only are instructors expected to be experts in all things fitness-related, but they are also expected to specialize and become innovators. The list of class types grows longer each day, with the latest trends including fusion classes that bring together such seemingly disparate activities as yoga and indoor cycling, Pilates and strength training. But remember, before instructors specialize and even create their own classes, it is essential that they first master the foundations of fitness and health.

The *ACE Group Fitness Instructor Manual,* Second Edition, was designed to serve the dual purpose of providing the core knowledge required to design safe and effective exercise classes and offering information on specialty areas that will help new instructors become more focused and thereby increase the demand for their services.

As with all ACE manuals, this new manual offers the most current, complete picture of the foundational knowledge, instructional techniques, and professional responsibilities group fitness instructors need to teach safe and effective exercise. Designed to serve as a study aid for the newly revised Group Fitness Instructor Certification Exam, it is also a comprehensive resource for new and veteran group fitness instructors.

It is important to note, however, that the scope of information presented in this manual will not exactly match the scope of information tested in the ACE certification exam. Exam candidates should refer to the Exam Content Outline in Appendix B for a detailed syllabus of information covered on the certification exam. In addition, ACE acknowledges various experience and skill levels among group fitness instructor exam candi-dates. As such, we encourage candidates lacking the practical skills and experience related to teaching group fitness classes to take advantage of ACE-approved training programs and products to prepare for the ACE examination.

The 12 chapters that comprise the *ACE Group Fitness Instructor Manual,* Second Edition, represent a comprehensive review of the knowledge group fitness instructors need to perform their jobs with a solid level of competency. Chapter 1, Exercise Physiology, covers the bioenergetics of exercise and the acute and long-term responses to aerobic exercise for both healthy partici-pants and persons with chronic disease, in addition to the fundamentals of exercise physiology with regard to the neuromuscular and cardiovascular-respiratory systems and environmental considerations.

Chapters 2 and 3, Fundamentals of Anatomy and Fundamentals of Applied Kinesiology, have been expanded to address the growing need in the fitness industry to develop a more robust knowl-edge base. After introducing and explaining common anatomical terminology, Chapter 2 provides an overview of the five major sys-tems of the body—cardiovascular, respira-tory, nervous, skeletal, and muscular. Chapter 3 begins by detailing the biome-chanical principles as they apply to human movement, before going on to break the human body down into muscle regions and explaining how various types of movement take place at specific joints in the body. This knowledge base is essential if a group fitness instructor is going to be able to explain how and why specific movements work or don't work in terms of applying to class or individual goals.

Chapter 4 provides an overview of nutrition

as it applies to health maintenance, weight control, and human performance. Other topics covered include ergogenic aids, eating disorders, and nutritional considerations during pregnancy.

Chapter 5, 6, and 7 offer the core of group fitness instruction. Chapter 5, Health Screening, presents the most up-to-date information related to the pre-exercise screening of participants, as well as guidelines for how to apply the findings. In Chapters 6 and 7, class format, teaching strategies and techniques, and music selection are discussed and then implemented in a detailed review of the critical components of designing and leading a group fitness class. Chapter 8, Adherence and Motivation, details the factors that impact exercise adherence and provides strategies to help you motivate your participants to get started and continue exercising.

Chapters 9 and 10 address one of the most challenging aspects of group fitness instruction: modifying overall class structure and individual movements for members of special populations. Chapter 9, Disabilities and Health Limitations, covers metabolic disorders, respiratory and pulmonary disorders, joint and bone disorders, autoimmune diseases, cardiac diseases, and human development and aging. Chapter 10 focuses exclusively on exercise and pregnancy, including the benefits and risks of exercising during pregnancy and specific guidelines for working with pregnant women.

The final two chapters provide information on the prevention, detection, and treatment of musculoskeletal injuries, basic emergency procedures, and the legal and professional responsibilities of group fitness instructors. While group fitness instructors may not need to draw upon this information on a daily basis, sound knowledge, judgment, and application of these principles are essential to your future success in this dynamic field.

Finally, the expanded Appendix section covers everything from ACE's Code of Ethics and the Exam Content Outline to an introduction to some of the many possible specialty areas (traditional aerobics, step training, kickboxing, group indoor cycling, aquatic exercise, yoga, Pilates, stability ball training, and group strength training) available in the ever-changing fitness industry.

Cedric X. Bryant, Ph.D.
Chief Science Officer

Daniel J. Green
Editor

Christine J. Ekeroth
Editor

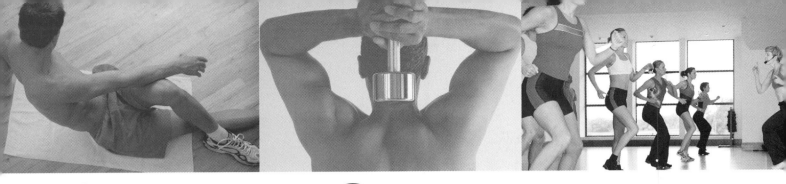

Chapter One

John P. Porcari, Ph.D., is a professor in the Department of Exercise and Sports Science and executive director of the La Crosse Exercise and Health Program at the University of Wisconsin–La Crosse. He is a fellow of the American College of Sports Medicine and of the American Association of Cardiovascular and Pulmonary Rehabilitation (AACVPR) and is a past president of AACVPR. Dr. Porcari's research interests have focused on the acute and chronic training responses to exercising on a variety of exercise modalities, particularly new fitness products. He has authored more than 75 peer-reviewed publications and made more than 120 national presentations dealing with health and fitness.

Carl Foster, Ph.D., is a professor in the Department of Exercise and Sports Science and director of the Human Performance Laboratory at the University of Wisconsin–La Crosse (UWL). He is a fellow of the American College of Sports Medicine (ACSM) and of the American Association of Cardiovascular and Pulmonary Rehabilitation. He also is the 2005–2006 President of ACSM. Dr. Foster's research interests range from high-performance physiology (he is the head of sports science for U.S. Speedskating) to clinical exercise physiology (he is the research director for the clinical exercise physiology graduate program at UWL). Dr. Foster has published more than 200 scientific papers and book chapters and 13 longer works (e.g., books, monographs, position stands, and videos).

IN THIS CHAPTER:

Exercise Physiology

By John P. Porcari and Carl Foster

The structure and function of the human body allow an extraordinarily wide range of possible movements requiring very complex interactions of neuromuscular coordination and metabolism. For example, a pole vaulter needs to be able to couple the coordination and agility to maneuver over the crossbar with the explosive burst of energy needed to sprint down the runway. At the other extreme, an ultramarathoner needs to be able to generate low levels of energy repetitively for prolonged periods of time.

Physical Fitness

Exercise Physiology

The study of **exercise physiology** allows an understanding of how the body responds to the varied demands placed on it by exercise. It is essential that the group fitness instructor understands the basics of exercise physiology so that he or she can design safe and effective exercise programs.

Physical Fitness

Before discussing the specific effects of exercise on the body, it is important to realize that there are several areas that contribute to overall "**physical fitness**" and, hence, different body systems that need to be trained appropriately. Physical fitness is a complex concept that has different meanings to different people. In this manual, physical fitness refers to the **capacity** of the heart, blood vessels, lungs, and muscles to function at a high level of efficiency. A person who is physically fit has an enhanced functional capacity that allows for a high quality of life. Although a somewhat vague phrase, quality of life generally implies an overall positive feeling and enthusiasm for life and the ability to do enriching and enjoyable activities without fatigue or exhaustion from routine and required activities. A high level of physical fitness allows people to comfortably perform their required daily tasks and enables them to participate in additional pleasurable activities for personal enjoyment. As physiological or functional capacity increases, one's capacity for physical activity or exercise also increases. In other words, a person can lift heavier weights or run farther or faster—in short, can participate in more strenuous activities. Being physically fit makes possible a lifestyle that the sedentary cannot enjoy. Increased physical fitness is often reflected by physiological adaptations, such as a lowered heart rate during a standard-

ized exercise test or an improved ability to mobilize and use body fuels. A high level of physical fitness implies optimal physical performance and good health.

There are five major components of physical fitness. It should be noted that the components are health-related as opposed to skill-related. The development of a high degree of **motor skill** is sometimes confused with physical fitness, but these two attributes are not necessarily related. A highly skilled person may have a low level of physical fitness, and the reverse may also be true. Motor skill (sometimes referred to as motor performance or motor fitness) is thought to be related to such attributes as **agility, balance, speed, power** and **coordination**—terms that defy precise definition but can profoundly affect a person's overall health or quality of life (e.g., balance deficits have been consistently linked to a greater risk of falling in older adults). Additional information on thsese skill-related components of fitness can be obtained on the ACE website (www.acefitness.org/FitFacts).

The five components of physical fitness are as follows:

1. **Muscular strength** is the maximal force a muscle or muscle group can exert during contraction. Muscular strength is essential for normal everyday functioning, and is required to lift and carry objects (e.g., groceries, suitcases) in daily life. Adequate muscular strength may become even more important as people age. In many cases, for instance, the elderly are not able to walk up stairs or get up out of a chair due to inadequate strength in the lower extremities.

2. **Muscular endurance** is the ability of a muscle or muscle group to exert force against a resistance over a sustained period of time. Muscular endurance is assessed by

measuring the length of time (duration) a muscle can exert force without fatigue or by measuring the number of times (**repetitions**) that a given task can be performed without fatigue. Many everyday activities require a significant amount of muscular endurance (e.g., walking up stairs, shoveling snow).

3. **Cardiovascular** or **cardiorespiratory endurance** (sometimes referred to as **aerobic power** or **aerobic fitness**) is the capacity of the heart, blood vessels, and lungs to deliver oxygen and nutrients to the working muscles and tissues during sustained exercise and to remove the metabolic waste products associated with fatigue. Efficient functioning of the cardiorespiratory system is essential for physical activities such as walking, running, swimming, and cycling. The performance of regular, moderately intense aerobic exercise is the key to developing and maintaining an efficient cardiorespiratory system.

4. **Flexibility** is the ability to move joints through their normal full **range of motion (ROM)**. An adequate degree of flexibility is important to prevent musculoskeletal injuries and to maintain correct body posture.

5. **Body composition** is the makeup of the body considered as a two-component model: **lean body mass** and **body fat**. The lean body mass consists of the muscles, bones, nervous tissue, skin, blood, and organs. These tissues have a high metabolic rate and make a direct and positive contribution to energy production during exercise. The primary role of body fat, or **adipose tissue,** is to store energy for later use. Body fat does not normally contribute in a direct sense to exercise performance. Body fat is further classified into **essential body fat** and storage body fat. Essential body fat is that amount of fat thought to be necessary for maintenance of life and reproductive function; 2 to 5% body

fat is generally thought to be essential for men, and 10 to 13% for women. (Percent body fat refers to the percentage of the total body weight that is fat.) Storage fat is contained in the fatty deposits or fat pads found under the skin (**subcutaneous fat**) and deep inside the body (**internal fat**). A large amount of storage fat is considered excess fat and results in the condition referred to as **obesity.**

Bioenergetics of Exercise

The body's cells require a continuous supply of energy to function. Ultimately, the food people eat supplies this energy. However, the cells do not directly use the energy contained in the food. Rather, they need a chemical compound called **adenosine triphosphate,** or **ATP.** ATP is the immediately usable form of chemical energy needed for all cellular function, including muscular contraction.

Foods are made up of carbohydrates, fats, and proteins. The process of digestion breaks these nutrients down to their simplest components (**glucose, fatty acids,** and **amino acids**), which are absorbed into the blood and transported to metabolically active cells, such as muscle, nerve, or liver cells. These components either immediately enter a metabolic pathway to produce ATP or are stored in body tissues for later use.

For example, excess glucose will be stored as **glycogen** in muscle or liver cells. Fatty acids that are not immediately used for ATP production will be stored as adipose tissue (body fat). In contrast, relatively little of the protein (amino acids) a person eats is used for energy production. Instead, it is used for the growth or repair of cellular structures or is excreted in waste products. Figure 1.1 summarizes the fate of carbohydrates, fats, and proteins.

Figure 1.1
Foods consumed ultimately produce the chemical energy required for cellular function.

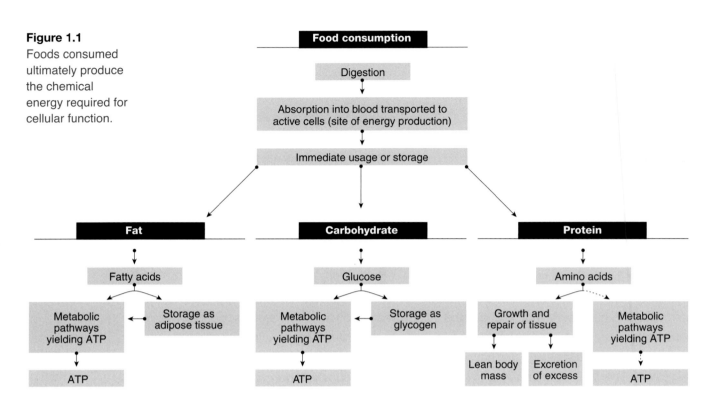

Stored ATP—The Immediate Energy Source

ATP is a complicated chemical structure made up of a substance called adenosine and three simpler groups of atoms called phosphate groups (P). Special high-energy bonds exist between the phosphate groups (Figure 1.2a). Breaking the terminal phosphate bond releases energy (E) that the cell uses directly to perform its cellular function

Figure 1.2
Breakdown of the ATP molecule

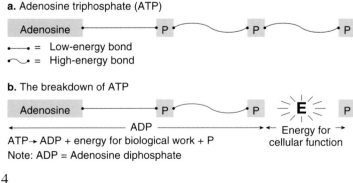

a. Adenosine triphosphate (ATP)

Adenosine — P ⁓ P ⁓ P

•——• = Low-energy bond
⁓ = High-energy bond

b. The breakdown of ATP

Adenosine — P ⁓ P ⁄E⁄ P

ADP ← Energy for cellular function →
ATP→ ADP + energy for biological work + P
Note: ADP = Adenosine diphosphate

(Figure 1.2b). The specific cellular function performed depends on the type of cell. In a muscle cell, the breakdown of ATP allows the mechanical work known as muscular contraction. If ATP is not available, muscle contraction stops.

While ATP can be stored within the cells, the amount stored and immediately available for muscle contraction is extremely limited, sufficient for only a few seconds of muscular work. Therefore, ATP must be continuously resynthesized. ATP can be resynthesized in several ways: immediately by the phosphagen system, somewhat more slowly with the **anaerobic** production of ATP from carbohydrate, or still more slowly with the aerobic production of ATP from either carbohydrate or fat. All three energy pathways are always active, but their relative activity varies from movement to movement, depending on the momentary level of muscular activity.

The Phosphagen System

Creatine phosphate (CP) is another high-energy phosphate compound found within muscle cells. Together, ATP and CP are referred to as the **phosphagens.** When ATP is broken down for muscular contraction, it is resynthesized very quickly from the break-down of CP. The energy released from break-ing the high-energy phosphate bond in CP is used to reconstitute ATP from **adenosine diphosphate (ADP)** and P (the phosphate group broken off from ATP), by-products of the initial reaction. This process is shown in Figure 1.3.

The total amount of ATP and CP stored in muscle is very small, and thus the amount of energy available for muscular contraction is extremely limited. There is probably enough energy available from the phosphagens for only about 10 seconds of all-out exertion. However, this energy is instantaneously avail-able for muscular contraction, and therefore is essential at the onset of physical activity and during short-term, high-intensity activities such as sprinting, performing a weight-lifting movement, or leaping across a stage.

Anaerobic Production of ATP From Carbohydrate

The anaerobic production of ATP from car-bohydrate is known as **anaerobic glycolysis. Anaerobic** literally means "without the pres-ence of oxygen," and **glycolysis** refers to the breakdown of glucose or its storage form, glycogen. Thus, anaerobic glycolysis is a metabolic pathway that does not require oxy-gen, the purpose of which is to transfer energy contained in glucose (or glycogen) to the for-mation of ATP.

Anaerobic glycolysis is capable of produc-ing ATP quite rapidly and thus is required when energy (ATP) is needed to perform activ-

Creatine phosphate (CP)

Creatine ⁓ P

CP → Creatine + energy for resynthesis of ATP + P

Creatine ≋E≋ P

←Energy→

ADP + energy from CP + P → ATP

Adenosine ·—·P·⁓·P·······P

Note: ⁓ = High-energy bond; P = Phosphate group; ·—· = Low-energy bond

Figure 1.3
The immediate resynthesis of ATP by CP

ities requiring large bursts of energy over somewhat longer periods of time than the phosphagen system allows. This metabolic pathway occurs within the cytoplasm of the cell and involves the incomplete breakdown of glucose (or glycogen) to a simpler substance called pyruvate. If exercise intensity is very high and adequate amounts of oxygen are not available, **pyruvate** is converted into **lactate,** as indicated in Figure 1.4a. Lactate may be transported out of the active cell and used for energy by other cells in the body.

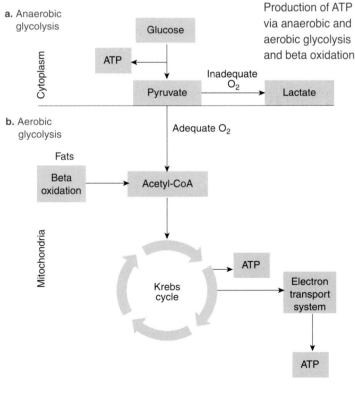

Figure 1.4
Production of ATP via anaerobic and aerobic glycolysis and beta oxidation

The formation of lactate poses a significant problem because it is associated with changes in muscle pH (acidity) and eventual muscle fatigue when it accumulates in large amounts. If the removal of lactate by the circulatory system cannot keep pace with its production in the active muscles, temporary muscle fatigue may occur with painful symptoms, usually referred to as "the burn." Thus, anaerobic glycolysis can only be used to a limited extent during sustained activity, but provides the main source of ATP for high-intensity exercise lasting up to a maximum of approximately three minutes.

Aerobic Production of ATP From Carbohydrate or Fat

The aerobic production of ATP is used for activities requiring sustained energy production. Since **aerobic** literally means "in the presence of oxygen," aerobic metabolic pathways require a continuous supply of oxygen delivered by the circulatory system. Without oxygen, these pathways cannot produce ATP.

The metabolic pathway, called **aerobic glycolysis** or **oxidative glycolysis,** occurs within highly specialized cell structures called the **mitochondria.** Mitochondria, which are often called the powerhouses of the cell, contain specific enzymes (**oxidative enzymes**) needed by the cell to utilize oxygen. This highly efficient metabolic process is limited mainly by the capacity of the cardiorespiratory system to deliver oxygen to the active cells. When sufficient oxygen is available, pyruvate is converted into acetyl-CoA, which enters the Krebs cycle and the electron transport system, produces substantial amounts of ATP (Figure 1.4b), and produces CO_2 and H_2O as easily removable waste products.

Aerobic pathways are also available to break down fatty acids (the digested component of dietary fat) for the production of ATP. This metabolic pathway, called **fatty acid oxidation,** or **beta oxidation,** also occurs within the mitochondria and requires a continuous supply of oxygen (as does aerobic glycolysis). The aerobic metabolism of fat yields a very large amount of ATP; therefore, fat is said to have a high caloric density. A calorie is a unit of energy. Fat yields 9 kilocalories of energy per gram compared to 4 kilocalories of energy per gram of glucose. That is why body fat is such an excellent source of stored energy (and so hard to get rid of).

At rest, the body uses both glucose and fatty acids for energy production via aerobic pathways. The cardiorespiratory system can easily supply the oxygen necessary for this low rate of energy metabolism. With exercise, however, supplying the required amount of oxygen rapidly enough becomes more difficult. Because glucose metabolism requires less oxygen than fatty acid metabolism, the body will use more glucose for energy production and less fat as exercise intensity increases. Table 1.1 provides a summary and comparison of the aerobic and anaerobic systems of ATP production.

Training

The various energy systems adapt to repetitive stress, meaning that they demonstrate a training effect. There is evidence that the concentrations of CP and ATP present in the muscle increase with training, particularly following high-intensity training that is likely to cause depletion of the phosphagens. Similarly, there is evidence to suggest that high-intensity training increases both the ability to transport lactate out of the muscle and the ability to buffer acid metabolites. There are profound adaptations to aerobic training, due to both central and peripheral changes. The ability of the heart to pump blood (cardiac output) increases, primarily as a result of an increase in stroke volume. The ability of the muscles to utilize oxygen to produce ATP also increases due to an increase in the number of mitochondria in the active muscles. Collectively, these changes result in an increase in an individual's aerobic capacity.

Muscles and Metabolism

Muscles are composed of several kinds of fibers that differ in their ability to utilize the metabolic pathways outlined above. **Fast-twitch (FT) fibers** are rather poorly equipped in terms of the oxygen delivery system, but have an outstanding capacity for the phosphagen system and a very high capacity for anaerobic glycolysis. Therefore, fast-twitch fibers are specialized for anaerobic metabolism. They are recruited by the nervous system predominantly for rapid, powerful movements such as jumping, throwing, and sprinting.

Slow-twitch (ST) fibers, on the other hand, are exceptionally well equipped for oxygen delivery and have a high quantity of aerobic, or oxidative, enzymes. Although they do not

Table 1.1
Comparison of Anaerobic and Aerobic Systems of ATP Production

Anaerobic System	Rate of ATP Production	Substrate(s)	Capacity of System	Major Limitation(s)	Major Use
Phosphagens (stored ATP & CP)	Very rapid rate	CP	Very limited ATP production	Very limited supply of CP	Very high-intensity, short-duration sprint activities. Predominates during activities of 1–10 seconds.
Anaerobic glycolysis (GLU → ATP + LA)	Rapid metabolic rate	Blood glucose Glycogen	Limited ATP production	Lactate by-product causes rapid fatigue	High-intensity, short-duration activities. Predominates during activities of 1–3 minutes.

Aerobic System	Rate of ATP Production	Substrate(s)	Capacity of System	Major Limitation(s)	Major Use
Aerobic glycolysis	Slow metabolic rate	Blood glucose Glycogen	Unlimited ATP production	Relatively slow rate of oxygen delivery to cells Glycogen storage	Lower-intensity, longer-duration endurance activities. Predominates during activities longer than 3 minutes.
Fatty acid oxidation	Slow metabolic rate	Fatty acids	Unlimited ATP production	Relatively slow rate of oxygen delivery to cells Large amount of O_2 needed	Lower-intensity, longer-duration endurance activities. Fatty acid oxidation predominates after about 20 minutes of continuous activity.

Note: ATP = Adenosine triphosphate; GLU = Glucose; LA = Lactate; CP = Creatine phosphate

have a highly developed mechanism for use of the phosphagens or anaerobic glycolysis, ST fibers have a large number of mitochondria and, consequently, are particularly well designed for aerobic glycolysis and fatty acid oxidation. Thus, ST fibers are recruited primarily for low-intensity, longer-duration activities such as walking, jogging, and swimming.

Most people have roughly equal percentages of both fiber types. Persons who excel in activities characterized by sudden bursts of energy, but who tire relatively rapidly, probably have a high percentage of fast-twitch fibers. Persons who are best at lower-intensity endurance activities probably have a large percentage of slow-twitch fibers. There are also a number of "intermediate" muscle fibers that have a fairly high capacity for both fast anaerobic and slow aerobic movements.

Muscle fiber distribution (fast twitch, intermediate, or slow twitch) is determined to a large extent by genetic makeup. This is not to say, however, that muscle fiber type is unresponsive to activity. All three types of muscle fiber are highly trainable; that is, they are capable of adapting to the specific metabolic demands placed on them. If a person engages regularly in low-intensity endurance activities, aerobic capacity will improve. Although all three types of muscle fiber will show some improvement in aerobic ability, the ST fibers will be most responsive to this kind of training and will show the largest improvement in aerobic capacity. If, on the other hand, short-duration, high-intensity exercise such as interval training is performed regularly, other metabolic pathways will be emphasized, and the capabilities of the FT fibers to perform anaerobically will be enhanced. ST fibers are less responsive to this kind of training.

It is important for group fitness instructors to have a thorough understanding of the different metabolic systems to develop specific exercise programs that will enable participants to achieve desired results. As discussed, exercise intensity and duration is directly related to the continuum of metabolic pathways and movement patterns. For example, including quick, explosive movements specific to the use of the phosphagens and anaerobic glycolysis in a workout will be ineffective if the goal of the exercise program is to develop cardiorespiratory endurance. This concept, known as **exercise specificity,** is one of the most important principles of exercise physiology.

The Neuromuscular System

Group fitness instructors need to understand how a motor skill is executed. Such an understanding requires a basic appreciation of the neuromuscular system, which includes both the nervous and musculoskeletal systems. The nervous system is responsible for coordinating movement, while the musculoskeletal system is responsible for carrying out the movement.

Basic Organization of the Nervous System

The basic anatomical unit of the nervous system is the **neuron,** or nerve cell. There are two kinds of neurons: sensory and motor. **Sensory neurons** convey electro-chemical impulses from sensory organs in the periphery (such as the skin) to the spinal cord and the brain (called the **central nervous system,** or **CNS**). **Motor neurons** conduct impulses from the CNS to the periphery. Because the motor neurons carry electrical impulses from the CNS to the muscle cells, they signal the muscles to contract or to relax and, therefore, regulate muscular movement. The endings of the motor neuron connect, or synapse, with muscle cells in the periphery of the body. This motor neuron–muscle cell synapse is called the neuromuscular junction, or **motor end plate** (Figure 1.5). The basic functional unit of the neuromuscular system is the **motor unit,** which consists of one motor neuron and the muscle cells that it innervates. Motor units are arranged according to muscle fiber type. A neuron capable of conducting nervous impulses very rapidly synapses with the cells of fast-twitch muscle fibers. The cells of slow-twitch muscle fibers are controlled by somewhat slower-conducting neurons.

Basic Organization of the Muscular System

The skeletal muscle is a complex tissue. Basically, muscle is surrounded by a layer of connective tissue called the **epimysium.** At the ends of a muscle, the epimysium thickens into a **tendon** that connects the muscle

to the bone. Sublayers of connective tissue further divide each muscle into bundles of individual muscle cells, and, finally, each individual muscle fiber is covered by the **endomysium** (Figure 1.6).

An individual muscle cell is composed of many thread-like protein strands called

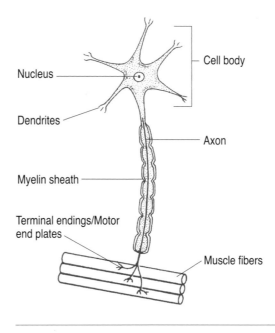

Figure 1.5
Basic anatomical structure of a motor neuron (or nerve cell) and motor end plate

Nucleus
Dendrites
Myelin sheath
Terminal endings/Motor end plates
Cell body
Axon
Muscle fibers

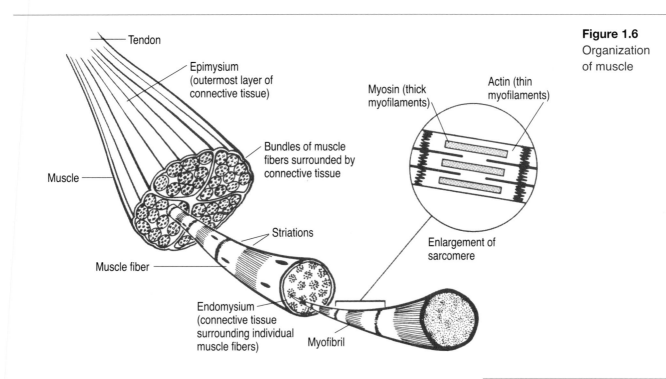

Figure 1.6
Organization of muscle

Tendon
Epimysium (outermost layer of connective tissue)
Muscle
Bundles of muscle fibers surrounded by connective tissue
Striations
Muscle fiber
Endomysium (connective tissue surrounding individual muscle fibers)
Myofibril
Myosin (thick myofilaments)
Actin (thin myofilaments)
Enlargement of sarcomere

myofibrils that contain the **contractile proteins.** The basic functional unit of the myofibril is the **sarcomere.** Within the sarcomere are two protein **myofilaments:** the thick myofilament is **myosin,** and the thinner myofilament is **actin** (see Figure 1.6). The myosin and actin myofilaments are arranged to interdigitate in a prescribed, regular way, resulting in a pattern of alternating light and dark bands, or striations, within the sarcomere. Tiny projections called cross-bridges extend from the myosin myofilaments toward the actin myofilaments.

According to the **sliding filament theory,** muscular contraction occurs when the cross-bridges extending from the myosin myofilaments attach (or couple) to the actin myofilaments and pull them past the myosin myofilaments. As the cross-bridges produce tension, the muscle shortens. The actual muscle shortening occurs as the actin myofilaments are pulled toward the center of the sarcomere, and the sarcomere shortens (Figure 1.7). The coupling of myosin and actin and the shortening process are dependent upon the availability of ATP to link actin and myosin and to provide the energy to allow shortening to occur.

Types of Muscular Contraction

What is described above is a form of **isotonic** muscular contraction, in that there is joint movement when the muscle is stimulated. Tension (or force) develops throughout the muscle as it contracts, but the tension

Figure 1.7
The sliding filament theory

Myofibril at rest

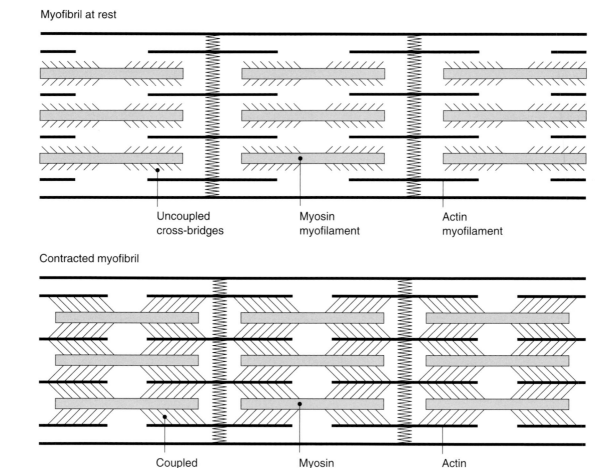

Uncoupled   Myosin   Actin
cross-bridges   myofilament   myofilament

Contracted myofibril

Coupled   Myosin   Actin
cross-bridges   myofilament   myofilament

The Neuromuscular System

changes with the total length of the muscle and the angle of the joint. The greatest force is generated at the muscle's optimal length, where the actin and myosin myofilaments are aligned so that the largest number of cross-bridges between the myofilaments is activated simultaneously. At all other lengths, fewer cross-bridges are simultaneously coupled to actin myofilaments and, therefore, less force can be developed. The relationship of muscle tension (force) to muscle length during an iso-tonic contraction is illustrated in Figure 1.8a.

There are two types of isotonic contraction: **concentric** and **eccentric.** A concentric contraction occurs when the muscle short-ens when it is stimulated. An eccentric con-traction is the opposite of a concentric con-traction in that the muscle develops tension as it lengthens against a resistance (rather than as it shortens against a resistance). This is sometimes called "negative work." Using walking up and down a flight of stairs as an example, going up the stairs requires the quadriceps muscle group to contract con-centrically (shortening and lifting the weight of the body against gravity), while going down the stairs requires the quadriceps to contract eccentrically (slowly lengthening and lowering the weight of the body with gravity). In typical weight-lifting movements, eccentric contractions usually follow concen-tric contractions.

Isometric muscular contractions occur when actual muscle shortening does not take place. Since no joint movement occurs, this type of contraction is sometimes referred to as a static contraction. An example of an iso-metric muscle contraction is holding a weight at arm's length or attempting to move an immovable object (e.g., exerting force out-ward against a door frame). Isometric exer-cises are often used during physical rehabili-

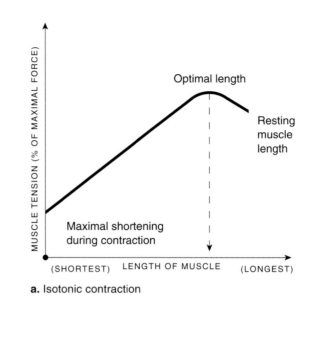

a. Isotonic contraction

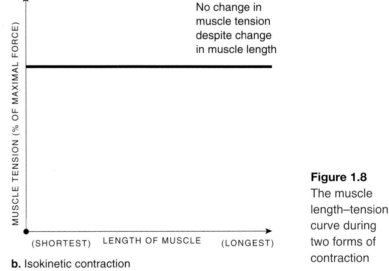

b. Isokinetic contraction

Figure 1.8
The muscle length–tension curve during two forms of contraction

tation and physical therapy when a joint has been injured. By contracting the muscles isometrically, an individual can maintain or increase muscular strength without aggra-vating the injured joint. It should be remem-bered, however, that because no joint movement is taking place, increases in strength are very specific to the joint angle at which the contractions are carried out and that contractions should be carried out at several joint angles.

Isokinetic contractions, in outward appearance, look much like isotonic contractions. In an isotonic contraction, however, tension within the muscle changes throughout the range of motion. To accomplish an isokinetic contraction, special equipment is required to alter the resistance offered to the muscle as it contracts at a constant velocity. This approach is sometimes referred to as "accommodating-resistance" or "variable-resistance" exercise. Isokinetic exercise enables maximal tension to develop in a muscle throughout its entire range of motion (Figure 1.8b). With isotonic exercise, the maximal amount of weight that can be lifted corresponds to a weight that can be lifted through the weakest point in the range of motion. Thus, the muscle is only developing maximal tension at that point and tension development (as a percentage of maximal tension) varies throughout the range of motion.

Muscular Strength and Endurance

Resistance-training programs can be designed to improve either muscular strength or muscular endurance. While there is considerable overlap in the training responses, there are several key differences. The sections below discuss how the principle of **specificity** applies to these two components of physical fitness.

Muscular Strength

Strength refers to the maximal tension or force produced by a muscle or muscle group. Strength is usually measured by determining how much weight can be lifted in a single effort. The one-repetition maximum (1-RM) test is determined through a trial-and-error procedure using either free weights (barbells and weights) or special machines (e.g., dynamometers,

selectorized equipment, multi-station gym). Most often, 1-RM tests are completed for the following muscle groups: (a) the bench press for the muscles of the chest and upper arms; (b) the arm curl for the muscles on the anterior aspect of the upper arms; and (c) the leg press or squat for the muscles of the upper legs and hips.

Programs designed specifically to develop muscular strength should use a high-intensity (80 to 90% of 1 RM), low-repetition format (fewer than eight repetitions), and the movements should be performed carefully at a controlled speed so there is a consistent application of force throughout the movement. Good posture and body mechanics are extremely important to avoid injury, as is breathing properly and avoiding the **Valsalva maneuver,** which occurs when the breath is held while a great deal of force is exerted. When the breath is held, the glottis in the back of the throat is closed. Exerting force with the glottis closed results in an increase in pressure within the chest cavity (intrathoracic pressure). This increase in pressure squeezes down on the large veins in the chest cavity, impeding venous return (blood flow back to the heart). If blood flow back to the heart is impeded, the heart has less blood to pump out. As a consequence, there is less flow of blood and oxygen to the brain, and dizziness and fainting may occur. It is generally recommended that people exhale when they are performing the concentric phase of a lift and inhale during the eccentric phase.

Movements requiring a high level of strength recruit both ST and FT muscle fibers. Because little total work is done, strength-training movements do not require or develop a high level of aerobic capacity because the muscles are using primarily the phosphagen (ATP-CP) system. And, because strength training is relatively stressful on the connective tissues and muscular structures of the body, it is usually recommended that heavy strength training be performed only two or three times per week. It is important that the muscles and supporting structures be given time to recover sufficiently between workouts. At the same time, strength training can help support bone health during aging.

Muscular **hypertrophy** is often associated with a strength-development program. This hypertrophy is the result of an increase in the size of individual muscle cells. The increase in size is due to a proliferation of actin and myosin myofilaments within the myofibrils, especially within the fast-twitch muscle fibers. One common misconception is that women will develop "large" muscles if they strength-train. Generally, women do not experience muscular hypertrophy to the same extent as men, because the male hormone testosterone is important in synthesizing the contractile proteins. Nevertheless, women will increase substantially in strength in response to a pro-gressive strength-training program.

Consistent with the **reversibility principle,** training adaptations will gradually decline if not reinforced by a maintenance program. With muscle disuse, as in paralysis, muscle **atrophy,** or wasting, occurs. Strength training even once per week appears to be sufficient to maintain strength gains and muscle size.

Muscular Endurance

Endurance refers to the ability to repeatedly contract a muscle or muscle group against resistance. Tests of muscular endurance usu-ally involve selecting a fixed percentage of the maximum strength (e.g., 70% of the 1 RM) and counting the number of repetitions that can be completed without resting. Sit-up or pull-up tests are other examples of muscular-endurance tests (not of strength tests, as is often thought).

It is usually recommended that muscular-endurance training be conducted using a moderate-resistance (40 to 70% of 1 RM), high-repetition (10 to 50 repetitions) format. Because this type of format is not as stress-ful to the muscles and connective tissue, muscular-endurance training can be com-pleted as often as three to five times per week for maximum results. If training for a particular sport, the speed of contraction should be matched to the rate required dur-ing performance.

Training for muscular endurance is specific to both ST and FT muscle fibers and motor units. Training increases the concentration of oxidative enzymes that extract oxygen from the blood in both types of fibers, thus making energy production more efficient. An increase in tissue **vascularity,** or an increase in the number and size of blood vessels, often accompanies this type of program. Increased vascularity enhances blood supply and, con-sequently, oxygen delivery to the myofibrils. It also aids in transporting metabolites, such as lactate, away from the contracting muscle.

Flexibility

Flexibility refers to the range of motion (ROM) possible about a joint. Flexibility is often related to age: Young children are usually extremely flexible, while the elderly gradually lose much of the flexibility they had as younger adults. With specific flexibility training, the muscles and connective tissues adapt by elongating, thus increasing the range of motion.

ROM can be limited by the bony structure of a joint, the ligamentous structure of a joint, or the musculotendinous structure of the muscle(s) spanning the joint. The bony structure of a joint is a self-limiting factor

13

that cannot be altered. A joint ligament (the fibrous band connecting bones) or joint capsule should not be stretched, because doing so leads to an unstable joint (joint laxity) and an increased risk of joint injury. Therefore, the only desirable way to alter that range of motion is by gently stretching the musculotendinous structures controlling the movement of the joint. These structures can sometimes become extremely taut, causing a reduction in the normal range of motion.

Flexibility may be related to the incidence of acute muscle injury due to strenuous exercise and also to **delayed onset muscle soreness (DOMS).** Acute muscle injuries such as muscle pulls or tears are more likely to occur if the muscle fibers or surrounding tissues are so taut and inflexible that a sudden stretch causes tissue injury. The exact cause of DOMS, which occurs 24 to 48 hours after strenuous exercise, is not known. Evidence suggests that it is caused by microscopic damage to muscle cell ultrastructure due to excessive mechanical force exerted by the muscle and connective tissues. DOMS is particularly associated with the eccentric phase of a movement, especially if the person is unaccustomed to the exercise. Stretching exercises performed before and after an exercise session may help to prevent soreness, and also to relieve soreness when it does occur, but not all of the evidence suggests this.

There are three types of stretching to increase flexibility: static stretching; dynamic, or ballistic, stretching; and proprioceptive neuromuscular facilitation. **Static stretching** involves holding a static (nonmoving) position so that a joint is immobilized in a position that places the desired muscles and connective tissues passively at their greatest possible length. A static stretch position should be held for 15 to 30 seconds to achieve optimal

results (Bandy & Irion, 1994; McHugh et al., 1992). Static stretching is best characterized as low-force, long-duration stretching and has repeatedly been shown to produce good results with little muscle soreness. In fact, static stretching is commonly used to reduce muscle soreness. Little risk of physical injury exists if static stretching is performed correctly. However, static stretching performed just before exercise has been shown to transiently reduce muscle strength.

Dynamic, or ballistic, stretching is characterized by rhythmic bobbing or bouncing motions representing relatively high-force, short-duration movements. **Ballistic stretching** motions, while seemingly effective, actually invoke stretch reflexes that oppose the desired stretching. Muscle stretch reflexes are involuntary motor responses controlled by the **muscle spindle,** a sensory organ located within the muscle. When a muscle spindle is stimulated, an impulse is propagated over a sensory nerve fiber. The nerve fiber synapses in the spinal cord with a motor neuron that returns to the muscle containing the muscle spindle (Figure 1.9a). This reflex causes the suddenly stretched muscle to respond with a corresponding contraction; the amount and rate of this contraction varies directly with the amount and rate of the movement causing the initial stretch. Thus, ballistic stretching evokes the opposite physiological response from the one desired—an increase in muscle tension.

A firm static stretch, on the other hand, invokes an inhibition of the stretch reflex by stimulating another sensory organ (with a higher threshold level) called the **Golgi tendon organ.** When stimulated, this organ causes an inhibition not only of the muscle in which the muscle spindle was stretched, but also of the entire muscle group (Figure 1.9b).

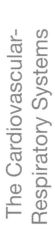

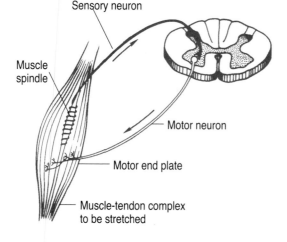

Sensory neuron

Muscle spindle

Motor neuron

Motor end plate

Muscle-tendon complex to be stretched

a. Simple muscle stretch-reflex arc: The stretch of the muscle spindle causes a reflex contraction.

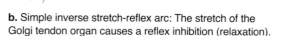

Sensory neuron

Golgi tendon organ

Inhibitory neuron

Motor neuron

Motor end plate

Muscle-tendon complex

b. Simple inverse stretch-reflex arc: The stretch of the Golgi tendon organ causes a reflex inhibition (relaxation).

Figure 1.9
Simple muscle reflexes

Thus, static stretching brings about a reduction in muscle tension—the desirable physiological response. In addition, static stretching is safer than ballistic stretching because it does not impose a sudden, possibly injurious force upon the tissues.

A third type of stretching, **proprioceptive neuromuscular facilitation,** or **PNF,** is a technique originally developed for rehabilitative purposes in physical therapy. PNF involves statically stretching a muscle immediately after maximally contracting it against resistance. Carefully controlled experiments using PNF have generally found it to be superior to either static or **dynamic stretching.** However, it is not practical in the majority of cases, as it requires a partner trained in the technique.

General flexibility exercises should be part of every physical-fitness program and should be included primarily during the cool-down phase of every exercise session. Some general principles specific to the enhancement of flexibility include the following:

• A low-level aerobic warm-up (such as walking and swinging the arms) should precede specific stretching exercises to increase blood flow.

• Stretching exercises should be performed without bouncing or jerking, which may injure connective tissues and stimulate the stretch reflex.

• Never attempt to stretch a muscle or muscle group beyond its normal range of motion.

• All stretching should be done gently and only to the extent that muscle tension is perceived; stretching should not be painful.

• Instructors should understand that their participants will vary greatly in their flexibility. Everyone is not equally flexible or equally responsive to flexibility training.

The Cardiovascular–Respiratory Systems

Cardiorespiratory endurance is defined as the capacity of the heart and lung systems to deliver blood and, hence, oxygen to the working muscles during sustained exercise. Oxygen is used to produce ATP to perform low- to moderate-intensity exercise for long periods. The capacity to perform aerobic exercise depends largely on the interaction of the

Exercise Physiology

cardiovascular system and the respiratory system to provide oxygen to the active cells so that carbohydrates and fatty acids can be converted to ATP for muscular contraction. These two systems also are important for the removal of metabolic waste products such as carbon dioxide and lactate, and for the dissipation of the internal heat produced by metabolic processes.

There are three basic processes that must interact to provide adequate blood and nutrients to the tissues:

1. Getting oxygen into the blood—a function of **pulmonary ventilation** coupled with the oxygen-carrying capacity of the blood

2. Delivering oxygen to the active tissues—a function of cardiac output

3. Extracting oxygen from the blood to complete the metabolic production of ATP—a function of localizing the delivery of cardiac output to the active muscles and the oxidative enzymes located within the active cells

See Chapter 2 for information on basic cardiovascular and pulmonary anatomy.

Oxygen-carrying Capacity

The oxygen-carrying capacity of blood is determined primarily by two variables: the ability to ventilate the lungs adequately and the hemoglobin content of the blood. Pulmonary **ventilation** is a function of both the rate and depth (**tidal volume**) of breathing. With the beginning of exercise, both tidal volume and breathing rate increase. This increase in ventilation volume brings more oxygen into the lungs, where it can be absorbed into the blood. In normal individuals, respiration does not limit exercise performance. However, individuals with **emphysema** (degradation of the alveoli) or **asthma** (constriction of the breathing pas-

sages) cannot move enough air through their lungs to adequately oxygenate the blood. As a result, the blood leaving the lungs is not sufficiently loaded with oxygen, and exercise capacity is diminished.

Hemoglobin (Hb) is a protein in red blood cells that is specifically adapted to bond (carry) oxygen molecules. When oxygen enters the lungs, it diffuses through the pulmonary membranes into the bloodstream, where it binds to hemoglobin. The oxygen is then carried within the bloodstream throughout the body. Persons with low hemoglobin concentrations cannot carry as much oxygen in their blood as persons with high hemoglobin concentrations. For instance, in individuals with **anemia** (less than 12 g of Hb per 100 mL of blood), the blood's oxygen-carrying capacity is severely limited, and they fatigue very easily. In most healthy persons, however, the oxygen-carrying capacity of the blood is not a limiting factor in the performance of aerobic exercise.

Oxygen Delivery

Probably the most important factor in cardiorespiratory endurance is the delivery of blood to the active cells, which is a function of **cardiac output.** Cardiac output is the product of **heart rate** (**HR;** beats per minute) and **stroke volume** (**SV;** the quantity of blood pumped per heart beat):

$$\text{Cardiac output} = \text{HR} \times \text{SV}$$

At rest, cardiac output averages about 5 liters (1.5 gallons) per minute. During maximal exercise, this number can increase to up to 30 to 40 liters (10 gallons) per minute in highly trained individuals. The increase in cardiac output is brought about by an increase in both HR and SV. HR generally increases in a linear fashion up to maximal levels, while SV increases up to approximately 40 to 50% of an individual's maximal capacity and then plateaus. The increase in SV is brought about by increases in both venous return and in the contractile force of the heart.

Also during exercise, blood flow patterns change according to metabolic need. Blood is shunted to the working muscles (to produce ATP for contraction) and to the skin (to dissipate the metabolic heat produced), while the amount of blood flowing to less active organs such as the kidneys and intestinal tract decreases.

Blood pressure is also very important in blood-flow distribution because it provides the driving force that pushes blood through the circulatory system. Blood pressure is influenced by many factors. **Systolic blood pressure** is a function of the force generated by the heart during its contraction phase (systole) and the resistance offered by the vessels to the blood flowing through them (peripheral resistance). Just as the strength of heart contractions can vary, some blood vessels (notably the smaller arteries called arterioles) can contract (**vasoconstriction**) or relax (**vasodilation**) and thus alter their resistance to blood flow, a fact important in determining the pattern of blood flow. During exercise, vasoconstriction occurs in the vessels of inactive organs (such as the intestine), and vasodilation occurs in vessels of active organs (muscles), thus redirecting blood flow to areas of the body where it is most needed. Similar to HR, systolic blood pressure increases in a linear fashion throughout the range of exercise intensities (Figure 1.10).

Diastolic blood pressure is a measure of the pressure in the arteries during the relax-

ation phase (diastole) of the heart cycle. Because of the vasodilation of the blood vessels within the working muscles, more blood is allowed to enter the muscles. As a result, less blood is "trapped" on the arterial side of the circulation. Diastolic blood pressure usually stays the same or decreases slightly during exercise (see Figure 1.10).

Oxygen Extraction

A third factor important in cardiorespiratory endurance is the extraction of oxygen from the blood at the cellular level for the aerobic production of ATP. The amount of oxygen extracted is largely a function of muscle fiber type and the availability of specialized oxidative enzymes. The slow-twitch muscle fibers are specifically adapted for oxygen extraction and utilization due to their high levels of oxidative enzymes. One of the most important adaptations to training is an increase in the number and size of the mitochondria, with a corresponding increase in the levels of oxidative enzymes used to aerobically produce ATP.

Figure 1.10
Normal responses to blood pressure during exercise

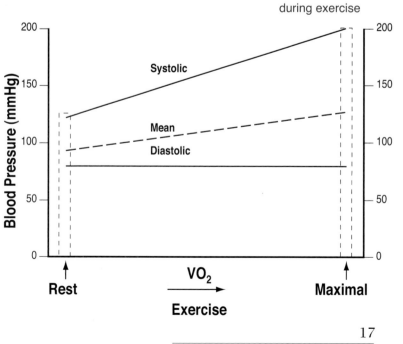

Acute Responses to Aerobic Exercise

Aerobic exercise is best characterized as large-muscle, rhythmic activities (e.g., walking, jogging, aerobic dance, swimming, cross-country skiing) that can be sustained without undue fatigue for at least 10 to 15 minutes. Such movement patterns depend on the oxidative metabolic pathways to create ATP, and the goal of the body is to be in a **steady state,** where the energy needs are being met aerobically. The other metabolic pathways (the phosphagen system and anaerobic glycolysis) are used only minimally to produce energy at the onset of these types of activity.

Figure 1.11 highlights the changes that take place. When aerobic exercise begins, the body rapidly responds to increase the quantity of oxygen available to produce the ATP necessary to meet the molecular demands. Cardiac output increases to deliver more blood to the active muscle cells. To meet this requirement, HR, SV, and systolic blood pressure increase immediately. Pulmonary ventilation also increases to provide more oxygen to the red blood cells in the lungs.

The bold line in Figure 1.11 indicates the level of **oxygen consumption** required at rest and the instantaneous increase that occurs with commencement of exercise (at upward arrow). The line returns to the resting level when exercise is abruptly stopped (at downward arrow). The actual oxygen consumption that results from the physiological responses to aerobic exercise is indicated by the sloping line in the figure. Notice that actual oxygen consumption does not immediately meet the physiological requirement for oxygen. Instead, an **oxygen deficit** occurs.

The physiological responses that occur with commencement of exercise take approximately two to four minutes to meet the increased metabolic demands for oxygen. During this time, the anaerobic metabolic systems—which are capable of producing ener-

Figure 1.11
Oxygen consumption during aerobic exercise

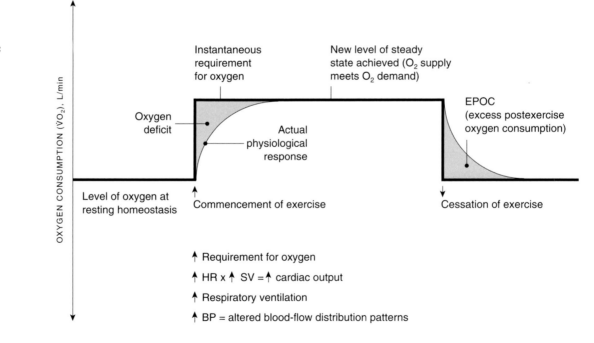

Note: HR = Heart rate; SV = Stroke volume; BP = Blood pressure

gy more rapidly—produce the energy needed to carry out the exercise. During this period, the phosphagens are depleted, and excess lactate is produced. When the cardiorespiratory systems have fully responded, a new level of oxygen consumption is achieved. If the exercise intensity is not too high relative to the body's ability to provide oxygen to the muscles, a steady state is achieved.

With cessation of exercise, the requirement for oxygen abruptly returns to the initial resting level. Again, however, the body responds more slowly. As cardiac output, blood pressure, and **respiratory ventilation** return to resting levels, oxygen consumption slowly declines as well, but is still elevated above resting levels. This is called **excess postexercise oxygen consumption (EPOC).** The energy produced during this time is used to replenish the depleted phosphagens, to eliminate accumulated lactate if it has not already been cleared from the blood, and to restore other homeostatic conditions.

If exercise intensity is so high that the body cannot meet all of the metabolic demands of the muscles aerobically (i.e., not reach a steady state), the muscles have to supplement ATP production via anaerobic metabolism. When this occurs, one is said to have exceeded the **anaerobic threshold (AT).** When someone exceeds their AT, lactate accumulates very rapidly in the blood, the oxygen deficit and corresponding EPOC are extremely high, and exercise cannot be performed for more than a few minutes (Figure 1.12). It is also at this point that hyperventilation begins to occur. As the body tries to buffer the lactate (remove it from the system), one of the by-products is carbon dioxide (CO_2). Carbon dioxide provides a powerful stimulus to the respiratory system, and the body increases respiration in an attempt to "blow off" the excess CO_2. This increase in respiration is often called the ventilatory threshold (VT) and is often used as an indirect indicator of the AT.

Figure 1.12
Oxygen consumption during anaerobic exercise

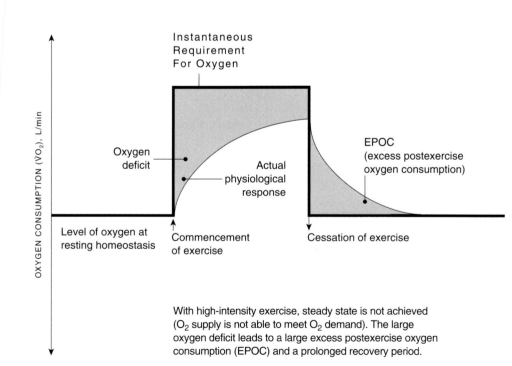

With high-intensity exercise, steady state is not achieved (O_2 supply is not able to meet O_2 demand). The large oxygen deficit leads to a large excess postexercise oxygen consumption (EPOC) and a prolonged recovery period.

Guidelines for Improving Cardiovascular–Respiratory Endurance

When developing an exercise program, it is important to individualize it for each participant. There are four basic variables to consider when developing an exercise program to improve cardiovascular-respiratory endurance:

1. Exercise **intensity**—how hard to exercise
2. Exercise **duration**—how long to exercise
3. Exercise **frequency**—how often to exercise
4. Exercise **mode**—what type of exercise

The following general recommendations are based upon well-established guidelines from the American College of Sports Medicine.

Intensity of Exercise

The principles of aerobic and anaerobic energy production make it clear that to improve cardiorespiratory endurance, the exercise needs to be conducted within an aerobic-training zone. Exercise at too great an intensity for a client's level of fitness will rely on the anaerobic systems, not the aerobic systems. Research shows that an acceptable exercise intensity for fitness improvement is in the range of about 40 to 85% of heart-rate reserve, which corresponds to approximately 60 to 95% of maximum heart rate. The ranges are broad because genetic factors, as well as initial fitness level, influence the degree of improvement. The higher a client's initial level of fitness, the higher the appropriate exercise intensity. Research also shows that very deconditioned individuals may improve aerobic fitness at intensities below the minimal intensities listed above.

Duration of Exercise

The recommended time that an individual should exercise aerobically ranges from 20 to 60 minutes. In general, the lower the intensity, the longer the duration needs to be. Individuals training at a low intensity should exercise for at least 30 minutes, while 20 to 30 minutes may be sufficient for individuals who are training at higher intensities. While it was previously thought that activity must be sustained for the minimum time to cause adequate aerobic **overload,** subsequent research has shown that three 10-minute sessions will lead to the same improvements as one 30-minute session if they are done at the same relative intensity (Franklin, 1999; Murphy & Hardman, 1998; Jakicic et al., 1995).

Because aerobic training is related to the oxygen cost of activity, there is an inverse relationship between intensity and duration. If intensity is increased, the duration can be decreased and a similar training effect will be achieved. Conversely, if the intensity is decreased, the duration must be increased to elicit the same training effect. In general terms, when the cells of the body consume 1 liter (about 1 quart) of oxygen per minute, about 5 kilocalories per minute have been expended (1 liter O_2/min $\cong$ 5 kcal/min). If 2 liters per minute are consumed, the expenditure would be about 10 kilocalories per minute. For example, walking costs approximately 5 kcal/min and jogging costs approximately 10 kcal/min. So jogging for 30 minutes would use about 300 kilocalories (10 x 30 = 300), which is the same as 60 minutes of walking (5 x 60 = 300). Therefore, walking for twice as long as jogging will result in approximately the same training effect. This is an especially important consideration for the deconditioned client.

Frequency of Exercise

The proper type of activity, done at the correct intensity and continued for a sufficient length of time, must be performed at least three days per week. While training three days per week may be sufficient, especially for those just beginning an exercise program, more frequent exercise, such as a brisk daily walk, is certainly acceptable. It also will lead to more rapid improvements. Keep in mind that it is important to allow for adequate rest and recovery to minimize the risks associated with training. Most experts encourage even competitive athletes to take at least one day per week for rest or a low-intensity recreational activity, such as a round of golf.

Interval training involves exercising at high intensity levels (80 to 100% of maximal HR) for relatively brief periods (usually 10 seconds to five minutes) with intervening rest or relief periods (walking, jogging) that allow HR to decline. The exercise periods often are "anaerobic" rather than "aerobic." For athletes in training, interval training may offer an advantage, because the higher intensity may more accurately simulate competitive conditions and result in improved performance. An athlete can thus maintain a faster pace before going into anaerobic metabolism. Generally, however, continuous exercise at lower levels of intensity is safer and more compatible with the goals of most individuals. Lower-intensity continuous training is less stressful to the musculoskeletal system and, therefore, more appropriate for middle-aged and older adults.

Mode of Exercise

To induce changes in aerobic capacity, it is recommended that the activity involve large muscle groups and be rhythmic in nature. Most traditional locomotive-type activities are considered to be good aerobic exercises (e.g., walking, running, cross-country skiing, swimming, rowing, cycling, stepping) because they utilize the large muscles of the body and can

be continued for prolonged periods. There is very little difference in the degree of aerobic improvement between various exercise modes, as long as they are conducted at the same relative intensity. Exercises that simultaneously utilize the upper and lower body (e.g., cross-country skiing, combined upper- and lower-body cycle ergometry) may have an added benefit, as they increase total-body muscular endurance and allow the work to be shared by both the upper and lower body, thus minimizing local muscular fatigue. This may allow more total work to be completed in a workout, resulting in greater total caloric expenditure.

It should be noted that the recommendations concerning intensity, frequency, duration, and mode of exercise relate specifically to improving aerobic capacity and are distinctly different than the recommendation by the Surgeon General that adults accumulate at least 30 minutes of moderate-intensity physical activity on most, if not all, days of the week. This "physical activity" can include everyday activities (e.g., gardening, mowing the lawn). Doing so will improve the overall health and well-being of the general population. If the guidelines provided by the American College of Sports Medicine are adhered to, the Surgeon General's recommendations also will be met.

Warm-up and Cool-down

The period of exercise at the desired target heart rate should be preceded by a warm-up of about five to 10 minutes. The warm-up should include limbering exercises to prepare the musculoskeletal system for the exercises to be performed. Static stretching—holding a steady stretch with the desired muscles at their greatest possible length—is beneficial to joints and muscles and may help to prevent injuries and muscle soreness. Warm-up activities should also include large-muscle movements to gradually increase HR, blood pressure, cardiac output, and respiratory ventilation to intermediate levels so that these mechanisms are not suddenly taxed. A proper warm-up may also reduce the incidence of exercise-induced cardiac abnormalities such as **arrhythmias** (abnormal heart rhythms) or **ischemia** (lack of blood flow to the heart muscle).

It is important to cool down gradually after a period of vigorous exercise. Abruptly stopping exercise after a vigorous workout may allow a large quantity of blood to pool in the lower extremities, reducing venous return. As a result, cardiac output is reduced and blood flow to the brain is diminished, which may cause dizziness or faintness. It is best to provide a series of movements during the cool-down period that allows the muscles and cardiorespiratory system to gradually return to their pre-exercise levels. A gradual cool-down also aids in the removal of accumulated **lactic acid** and may prevent cardiac arrhythmias following strenuous exercise. When heart rates are near resting levels, muscle stretching and limbering exercises should again be performed to reduce the risk of developing DOMS. Probably the most effective time to perform flexibility exercises is when muscles are warm and body temperature is elevated after exercise.

Use of Hand or Ankle Weights With Aerobic Exercise

Individuals often seek ways to increase the intensity of an aerobic workout. Adding extra weight in the form of hand, wrist, or ankle weights increases the total mass that must be moved, so it seems logical that using extra weight would be beneficial in boosting the physiological demands of an activity. Research on the use of hand or wrist weights during a variety of different aerobic activities (e.g., walking, traditional aerobics, step aerobics) is very consistent and indicates that the use of 1- to 3-pound (450 to 1350 g) weights can increase heart rate by five to 10 beats per minute and oxygen consumption (as well as caloric expenditure) by about 5 to 15% compared to performing the same activity without weights. Weights greater than 3 pounds (1350 g) are not generally recommended, because they may put undue stress on the arm and shoulder muscles. Additionally, wrist weights are preferred over hand weights because they don't have to be gripped, which can cause an elevated blood-pressure response in some people.

The beneficial effect of ankle weights is lower than that of either hand or wrist weights. Weights ranging from 1 to 3 pounds (450 to 1350 g) can increase HR by an average of three to five beats per minute and oxygen consumption by 5 to 10% over unweighted conditions. A potential drawback to the use of ankle weights is that they may alter the biomechanics of the lower limbs, leading to injury. As a consequence, ankle weights are not generally recommended for use during aerobic exercise activities.

Long-term Adaptations to Aerobic Exercise for Healthy Participants

When performed appropriately, a regular program of aerobic exercise can have significant physiological benefits in as little as eight to 12 weeks. Changes to the cardiorespiratory system include improvements in cardiac efficiency (increased SV and a lower HR), increased respiratory capacity, and, ultimately, an increase in maximal oxygen consumption ($\dot{V}O_2$max). These improvements provide individuals with a greater physiological reserve and allow them to perform everyday activities with less stress and strain. Regular exercise has also been shown to result in lowered blood pressure in moderately hypertensive individuals. This results in less work for the heart muscle and puts less stress on the blood vessels.

The benefits of aerobic exercise are not limited to the cardiovascular and respiratory systems. Studies have shown that weightbearing exercise promotes improved bone density, an extremely important consideration in the prevention of osteoporosis after age 50 to 60, particularly in women. Improvements in the control of blood glucose and blood lipids (e.g., cholesterol, triglycerides) are also associated with consistent physical activity. One of the main reasons many people exercise is to control body weight. Exercise obviously burns calories, but, just as importantly, exercise serves to maintain or increase lean body mass, which is vital for maintaining resting metabolic rate. It is the decrease in muscle mass that contributes to the fall in metabolic rate as people age. Finally, the psychological benefits of exercise cannot be overlooked. Exercise has long been associated with lower levels of anxiety and depression and a higher quality of life.

Long-term Adaptations to Aerobic Exercise for Persons With Chronic Disease

A well-planned aerobic-exercise program also can provide significant health benefits to persons with chronic diseases such as diabetes, osteoarthritis, obesity, pulmonary disease, and coronary heart disease.

Individuals with type 2 diabetes have difficulty utilizing glucose (carbohydrates) for energy, due to either a lack of insulin or the body's inability to utilize the available insulin (insulin resistance). Most of the time, individuals with type 2 diabetes are overweight. Treatment of type 2 diabetes usually involves a three-pronged approach: diet, weight loss, and exercise. Exercise enables carbohydrates to be used more effectively by promoting glucose uptake from the blood, thereby reducing insulin resistance. Exercise also helps to promote weight loss. Exercise programming for persons with type 2 diabetes is rarely dangerous or difficult. Exercise for individuals with type 1 diabetes is much more complex and is beyond the scope of this book. Any program of exercise for individuals with type 1 diabetes must be performed under the guidance of a physician. The person with type 1 diabetes needs to understand the interactions between exercise, glucose uptake, insulin, and carbohydrate consumption, because exercise can result in **hypoglycemia,** or hazardously low blood sugar, if done inappropriately.

Osteoarthritis is a gradual, progressive degeneration of joint structures that makes even normal movements painful. It has been speculated that high-impact exercise early in life contributes to the incidence of arthritis later on. However, research has found no association between exercise intensity and the incidence of arthritis, other than the tendency for arthritic pain to occur in areas of the body that have experienced earlier athletic injury. In fact, lifelong exercisers have been found to have less osteoarthritis than nonexercisers. Maintenance of good flexibility and the development of moderate levels of muscular strength have been found to stabilize the joints and provide relief for the minor aches and pains of arthritis. An exercise program for individuals with arthritis should focus on non-weightbearing exercise modalities (e.g., stationary cycling, water-based exercise) and should avoid high-impact stress on the knees, hips, and lower back.

Obesity (the condition of having excess body fat) has become a major health-related problem in the industrialized world. Excess body weight is associated with a number of chronic diseases, including **hypertension,** diabetes, and coronary artery disease. The most effective way to lose body weight and body fat is through a sound program of caloric restriction and low- to moderate-intensity aerobic exercise. Dieting alone is not effective. While severe dieting can lead to weight loss, the loss is frequently from the lean body mass (mainly the muscles) rather than from the fat mass of the body, which results in a decrease in metabolic rate. An exercise program for the obese or overweight client should focus on burning the maximum number of calories per session and avoiding musculoskeletal injuries. The goal should be to perform longer-duration (building up to 45 to 60 minutes per day), low- to moderate-intensity (40 to 60% of **heart-rate reserve**) exercise five to six days per week. Nonweightbearing or low-impact activities should also be stressed (e.g., walking, stationary cycling, aquatic exercise).

People with pulmonary disease are severely limited by the amount of air they can move into and out of their lungs. The blood does not get adequately oxygenated and exercise capacity is very low. The most common forms of pulmonary disease are emphysema, bronchitis, and asthma. Emphysema and chronic bronchitis are usually the result of long-term cigarette smoking, whereas the exact cause of asthma is unknown. Asthma occurs when the bronchi (large breathing passages) become constricted (bronchospasm), and the onset of symptoms is usually related to irritants such as tobacco smoke, animal dander, and cold air. Some people also experience exercise-induced asthma (EIA). The most widely accepted hypothesis for the cause of EIA is that airway cooling irritates the lining of the respiratory tree and causes the bronchospasm. It was once thought that individuals with pulmonary disease should not exercise. However, a regular program of aerobic exercise has been proven to decrease the amount of dyspnea (shortness of breath) in individuals with emphysema and bronchitis and increase their quality of life. People with asthma should also be encouraged to exercise and to have bronchodilator medications readily available if symptoms become severe. All patients with pulmonary disease should be under the care of a physician.

Coronary heart disease (CHD) involves partial or total closure of the coronary arteries, which results in symptoms or signs of ischemia (lack of blood flow to the heart muscle). The American Heart Association has identified a number of factors that increase the risk of **cardiovascular disease.** The primary **risk factors** are hypertension (elevated blood pressure), cigarette smoking, elevated blood lipid levels, and physical inactivity. Secondary risk factors include family history of heart disease, obesity, diabetes, being male, age over 65 for women and over 55 for men, and a high level of emotional stress. Obviously, little can be done to change one's age, gender, or family health history, but lifestyle changes can significantly alter the other risk factors. Regular participation in a well-planned aerobic exercise program has been shown to reduce high blood pressure, serum lipid levels, body fat, emotional stress, and cardiovascular mortality. Safety is a primary issue when developing exercise programs for individuals with cardiac disease. Patients should be under the care of a physician and may require an exercise stress test to guide the exercise program design.

Hormonal Responses to Exercise

The endocrine system plays a major role in regulating the body's response to exercise and training by releasing various hormones via glandular secretion. After binding to specific receptors on a target cell, these hormones perform a number of functions in the body, such as regulating cellular metabolism, facilitating the cardiovascular responses to exercise, and modulating protein synthesis. The hormonal response to exercise is very complex, and the integrated response of the various systems provides the changes necessary to help the body make the acute and chronic adaptations to exercise training. A brief description of the major hormonal responses to exercise is presented below.

- **Growth hormone (GH)** is secreted by the anterior pituitary gland and facilitates protein synthesis in the body. Many effects of growth hormones are mediated by **insulin-like growth factors** (IGF I and IGF II), which are synthesized in the liver as a result of GH release during exercise.
- **Antidiuretic hormone (ADH),** which is also called **vasopressin,** is released by the posterior pituitary gland during exercise. As its name implies, its primary function is to reduce urinary excretion of water. By conserving water during exercise, it helps to prevent dehydration.
- **Epinephrine** and **norepinephrine** are called **catecholamines** and are released by the adrenal medulla. They are released

as part of the sympathetic response to exercise (the "fight or flight" mechanism) and play two major roles. One role is to increase cardiac output by increasing heart rate and contractility during exercise. The second role is to cause **glycogenolysis** (glycogen breakdown) in the liver, so that more glucose can be released into the bloodstream for use by the actively working muscles.

- **Aldosterone** and **cortisol** are two of the main hormones released by the adrenal cortex. Aldosterone plays a role in limiting sodium excretion in the urine, which serves to maintain electrolyte balance during exercise. Cortisol is a glucocorticoid and plays a major role in maintaining blood glucose during prolonged exercise by promoting protein and triglyceride breakdown.
- **Insulin** and **glucagon** are both secreted by the cells of the **islets of Langerhans** in the pancreas, yet they have opposite effects. When blood glucose is high (e.g., after a meal), insulin is released from the **beta cells** in the islets of Langerhans to facilitate glucose removal from the blood and return blood glucose to a normal range. When blood glucose levels are low (e.g., during prolonged endurance exercise), glucagon is released from the **alpha cells** in the islets of Langerhans to stimulate glucose release from the liver to increase blood glucose. Glucagon also causes the release of free fatty acids from adipose tissue so that they can be used as fuel.
- **Testosterone** (released by the testes) and **estrogen** (released by the ovaries) are the primary male and female sex hormones, respectively. Testosterone is responsible for the masculine characteristics associated

with manhood (**androgenic** effects) and also has **anabolic** (muscle-building) effects. Because of their potent anabolic effects, testosterone and its derivatives are often abused in attempts to enhance athletic performance. Estrogen is responsible for the feminine characteristics associated with being a woman and also plays a major role in bone formation and maintenance. High levels of chronic exercise training have been shown to decrease estrogen levels to the point where some female athletes no longer have their menstrual cycle (**amenorrhea**). Amenorrhea has been associated with **osteoporosis** and increased risk of bone fractures.

Environmental Considerations When Exercising

Exercising under extreme environmental conditions can add significant stress to the cardiovascular system. Special precautions need to be taken when exercising in the heat or cold, at high altitude, or in the presence of pollution.

Exercising in the Heat

Considerable metabolic heat is produced during exercise. To reduce this internal heat load, venous blood is brought to the skin surface (peripheral vasodilation) to be cooled. When the sweat glands secrete water onto the skin, it is evaporated, which serves to cool the underlying blood. If environmental conditions are favorable, these mechanisms will adequately prevent the body temperature from rising more than about 2 to 3° F, even during heavy exercise.

When exercising in the heat, however, dissipating internal body heat is difficult, and external heat from the environment may significantly add to the total heat load. This results in

a higher-than-normal heart rate at any given level of exercise. For example, if someone walks at 3 miles per hour and their heart rate is normally 125 beats per minute, walking at the same speed in the heat may result in a heart rate of 135 to 140 beats per minute. Thus, exercisers (regardless of the type of exercise performed) need to decrease their absolute workload in the heat to stay within their target HR zone.

This elevated HR comes about primarily for two reasons. First, as the body tries to cool itself, the high degree of vasodilation in the vessels supplying the skin reduces venous return of blood to the heart and SV declines. The heart attempts to maintain cardiac output by elevating HR. Second, sweating results in a considerable loss of body water. If lost fluids are not replenished, dehydration eventually results, and blood volume declines. This will also decrease venous return to the heart. Again, the body responds with a higher HR to maintain cardiac output.

The most stressful condition in which to exercise is a hot, humid environment. When the air contains a large quantity of water vapor, sweat will not evaporate readily. Since it is the evaporative process that cools the body, adequate cooling may not occur in humid conditions. Under these conditions, heat exhaustion and heat stroke become dangerous possibilities. Heat exhaustion usually develops in unacclimatized individuals and is typically a combination of inadequate circulatory adjustments to exercise coupled with fluid loss. Heat stroke is a complete failure of the heat-regulating mechanisms, with core temperature exceeding 105° F (41° C). Both conditions require immediate medical attention. Symptoms of heat exhaustion and heat stroke, as well as treatment options, are presented in Table 1.2. Table 1.3 combines measures of heat and humidity

Table 1.2
Heat Exhaustion and Heat Stroke

	Signs and Symptoms	Treatment
Heat Exhaustion	Weak, rapid pulse	Stop exercising
	Low blood pressure	Move to a cool, ventilated area
	Headache	Lay down and elevate feet 12–18 inches
	Nausea	Give fluids
	Dizziness	Monitor temperature
	General weakness	
	Paleness	
	Cold clammy skin	
	Profuse sweating	
	Elevated body core temp (<104° F or 40° C)	
Heat Stroke	Hot, dry skin	Stop exercising
	Bright red skin color	Remove as much clothing as feasible
	Rapid, strong pulse	Try to cool body immediately in any way possible (wet towels, ice packs/baths, fan, alcohol rubs)
	Labored breathing	Give fluids
	Elevated body core temp (>105° F or 41° C)	Transport to emergency room immediately

Table 1.3
Heat Index

TEMPERATURE (°F) (°C given in parentheses)

RELATIVE HUMIDITY %	70 (21)	75 (24)	80 (27)	85 (29)	90 (32)	95 (35)	100 (38)	105 (41)	110 (43)	115 (46)	120 (49)
	APPARENT TEMPERATURE* (°F) (°C given in parentheses)										
0	64 (18)	69 (21)	73 (23)	78 (26)	83 (28)	87 (31)	91 (33)	95 (35)	99 (37)	103 (39)	107 (42)
10	65 (18)	70 (21)	75 (24)	80 (27)	85 (29)	90 (32)	95 (35)	100 (38)	105 (41)	111 (44)	116 (47)
20	66 (19)	72 (22)	77 (25)	82 (28)	87 (31)	93 (34)	99 (37)	105 (41)	112 (44)	120 (49)	130 (54)
30	67 (19)	73 (23)	78 (26)	84 (29)	90 (32)	96 (36)	104 (40)	113 (45)	123 (51)	135 (57)	148 (64)
40	68 (20)	74 (23)	79 (26)	86 (30)	93 (34)	101 (38)	110 (43)	123 (51)	137 (58)	151 (66)	
50	69 (21)	75 (24)	81 (27)	88 (31)	96 (36)	107 (42)	120 (49)	135 (57)	150 (66)		
60	70 (21)	76 (24)	82 (28)	90 (32)	100 (38)	114 (46)	132 (56)	149 (65)			
70	70 (21)	77 (25)	85 (29)	93 (34)	106 (41)	124 (51)	144 (62)				
80	71 (22)	78 (26)	86 (30)	97 (36)	113 (45)	136 (58)					
90	71 (22)	79 (26)	88 (31)	102 (39)	122 (50)						
100	72 (22)	80 (27)	91 (33)	108 (42)							

How to Use Heat Index
1. Locate temperature across top
2. Locate relative humidity down left side
3. Follow across and down to find Apparent Temperature
4. Determine Heat Stress Risk on chart at right

Note: This Heat Index chart is designed to provide general guidelines for assessing the potential severity of heat stress. Individual reactions to heat will vary. In addition, studies indicate that susceptibility to heat disorders tends to increase among children and older adults. Exposure to full sunshine can increase Heat Index values by up to 15° F.

Apparent Temperature		Heat Stress Risk with Physical Activity and/or Prolonged Exposure
90–105	(32–41)	Heat cramps or heat exhaustion possible
105–130	(41–54)	Heat cramps or heat exhaustion likely; Heat stroke possible
130–151	(54–66)	Heat stroke highly likely

*Combined index of heat and humidity and what it feels like to the body

into a simple-to-use **heat index**. The heat index provides guidelines regarding when exercise can be safely undertaken, and when it should be avoided.

Below are some additional tips for exercising in the heat:

• **Begin exercising gradually in the heat.** Becoming acclimatized to exercising in the heat takes approximately one week to 10 days. Start by exercising for short periods of time each day.

• **Always wear lightweight, well-ventilated clothing.** Cotton materials are cooler; most synthetics retain heat. Wear light-colored clothing if exercising in the sun; white reflects heat better than other colors.

• **Never wear impermeable or nonbreathable garments.** The notion that wearing rubber suits or nonbreathable garments adds to weight loss is a myth. Wearing impermeable clothing is a dangerous practice that could lead to significant heat stress and heat injury.

• **Replace body fluids as they are lost.** Drink fluids at regular intervals while exercising, but avoid overhydration, which, although relatively rare, can be as dangerous as dehydration. Frequent consumption of small amounts of fluid, designed to minimize sweat-related weight loss, is the best approach.

• **Recording daily body weight is an excellent way to prevent accumulative dehydration.** For example, if 5 pounds (2.25 kg) of body water is lost during aerobic exercise, this water should be replaced before exercising again the next day. If lost water has not been regained, exercise should be curtailed until the body is adequately rehydrated.

Exercising in the Cold

The major problems encountered when exercising in the cold are associated with an excessive loss of body heat, which can result in hypothermia or frostbite. Additionally, the cold can cause a generalized vasoconstriction that can increase peripheral resistance and blood pressure. This may cause problems in people who are hypertensive or who have heart disease. Following exercise, chilling can occur quickly if the body surface is wet with sweat and heat loss continues.

Heat loss from the body becomes greatly accelerated when there is a strong wind. The windchill factor can be quite significant. Similar to the heat index chart, Table 1.4 provides the various combinations of temperature and wind velocity that can be used as guidelines when deciding if it is safe to exercise in the cold.

Below are some additional tips for exercising in the cold:

• **Wear several layers of clothing.** By layering clothing, an exerciser can remove and replace garments as needed. When exercise intensity is high, remove outer garments. Then, during periods of rest, warm-up, cool-down, or low-intensity exercise, put them back on. A head covering is also important, because considerable body heat radiates from the head.

• **Allow for adequate ventilation of sweat.** Sweating during heavy exercise can soak inner garments. If evaporation does not readily occur, the wet garments will continue to drain the body of heat during rest periods, when retention of body heat is important.

• **Select garment materials that allow the body to give off body heat during exercise and retain body heat during inactive periods.** Cotton is a good choice for exercising in the heat because it readily soaks up sweat and allows evaporation; for those same reasons, however, cotton is a poor choice for exercising in the cold. Wool is an excellent choice when exercising in the

Table 1.4
Windchill Factor Chart

Estimated wind speed (in mph) (km/h given in parentheses)	ACTUAL THERMOMETER READING (°F) (°C given in parentheses)											
	50 (10)	40 (4)	30 (-1)	20 (-7)	10 (-12)	0 (-18)	-10 (-23)	-20 (-29)	-30 (-34)	-40 (-40)	-50 (-46)	-60 (-51)
	EQUIVALENT TEMPERATURE (°F) (°C given in parentheses)											
calm	50 (10)	40 (4)	30 (-1)	20 (-7)	10 (-12)	0 (-18)	-10 (-23)	-20 (-29)	-30 (-34)	-40 (-40)	-50 (-46)	-60 (-51)
5 (8)	48 (9)	37 (3)	27 (-3)	16 (-9)	6 (-14)	-5 (-21)	-15 (-26)	-26 (-32)	-36 (-38)	-47 (-44)	-57 (-49)	-68 (-56)
10 (16)	40 (4)	28 (-2)	16 (-9)	4 (-16)	-9 (-23)	-24 (-31)	-33 (-36)	-46 (-43)	-58 (-50)	-70 (-57)	-83 (-64)	-95 (-71)
15 (24)	36 (2)	22 (-6)	9 (-13)	-5 (-21)	-18 (-28)	-32 (-36)	-45 (-43)	-58 (-50)	-72 (-58)	-85 (-65)	-99 (-78)	-112 (-80)
20 (32)	32 (0)	18 (-8)	4 (-16)	-10 (-23)	-25 (-32)	-39 (-39)	-53 (-47)	-67 (-55)	-82 (-63)	-96 (-71)	-110 (-79)	-124 (-87)
25 (40)	30 (-1)	16 (-9)	0 (-18)	-15 (-26)	-29 (-34)	-44 (-42)	-59 (-51)	-74 (-59)	-88 (-67)	-104 (-76)	-118 (-83)	-133 (-92)
30 (48)	28 (-2)	13 (-11)	-2 (-19)	-18 (-28)	-33 (-36)	-48 (-44)	-63 (-53)	-79 (-62)	-94 (-70)	-109 (-78)	-125 (-87)	-140 (-96)
35 (56)	27 (-3)	11 (-12)	-4 (-20)	-20 (-29)	-35 (-37)	-51 (-46)	-67 (-55)	-82 (-63)	-98 (-72)	-113 (-81)	-129 (-89)	-145 (-98)
40 (64)	26 (-3)	10 (-12)	-6 (-21)	-21 (-29)	-37 (-38)	-53 (-47)	-69 (-56)	-85 (-65)	-100 (-73)	-116 (-82)	-132 (-91)	-146 (-99)

[Wind speeds greater than 40 mph (64 km/h) have little additional effect.]	GREEN	YELLOW	RED
	LITTLE DANGER (for properly clothed person). Maximum danger of false sense of security.	INCREASING DANGER Danger for freezing of exposed flesh.	GREAT DANGER

cold because, even when it is wet, it maintains body heat. Newer, synthetic materials (e.g., polypropylene) are also excellent choices, as they wick sweat away from the body, thus preventing heat loss. When windchill is a problem, nylon materials are good for outerwear. Gore-Tex®-like materials, although much more expensive than nylon, are probably the best choice for outerwear because they can block the wind, are waterproof, and allow moisture to move away from the body.

• **Replace body fluids in the cold, just as in the heat.** Fluid replacement is vitally important when exercising in cold air. Large amounts of water are lost from the body during even normal respiration and this effect becomes magnified when exercising. Because sweat losses may not be as obvious as when exercising in the heat, monitoring of body weight over several days is recommended. (See Chapter 4 for recommended fluid intakes.)

Exercising at Higher Altitudes

At moderate-to-high altitudes, the **partial pressure*** of oxygen in the air is reduced. Because there is less pressure to drive the oxygen molecules into the blood in the lungs, the oxygen carried in the blood is reduced. Therefore, a person exercising at high altitude will not be able to deliver as much oxygen to the exercising muscles and exercise intensity will have to be reduced (e.g., the person will have to walk or run slower) to keep his or her HR in a target zone.

Signs and symptoms of altitude sickness include shortness of breath, headache, light-

---

* Partial pressure is the pressure of each gas in a multiple-gas system such as air, which is composed of nitrogen, oxygen, and carbon dioxide.

headedness, and nausea. Generally, altitude sickness can be avoided by acclimatizing oneself properly. This means gradually increasing exercise and activity levels over the span of several days. Using a prolonged warm-up and cool-down and incorporating frequent exercise breaks at a lower intensity should help most people acclimate to exercising at higher altitudes.

Air Pollution

Some areas of the country have a high degree of airborne pollutants (smog) that can adversely affect exercise performance. These pollutants are the result of the combustion of fossil fuels and primarily include ozone, sulfur dioxide, and carbon monoxide. When these airborne particles are inhaled, they can have a number of deleterious effects on the body, such as irritating the airways and decreasing the oxygen-carrying capacity of the blood, both of which hamper performance. In individuals with cardiovascular disease, prolonged exposure to air pollution can even induce ischemia and angina. The overall physiological effects are determined by the degree (or dose) of pollutants to which an individual is exposed. This dose is related to the amount of pollutants in the air, the length of exposure, and the amount of air breathed. Practical suggestions to minimize the effects of air pollution include exercising early in the morning to avoid the build-up of

pollutants associated with increased vehicular traffic, and avoiding high-traffic, urban areas. Similar to when exercising in the heat or at altitude, exercise pace may need to be reduced to keep HR in the appropriate training range. Under extreme conditions, exercising indoors is probably the best choice.

Summary

This chapter is designed to provide the group fitness instructor with basic principles of exercise physiology. Considerable space has been devoted to the presentation of aerobic and anaerobic metabolism, because the principle of specificity clearly dictates that physiological adaptations are specific to encountered stresses. The group fitness instructor must understand the various methods of applying progressive overload and the physiological adaptations that result. Too often, the exercising public falls victim to the poor advice of exercise teachers, coaches, and other "experts" who fail to apply the concept of exercise specificity because they simply do not understand basic principles.

A large amount of information has been given in a relatively small amount of space. The emphasis has been on basic understanding rather than on detailed explanation. Students of this material are strongly encouraged to seek further knowledge of exercise physiology and the principles of physical fitness and human movement through more advanced study.

References

Bandy, W.D. & Irion, J.M. (1994). The effect of time on static stretch on the flexibility of the hamstring muscles. *Physical Therapy,* 74: 845–850; discussion 850–852.

Franklin, B.A. (1999). Exercise adds up like loose change. *ACSM's Health and Fitness Journal,* 3, 4, 38–39.

Jakicic, J.M. et al. (1995). Prescribing exercise in multiple short bouts versus one continuous bout: Effect on adherence, cardiorespiratory fitness, and weight loss in overweight women. *International Journal of Obesity,* 19, 12, 893–901.

McHugh, M.P. et al. (1992). Viscoelastic stress relaxation in human skeletal muscle. *Medicine & Science in Sports & Exercise,* 24: 1375–1382.

Murphy, M.H. & Hardman, A.E. (1998). Training effects of short and long bouts of brisk walking in sedentary women. *Medicine & Science in Sports & Exercise,* 30, 1, 152–157.

Suggested Reading

Alter, M.J. (1996). *Science of Flexibility* (2nd ed.). Champaign, Ill.: Human Kinetics.

American College of Sports Medicine (2006). *ACSM's Guidelines for Exercise Testing and Prescription* (7th ed.). Philadelphia: Lippincott Williams & Wilkins.

American College of Sports Medicine (1998). Position stand: The recommended quantity and quality of exercise for developing and maintaining cardiorespiratory and muscular fitness and flexibility in healthy adults. *Medicine & Science in Sports & Exercise,* 30, 975–991.

Fleck, S.J. & Kraemer, W.J. (2004). *Designing Resistance Training Programs.* Champaign, Ill.: Human Kinetics.

Howley, E.T. & Franks, B.D. (2003). *Health Fitness Instructor's Handbook* (5th ed.). Champaign, Ill.: Human Kinetics.

Plowman, S.A. & Smith, D.L. (2002). *Exercise Physiology for Health, Fitness, and Performance* (2nd ed.). Boston: Allyn and Bacon.

Pollock, M.L. et al. (1998). The recommended quantity and quality of exercise for developing and maintaining cardiorespiratory and muscular fitness, and flexibility in healthy adults. *Medicine & Science in Sports & Exercise,* 30, 6, 975–991.

Chapter Two

Rod A. Harter, Ph.D., A.T.C., F.A.C.S.M., is an associate professor in the Department of Nutrition and Exercise Sciences at Oregon State University in Corvallis. Dr. Harter is a certified athletic trainer and a fellow of the American College of Sports Medicine. His areas of specialization include kinesiology, biomechanics, and sports medicine.

Fundamentals of Anatomy

By Rod A. Harter

A strong background in human anatomy is essential for all fitness professionals for several reasons. Understanding the structure and function of the major systems in the body is crucial for the design of system-specific group fitness activities, as well as individualized adaptations and modifications based on varying levels of physical capacity. Current knowledge of the structure and function of bones, muscles, and ligaments, among other anatomical components, is critical for successful communication with clients and professional colleagues. Developing a comprehensive base of knowledge about human anatomy will enable instructors to correctly demonstrate and explain the numerous group fitness activities.

Fundamentals of Anatomy

The objective of this chapter is to explain how the parts of the body work together to provide the functional capacity, stability, **mobility,** and strength needed for effective human movement in sport, recreation, and the activities of daily living.

Anatomical Terminology

When studying anatomy for the first time, most people will likely encounter terms that are unfamiliar to them. Use of the correct anatomical terms for position, location, and direction is essential when describing a particular movement, exercise, or activity to a participant or colleague. The majority of anatomical terms have their origins in the Latin and Greek languages, and are typically very descriptive. The words used to name the more than 650 muscles in the human body typically describe the muscle's location, shape, or action. Consider the anterior tibialis muscle as an example. Anterior means "toward the front," while tibialis refers to the tibia, the larger of the two long bones in the lower leg. In

this case, by knowing the meanings of the root words, an instructor understands both the anatomical term and the location of this muscle—the anterior tibialis muscle is found on the front part of the tibia. As a general rule in anatomy, when there is a directional term included in the name of a structure (e.g., anterior, posterior), it typically means that there is a complementary structure (e.g., bone, muscle, ligament) nearby. In this case, the complementary structure to the anterior tibialis is the posterior tibialis, a muscle located on the opposite side (back) of the lower leg.

To help readers avoid having to refer continually to a medical dictionary to define the terms used throughout this chapter, a summary of commonly used anatomical terms is presented in Table 2.1. Other important terms that describe anatomical positions are defined in Table 2.2. A representation of **anatomical position,** a starting or reference position used to describe and define all human movement, is given in Figure 2.1, along with the anatomical planes of motion.

Figure 2.1
Anatomical reference position and planes of motion

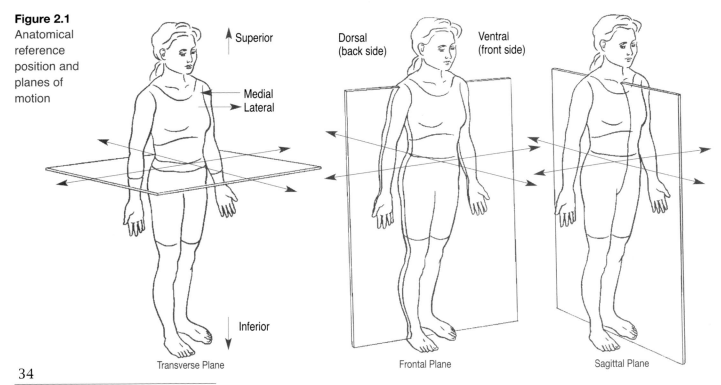

Superior

Medial
Lateral

Inferior

Transverse Plane

Dorsal (back side)

Ventral (front side)

Frontal Plane

Sagittal Plane

ACE GROUP FITNESS INSTRUCTOR MANUAL

Table 2.1
Anatomical, Directional, and Regional Terms

Term	Definition	Term	Definition
Anterior (ventral)	Toward the front	Palmar	The anterior or ventral surface of the hands
Posterior (dorsal)	Toward the back	Sagittal plane	A longitudinal (imaginary) line that divides the body or any of its parts into right and left halves
Superior	Toward the head		
Inferior	Away from the head		
Medial	Toward the midline of the body		
Lateral	Away from the midline of the body	Mediolateral axis	The transverse axis of rotation about which sagittal plane movement occurs; perpendicular to the sagittal plane
Proximal	Toward the attached end of the limb, origin of the structure, or midline of the body		
Distal	Away from the attached end of the limb, origin of the structure, or midline of the body	Frontal plane	A longitudinal (imaginary) section that divides the body or any of its parts into anterior and posterior halves
Cervical	Regional term referring to the neck	Anteroposterior axis	The front-to-back axis of rotation about which frontal plane movement occurs; perpendicular to the frontal plane
Thoracic	Regional term referring to the portion of the body between the neck and abdomen; also known as the chest (thorax)		
Lumbar	Regional term referring to the low back; the portion between the abdomen and the pelvis	Transverse plane	Also known as the horizontal plane; an imaginary line that divides the body or any of its parts into superior and inferior halves
Plantar	The sole, or bottom, of the feet		
Dorsal	The top surface of the feet and hands	Longitudinal axis	The vertical axis of rotation about which transverse plane motion occurs; perpendicular to the transverse plane

Table 2.2
Common Anatomical Terminology

Root	Meaning	Term	Definition
Arthro	Joint	Arthritis	Inflammation in a joint
Bi	Two, both	Bilateral	On both sides
Brachium	Arm	Brachialis	Muscle of the arm
Cardio	Heart	Cardiology	The study of the heart
Cephalo	Head	Cephalic	Pertaining to the head
Chondro	Cartilage	Chondroectomy	Excision of a cartilage
Costo	Rib	Costochondral	Pertaining to a rib and its cartilage
Dermo	Skin	Dermatitis	Inflammation of the skin
Hemo, hemato	Blood	Hemorrhage	Internal or external bleeding
Ilio	Pelvis or hip	Ilium	The wide, upper part of the pelvic bone
Myo	Muscle	Myocitis	Inflammation of a muscle
Os, osteo	Bone	Osteopenia	Loss of bone mineral
Pulmo	Lung	Pulmonary artery	Vessel that brings blood to the lungs
Thoraco	Chest	Thorax	Chest
Tri	Three	Triceps brachii	Three-headed muscle on the arm

Fundamentals of Anatomy

In the following sections, the functions of the five major systems in the human body that are most pertinent to exercise and physical activity will be reviewed in a summary manner. These systems are the cardiovascular system, the respiratory system, the nervous system, the skeletal system, and the muscular system.

Cardiovascular System

Oxygen is required for energy production, and thus sustains cellular activity (cellular metabolism) in the human body. A by-product of this cellular activity is carbon dioxide. High levels of carbon dioxide in the cells produce acidic conditions that are very poisonous to cells; thus, excess carbon dioxide must be eliminated rapidly. The cardiovascular and respiratory systems are primarily responsible for this function.

The cardiovascular system is composed of the blood, the blood vessels, and the heart. The cardiovascular system distributes oxygen and nutrients to the cells, carries carbon dioxide and metabolic wastes from the cells, protects against disease, helps regulate body temperature, and prevents serious blood loss after injury through the formation of clots.

Blood is composed of two parts: formed elements, which include different types of living blood cells—white blood cells, red blood cells, and platelets—and plasma, the nonliving liquid portion of blood. Plasma is composed of approximately 92% water and 8% dissolved solutes. There are more than 100 different types of dissolved solutes in plasma; the most abundant of these are plasma proteins. In adults, blood accounts for about 8% of body weight; an average-sized healthy woman has about 4 to 5 liters, while an average-sized healthy man has approximately 5 to 6 liters of blood.

Types of Blood Vessels

There are two types of blood vessels: **arteries,** which carry blood away from the heart, and **veins,** which transport blood toward the heart (Figures 2.2 and 2.3). Arteries are thicker than veins, and their muscular walls help propel blood. Unlike arteries, veins contain valves that prevent blood from flowing backward. The largest arteries are those nearest the heart. As blood flows farther away from the heart, the arteries branch into smaller arteries called **arterioles,** which deliver the blood to even smaller structures known as **capillaries.** These microscopic blood vessels branch to form an extensive network throughout the **distal** tissues. The critical exchange of nutrients and metabolic waste products takes place here in the capillary beds. Capillary blood, now depleted of oxygen and nutrients from the trip from the heart to the periphery, reaches the end of the line and then begins the long journey back to the heart via small vessels called **venules.** Within the body's closed circulatory system, the venules are a continuation of the capillaries, and these tiny structures ultimately join together to form veins. As the blood is carried closer and closer to the heart, the veins become larger, carrying a greater volume of blood.

The Heart

The human heart is a hollow, muscular organ at the center of the cardiovascular system. In the adult, the heart is about the same size as the closed fist and lies to the left of center, behind the sternum and between the lungs. The heart itself is divid-

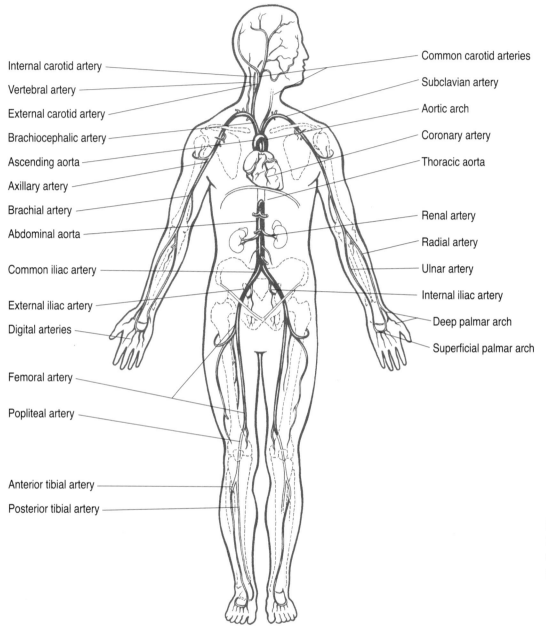

Internal carotid artery

Vertebral artery

External carotid artery

Brachiocephalic artery

Ascending aorta

Axillary artery

Brachial artery

Abdominal aorta

Common iliac artery

External iliac artery

Digital arteries

Femoral artery

Popliteal artery

Anterior tibial artery

Posterior tibial artery

Common carotid arteries

Subclavian artery

Aortic arch

Coronary artery

Thoracic aorta

Renal artery

Radial artery

Ulnar artery

Internal iliac artery

Deep palmar arch

Superficial palmar arch

Figure 2.2
Major arteries
of the body
(anterior view)

ed into four chambers that receive circulating blood. The two upper chambers are called the right and left **atria,** while the two lower chambers of the heart are known as the right and left **ventricles** (Figure 2.4).

The heart can be described as an efficient combination of four separate pumps: two primer pumps, the atria, and two power pumps, the ventricles. Knowledge of the sequence of blood flow through the heart is fundamental to understanding the cardiovascular system. The right atrium receives blood from all parts of the body except the lungs. The superior vena cava, the large vein that drains blood from body parts **superior** to (above) the heart (e.g., head, neck, arms), and its counterpart, the inferior vena cava, which brings blood from the parts of the body **inferior** to (below) the heart (e.g., legs, abdominal region), transport blood to the

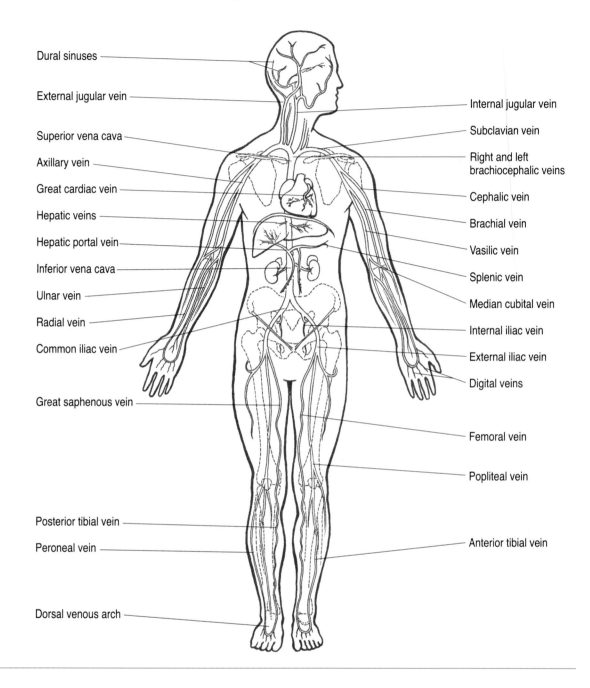

- Dural sinuses
- External jugular vein
- Superior vena cava
- Axillary vein
- Great cardiac vein
- Hepatic veins
- Hepatic portal vein
- Inferior vena cava
- Ulnar vein
- Radial vein
- Common iliac vein
- Great saphenous vein
- Posterior tibial vein
- Peroneal vein
- Dorsal venous arch

- Internal jugular vein
- Subclavian vein
- Right and left brachiocephalic veins
- Cephalic vein
- Brachial vein
- Vasilic vein
- Splenic vein
- Median cubital vein
- Internal iliac vein
- External iliac vein
- Digital veins
- Femoral vein
- Popliteal vein
- Anterior tibial vein

Figure 2.3
Major veins of
the body
(anterior view)

right atrium. During contraction of the heart, blood accumulates in the right atrium. With relaxation of the heart, blood from the right atrium flows into the right ventricle; during contraction, blood is pumped into the pulmonary trunk. The pulmonary trunk then divides into right and left pulmonary arteries, which transport blood to the lungs, where carbon dioxide is released and oxygen is acquired. This freshly oxygenated blood returns to the heart via four pulmonary veins that empty into the left atrium. The blood then passes into the left ventricle. During the contraction phase of the heart, blood is pumped from the left ventricle into the ascending **aorta.** From this point, the blood is distributed to all body parts (except the lungs) by several large arteries.

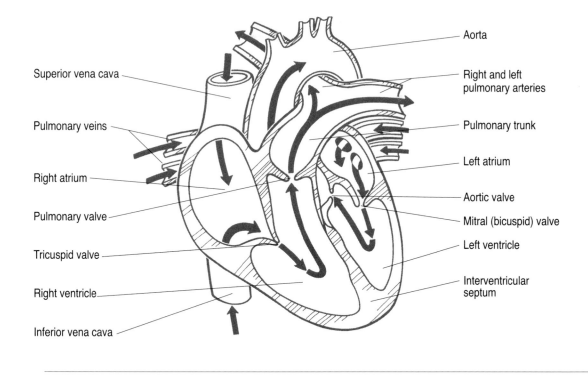

Aorta

Superior vena cava

Right and left
pulmonary arteries

Pulmonary veins

Pulmonary trunk

Left atrium

Right atrium

Aortic valve

Pulmonary valve

Mitral (bicuspid) valve

Left ventricle

Tricuspid valve

Interventricular
septum

Right ventricle

Inferior vena cava

Figure 2.4
Anatomy of the
heart and pattern
of blood flow
through it

Respiratory System

The respiratory system supplies oxygen, eliminates carbon dioxide, and helps regulate the acid-base balance (pH) of the body. The respiratory system is composed of the lungs and the series of passageways (e.g., mouth, throat, trachea, bronchi) leading to and from the lungs. The process of **respiration** is the overall exchange of gases (e.g., oxygen, carbon dioxide, nitrogen) between the atmosphere, the blood, and the cells.

There are three general phases of respiration: external, internal, and cellular. External respiration is the exchange of oxygen and carbon dioxide between the atmosphere and the blood within the large capillaries in the lungs. Internal respiration involves the exchange of those gases between the blood and the cells of the body. Cellular respiration involves the utilization of oxygen and the production of carbon dioxide by the metabolic activity within cells.

When the body is at rest, air enters the respiratory system via the nostrils and is warmed as it passes through a series of nasal cavities lined by a mucous membrane covered with cilia (small hairs) that filter out small particles. From the nasal cavity, inspired air next enters the pharynx (throat), which lies just **posterior** to the nasal and oral (mouth) cavities. The pharynx serves as a passageway for air and food and also provides a resonating chamber for speech sounds. During vigorous physical activity, mouth breathing predominates and air taken in via the mouth is not filtered to the same extent as air taken in through the nostrils.

The larynx, or voice box, is the enlarged upper (**proximal**) end of the trachea (windpipe). The larynx conducts air to and from the lungs via the pharynx. An easy landmark for locating the larynx is the thyroid **cartilage,** or Adam's apple. The trachea is a tubular airway approximately 4 or 5 inches long (about 12 to 14 centimeters) kept open by a series of C-shaped cartilages that have a function similar to the wire rings in a vacuum cleaner hose. The trachea extends from the larynx to approximately the level of the fifth thoracic vertebra, where it divides into the right and left **primary bronchi.** After this division, each primary bronchus enters a lung and divides into smaller secondary bronchi, one for each lobe of the lung (five total). The secondary bronchi branch into many tertiary bronchi, and these tubes branch several times further, eventually forming tiny terminal **bronchioles.** The terminal bronchioles have microscopic branches called respiratory bronchioles that, in turn, subdivide into several alveolar ducts (plural = **alveoli**). The actual

exchange of respiratory gases, such as oxygen and carbon dioxide, between the lungs and the blood occurs at this anatomic level. Lungs contain an estimated 300 million alveoli that provide an extremely large surface area (approximately 750 square feet or 70 square meters) for the exchange of gases. The continuous branching of the trachea resembles a tree trunk and its branches, and thus is commonly referred to as the **bronchial tree** (Figure 2.5).

The final components of the respiratory system are the lungs—paired, cone-shaped organs located in the thoracic cavity. The right lung has three lobes, while the left lung has only two. The diaphragm is the muscle that forms the floor of the thoracic cavity,

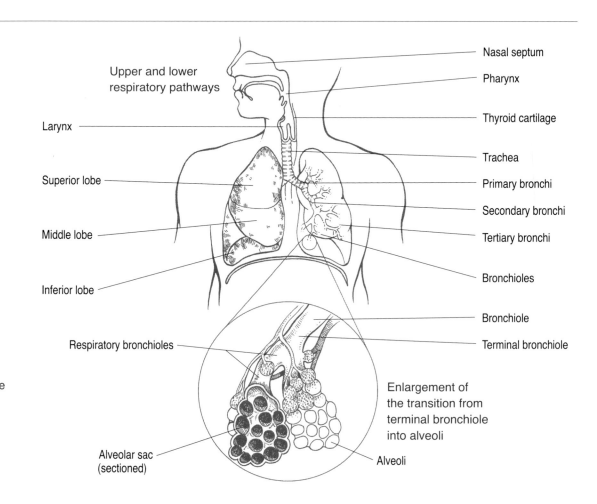

Figure 2.5
The bronchial tree

Upper and lower respiratory pathways

Larynx

Superior lobe

Middle lobe

Inferior lobe

Respiratory bronchioles

Alveolar sac (sectioned)

Nasal septum

Pharynx

Thyroid cartilage

Trachea

Primary bronchi

Secondary bronchi

Tertiary bronchi

Bronchioles

Bronchiole

Terminal bronchiole

Enlargement of the transition from terminal bronchiole into alveoli

Alveoli

contracts during inspiration, and relaxes to allow expiration. The lungs are separated by a space known as the mediastinum, which contains the heart, the esophagus (the tube that connects the throat with the stomach), and a portion of the trachea.

Nervous System

The nervous system is considered the body's control center and network for internal communication. The nervous system has two main classes of cells: approximately 10,000 million nerve cells, or neurons, and 10 to 50 times as many glial cells, or glia. Neurons rapidly conduct electrical impulses throughout the body to coordinate movement and other essential functions. The literal meaning of the Greek root glia is "glue," but these cells do not typically hold neurons together. While no evidence exists to suggest that glia are directly involved in the electrical signaling process, they perform a vital function by surrounding (insulating and protecting) the neurons (Kandel, Schwartz, & Jessell, 2000).

Rather than focusing on the cellular-level functions of neurons and glia, group fitness instructors should be primarily interested in the nervous system's role in creating and controlling movement. A skeletal muscle cannot contract until it receives a stimulus from either an internal source (e.g., a nerve impulse) or an external source (e.g., therapeutic electrical muscle stimulation). Without the central control provided by the specialized sections of the brain, coordinated human movements are impossible.

The cells of the nervous system are organized into two functional divisions (voluntary and autonomic nervous systems) and two structural divisions (central and peripheral nervous systems). The voluntary nervous system is by definition under volitional con-

trol, with the exception of reflexive movements. In contrast, the autonomic nervous system is not under conscious (voluntary) control and includes the portions of the nervous system that control the heart, visceral muscles, and endocrine glands. The two structural divisions of the nervous system are the central nervous system (CNS) and the peripheral nervous system (PNS). The brain and the spinal cord combine to form the CNS and are totally enclosed within bony structures. The skull protects the brain, while the spinal cord is protected by the vertebral canal of the spinal column. The CNS is the control center of the nervous system, as it receives input from the PNS, integrates this information, and formulates appropriate responses to the input. The PNS is made up of nerves that connect the extremities and their **receptors** within the CNS. The PNS includes 12 pairs of cranial nerves, two of which arise from the brain, while the remaining 10 pairs begin in the brain stem. The PNS also includes 31 pairs of spinal nerves that originate from the spinal cord. The spinal nerves include eight cervical pairs, 12 thoracic pairs, five lumbar pairs, five sacral pairs, and one coccygeal pair (Figure 2.6). These nerves are named and numbered according to region and the vertebral level at which they emerge from the spinal cord. For example, the fifth cervical nerve (written as C5) exits the spinal cord at the level of the fifth cervical vertebra.

Cells within the human nervous system carry messages known as nerve impulses that originate in either the CNS or in specialized nerve cells called receptors, which are located throughout the body. Different types of receptors are sensitive to pain, temperature, pressure, and changes in body position. Sensory nerve cells carry

Fundamentals of Anatomy

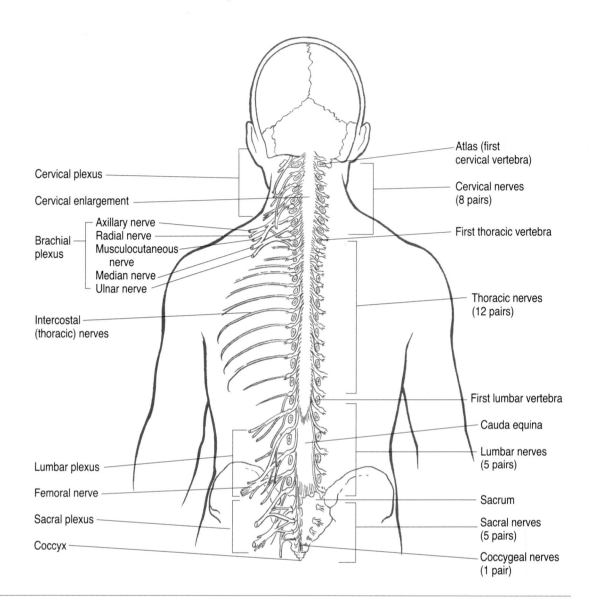

Cervical plexus

Cervical enlargement

Brachial plexus
— Axillary nerve
— Radial nerve
— Musculocutaneous nerve
— Median nerve
— Ulnar nerve

Intercostal (thoracic) nerves

Lumbar plexus

Femoral nerve

Sacral plexus

Coccyx

Atlas (first cervical vertebra)

Cervical nerves (8 pairs)

First thoracic vertebra

Thoracic nerves (12 pairs)

First lumbar vertebra

Cauda equina

Lumbar nerves (5 pairs)

Sacrum

Sacral nerves (5 pairs)

Coccygeal nerves (1 pair)

Figure 2.6
Spinal cord and spinal nerves (posterior view)

afferent impulses from the peripheral receptors to the spinal cord and brain. Motor nerve cells carry efferent impulses from the CNS to the extremities in response to the imposed physical demands of physical activity and/or perceived changes in the body's internal or external environment (i.e., physical pain or dangerous situations).

The anterior branches of the second through twelfth thoracic spinal nerves (T2 to T12 nerve roots) individually innervate muscles and other structures, such as the internal organs. In all other cases, the anterior branches of the spinal nerves combine with adjacent nerves to form one of the four networks of nerves or plexuses.

There are four major nerve plexuses in the human body: the cervical plexus, the brachial plexus, the lumbar plexus, and the sacral plexus. The C1 through C4 nerve roots join to create the cervical plexus, which innervates the head, neck, upper chest, and shoulders. The nerves of the brachial plexus (C5 to T1) provide motor and sensory functions for the shoulder all the way down to the fingers of the hand.

The brachial plexus has a unique anatomical feature, an "extra" nerve root; specifically, there is a pair of C8 nerve roots, but no C8 vertebra exists. The L1 to L4 nerve roots, which form the lumbar plexus, innervate the abdomen, groin, genitalia, and anterolateral aspect of the thigh, while the nerves of the sacral plexus (L4 to S4) supply the large muscles of the buttocks, posterior thigh, and the entire lower leg, ankle, and foot. Table 2.3 provides a summary of the primary spinal nerve roots that provide the

Table 2.3
Selected Spinal Nerve Roots and
Major Muscles Innervated

Nerve Root	Muscles Innervated
C3	Trapezius, longus capitis, longus cervicis, scalenus medius
C4	Diaphragm, trapezius, levator scapulae, scalenus anterior and medius
C5	Biceps brachii, deltoid, rhomboid major and minor, supraspinatus, infraspinatus
C6	Serratus anterior, latissimus dorsi, brachioradialis, extensor carpi radialis longus and brevis, extensor carpi ulnaris, supinator
C7	Triceps brachii, flexor carpi radialis, flexor carpi ulnaris
C8	Extensor pollicis longus and brevis, adductor pollicis longus
T1	Intrinsic muscles of the hand (lumbricals, interossei)
L2	Psoas major and minor, adductor magnus, adductor longus, adductor brevis
L3	Rectus femoris, vastus lateralis, vastus medialis, vastus intermedius, psoas major and minor
L4	Tibialis anterior, tibialis posterior
L5	Extensor hallucis longus, extensor digitorum longus, peroneus longus and brevis, gluteus maximus, gluteus medius
S1	Gastrocnemius, soleus, biceps femoris, semitendinosus, semimembranosus, gluteus maximus
S2	Gluteus maximus, flexor hallucis longus, flexor digitorum longus
S4	Bladder, rectum

motor functions for specific muscles (known as myotomes) and the areas of cutaneous sensation (referred to as dermatomes) attributed to each of these plexuses.

Neurological Factors Affecting Movement

Voluntary human movement is regulated and controlled by complex interactions within the central and peripheral nervous systems. The capacity for somatosensation is achieved through integration of three sources of input—the eyes (visual system), inner ear (vestibular system), and body (somatic system). Of particular interest and importance is the feedback received by the CNS from specific somatosensory receptors found in muscles (muscle spindle afferents, or MSAs), tendons (Golgi tendon organs, or GTOs), ligaments and joint capsules (Ruffini endings and Pacinian corpuscles), and the skin (Merkel discs and Meissner corpuscles). Each type of these microscopic sensory organs is stimulated into action by some form of mechanical deformation. Taken as a whole, these receptors are known as **proprioceptors,** and they provide near-instantaneous information about static body position and the direction and velocity of movement.

Effective learning and performance of the movement patterns taught by group fitness instructors depend on input from the participant's sensory pathways to his or her brain. The brain interprets this sensory information and a specific motor response is formulated in regard to the magnitude, direction, and rate of change of body movement. Sensory receptors can provide a conscious or **kinesthetic awareness** of body and limb position; first-hand evidence of this neurological capability can be seen

Fundamentals of Anatomy

when class participants follow the instructor's lead, mirroring him or her perfectly.

Kinesthesia is the conscious awareness of the position of body parts and the amount, direction, and velocity of joint movement. This information comes primarily from the previously defined proprioceptors that are located in the muscles, tendons, ligaments, and joint capsules. This type of perception allows a person to initiate and modify movement patterns; it also affects his or her perception of posture. When poor posture is habitual, the person may perceive a wrong alignment as being correct. To change that erroneous perception, additional input must be given to the sensory receptors. For example, to correct a chronic slouching (rounded shoulders) posture, the individual must repeatedly perform resistance exercises to strengthen the muscles that retract the shoulder blades (scapulae). In this way, the person develops the muscle tone and endurance required to maintain the appropriate posture and the receptors are re-educated to learn what normal posture feels like.

When a person is performing a complex physical activity, such as an inclined bench press, the central and peripheral nervous systems work together to initiate, guide, and monitor all aspects of the specific activity. In this example, the nerve receptors in the periphery, located in the arm and shoulder region, provide continuous information (feedback) to the CNS regarding the amount of resistance encountered, limb position, pressure sensed on the palms of the hands, and so on. This communication between central and peripheral nervous systems, utilizing the motor and sensory nerve pathways, is essential to learn, modify, and successfully perform both simple and complex physical activities.

Reflex Activity

Sensory receptors are also involved in unconscious reflexes that deserve brief mention here. Two important types of proprioceptors are located in the muscles (MSAs) and tendons (GTOs). Muscle spindle afferents are sensitive to high levels of, and/or rapid increases in, tension within the muscle and respond to this stimulus by triggering the **stretch reflex,** a protective activation of the muscle being stretched to prevent injury. Similarly, the GTOs located in the proximal and distal tendons of a muscle respond to tension, but their reflex action is to induce relaxation within the muscle in which they reside, diminishing the amount of tension in the tendon and preventing injury. Both reflex actions are protective and have important applications for the group fitness instructor utilizing stretching exercises as part of the warm-up and cool-down phases of a class. Activation of the stretch reflex can and should be avoided by using slow, controlled, static stretching techniques. Conversely, the GTO reflex is a desired response during flexibility exercises and is activated by holding a static stretch position for at least 15 seconds, causing the GTOs to fire and inhibit the muscle being stretched, thus permitting additional **range of motion** and stretching.

Skeletal System

As infants, human skeletons consist of approximately 270 bones; through the process of growth and development a number of these bones fuse together, so that eventually the adult skeleton has only 206 movable bones. The human skeletal system (Figure 2.7) can be divided into two sections: the **axial skeleton** (80 bones that comprise the head, neck, and trunk); and the **appendicular skeleton** (126 bones that form the extremities) (Table 2.4). The 206 bones that form the human skeleton perform five basic, yet important, functions. First, the skeletal system provides protection for many of the vital organs, such as the heart, brain, and spinal cord. Second, the skeleton provides support for the soft tissues so that erect posture and the form of the body can be maintained. Third, the bones provide a framework of **levers** to which muscles are attached. When particular muscles are stimulated, long bones act as levers to produce movement. Fourth, the red marrow of bone is responsible for the production of certain blood cells, namely red blood cells, some types of white blood cells, and platelets. Fifth, bones serve as storage areas for calcium, phosphorus, potassium, sodium, and other minerals. Due to their high mineral content, bones often remain intact for thousands of years after death. Fat is also stored within the middle section of long bones in the medullary cavity (Figure 2.8).

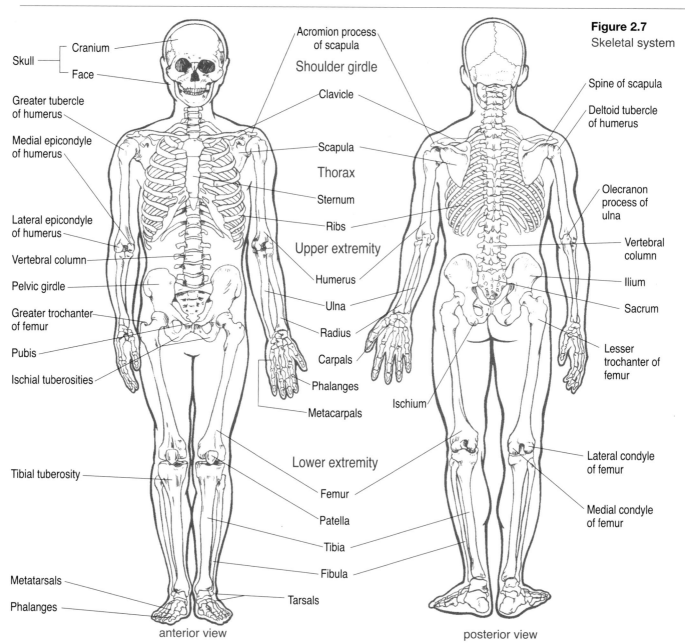

Figure 2.7
Skeletal system

Skull — Cranium / Face

Greater tubercle of humerus

Medial epicondyle of humerus

Lateral epicondyle of humerus

Vertebral column

Pelvic girdle

Greater trochanter of femur

Pubis

Ischial tuberosities

Tibial tuberosity

Metatarsals

Phalanges

Acromion process of scapula
Shoulder girdle
Clavicle
Scapula
Thorax
Sternum
Ribs
Upper extremity
Humerus
Ulna
Radius
Carpals
Phalanges
Metacarpals
Lower extremity
Femur
Patella
Tibia
Fibula
Tarsals

Spine of scapula
Deltoid tubercle of humerus
Olecranon process of ulna
Vertebral column
Ilium
Sacrum
Lesser trochanter of femur
Lateral condyle of femur
Medial condyle of femur

Ischium

anterior view

posterior view

Fundamentals of Anatomy

Bones may also be classified according to their shape: long, short, flat, irregular, or sesamoid. Long bones are those in which the length exceeds the width and the thickness. Most of the bones in the lower and upper

Table 2.4
Bones in the Axial and Appendicular Skeletons

Axial Skeleton	Number of Bones
Skull	
Cranium	8
Face	14
Hyoid	1
Vertebral Column	26
Thorax	
Sternum	1
Ribs	24
(Auditory ossicles)*	6
	80

Appendicular Skeleton	Number of Bones
Lower Extremity	
Phalanges	28
Metatarsals	10
Tarsals	14
Patella	2
Tibia	2
Fibula	2
Femur	2
Pelvic Girdle	
Hip or pelvis (os coxae = ilium, ischium, pubis)	2
Shoulder Girdle	
Clavicle	2
Scapula	2
Upper Extremity	
Phalanges	28
Metacarpals	10
Carpals	16
Radius	2
Ulna	2
Humerus	2
	126

*Note: The auditory ossicles, three per ear, are not considered to be part of the axial or appendicular skeletons, but rather a separate group of bones. They were placed in the axial skeleton group for convenience.

extremities are long bones, including the femur, tibia, fibula, and metatarsals in the lower limbs, and the humerus, radius, ulna, and metacarpals in the upper extremity. Each long bone has a shaft called a **diaphysis,** and on each end, usually wider than the shaft, is an **epiphysis.** During childhood and adolescence, these cartilaginous epiphyses are active as growth plates that permit normal longitudinal bone growth to take place. By the time the human skeleton fully matures at young adulthood (age range: 18 to 21 years), the epiphyses have changed from cartilage into fully ossified bone, and no further longitudinal growth in long bones takes place.

The outer surface of the diaphysis of a long bone is surrounded by a **connective tissue** sheath known as **periosteum** (see Figure 2.8). The periosteum has two layers, an outer layer that provides sites of attachment for muscles and tendons, and an inner layer that, when disrupted by fracture or trauma, signals the release of osteoblasts (bone-forming cells) to create new bone and repair the fracture. The anatomical complement to the periosteum is the **endosteum,** a soft-tissue lining of the internal surface of the diaphysis in the medullary canal. The primary function of the endosteum is to resorb old and/or unneeded bone through the action of osteoclasts (bone-resorbing cells). Throughout much of a person's lifetime, the ongoing, typically balanced activity of the osteoblasts and osteoclasts results in the constant remodeling of bones and helps to sustain the circumferential dimensions of long bones. Upon reaching middle age and, for women specifically, menopause, significant reductions in the level of the reproductive hormone estrogen negatively affect the metabolic activity in bone. In time, these changes may cause severe reductions in bone mineral den-

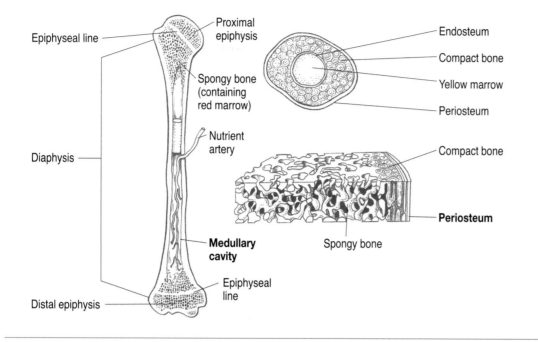

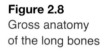

Figure 2.8
Gross anatomy
of the long bones

sity (osteopenia) and, ultimately, osteoporosis and spontaneous fractures of the vertebrae and femur, among others.

Short bones have no long axis and are approximately equal in length and width. This type of bone is found in the hands (carpals) and the feet (tarsals).

Flat bones are partially described by their name; they tend to be thin but are usually curved rather than flat. The bones of the skull, the ribs, the sternum, and the scapulae (shoulder blades) are examples.

Irregular bones are bones of various shapes that do not fall into any of the other categories (e.g., **vertebrae,** ilium, ischium, pubis).

Sesamoid bones, literally "seed-like" bones, are few in number and are found embedded within tendons. The largest sesamoid bone, the patella (kneecap), significantly increases the efficiency of the quadriceps femoris by improving the mechanical advantage for knee extension.

Human bone contains an inorganic component composed of mineral salts, primarily calcium and potassium; an organic component

made of **collagen,** a complex protein that is found in various forms in bone and other connective tissues; and water. According to **Wolff's Law,** bone is capable of adjusting its size and strength in proportion to the amount of stress placed on it. When young, healthy people participate in exercise programs for extended periods of time, their bones typically become more dense through increased deposition of mineral salts and the number of collagen fibers. On the other hand, if bones are not subjected to mechanical stresses, as in individuals with sedentary lifestyles or in the absence of gravitational loading, such as the microgravity environment in outer space or through nonweightbearing exercises like swimming, bones will become less dense over time as mineral is withdrawn from bone. An easy way to remember this important principle is with the saying, "form follows function." Simply stated, the form that bone will take (strong or weak) is in direct response to the recent functional demands placed on that bone. When Wolff's Law was

Skeletal
System

written in 1892, little was known about the important influences that genetics, nutrition, hormonal levels (estrogen and testosterone), and use of tobacco and alcohol have on bone. The modern understanding of these and other factors points out the limitations of Wolff's Law—mechanical loading is important to bone health, but is by no means the only factor that influences its density and material strength.

This knowledge has important implications for the group fitness instructor, who must have the bone health of his or her class participants in mind when creating specific conditioning and resistance-exercise programs. Group fitness instructors should emphasize the positive influence on bone health as one of the main reasons for their clients to begin or continue with their regular participation in physical activity. Since the lower levels of the hormone estrogen that accompany **amenorrhea** (two or fewer menstrual periods per year) and menopause in women lead to substantial bone mineral loss, it is important to assist participants in developing strength-building programs.

Axial Skeleton

As previously stated, the axial skeleton consists of the 80 bones that form the skull, the vertebral column, and the thorax (chest). This portion of the skeletal system provides the main structural support for the body while also protecting the central nervous system and vital organs in the thorax (e.g., heart, lungs). Of primary importance is the adult vertebral column, consisting of 33 vertebrae divided into five groups and named according to the region of the body in which they are located. The upper seven are **cervical vertebrae,** followed in descending

order by 12 **thoracic vertebrae,** five **lumbar vertebrae,** five **sacral vertebrae** fused into one bone as the sacrum, and four coccygeal vertebrae fused together into one bone called the **coccyx.** The sacral vertebrae and coccygeal vertebrae become fused in the adult, so there are only 24 movable vertebrae (Figure 2.9).

Appendicular Skeleton

The appendicular skeleton is composed of the bones of the lower and upper limbs and the bones by which the legs and arms attach to the axial skeleton—the pelvic (hip) and pectoral (chest) girdles. The pelvic girdle consists of two large hip bones known collectively as the os coxae, with each side made up of an ilium, an ischium, and a pubis (see Figure 2.7). The two pectoral girdles, each consisting of a clavicle (collarbone) and scapula (shoulder blade), attach the bones of the upper extremities to the axial skeleton at the sternum. Since the sternoclavicular joints are the only direct bone-to-bone links between the upper extremities and the axial skeleton, several trade-offs exist from this configuration. Most importantly, the pectoral girdle does not provide very strong support for the upper extremity. However, the girdle does permit a wide range of movements at the shoulder, making it the most mobile joint in the body.

Articulations (Joints)

An **articulation,** or joint, is the point of contact or connection between bones or between bones and cartilage. Ligaments— the dense, fibrous strands of connective tissue that link together the bony segments— maintain the stability and integrity of all joints. Some joints permit large ranges of

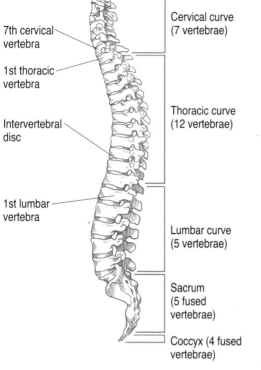

7th cervical vertebra

1st thoracic vertebra

Intervertebral disc

1st lumbar vertebra

Cervical curve (7 vertebrae)

Thoracic curve (12 vertebrae)

Lumbar curve (5 vertebrae)

Sacrum (5 fused vertebrae)

Coccyx (4 fused vertebrae)

Figure 2.9
Vertebral column (lateral view)

motion in several directions, while other joints permit virtually no motion at all. The various joints in the body can be classified into two general categories according to (a) the structure of the joints and (b) the type of movement allowed by the joints.

Structural Classification of Joints

When classifying joints according to their structure, two main characteristics differentiate the types of joints: (a) the type of connective tissue that holds the bones of the joint together and (b) the presence or absence of a joint cavity. There are three major structural categories of joints: fibrous, cartilaginous, and synovial. Fibrous joints have no joint cavity and include all joints in which the bones are held tightly together by fibrous connective tissue. Very little space separates the ends of the bones of these joints; as a result, little or no movement occurs. Examples include the

joints, or sutures, between the bones of the skull, the joint between the radius and ulna, and the joint between the distal tibia and fibula (Figure 2.10).

As the name implies, cartilaginous joints connect bones that are slightly separated by an intervening cartilage. No joint cavity exists and, similar to fibrous joints, little or no motion is possible. Familiar examples include intervertebral disks that separate the bodies of vertebrae that comprise the spinal column and the joints formed by the cartilages that connect the ribs to the sternum (breastbone) (Figure 2.11).

The vast majority of the joints in the human body are synovial joints. These joints all have a space, or joint cavity, between the bones forming the joint. Having space between these bones allows more movement to occur at that joint. The capacity for movement of synovial joints is limited by the shapes of the bones of the joint and the soft tissues, such as ligaments, joint capsules, tendons, and muscles, that surround the joint. Synovial joints have five distinguishing features that set them apart structurally from the other types of joints. First, as previously described, all synovial joints have a joint cavity. Second,

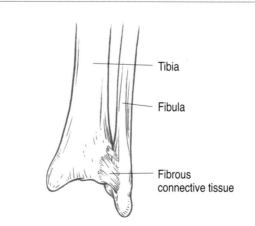

Tibia

Fibula

Fibrous connective tissue

Figure 2.10
Example of a fibrous joint—distal tibiofibular joint

49

Fundamentals of Anatomy

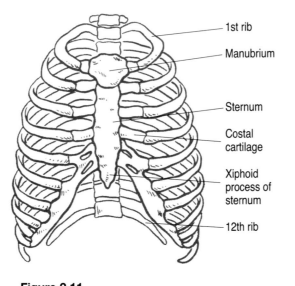

1st rib

Manubrium

Sternum

Costal
cartilage

Xiphoid
process of
sternum

12th rib

Figure 2.11

Example of a cartilaginous joint—
sternocostal joint

a ligamentous joint capsule made of dense, fibrous connective tissue surrounds each synovial joint. Third, the ends of the bones in synovial joints are covered with a thin layer of articular cartilage. This articular cartilage is made of hyaline ("glass-like") cartilage, and while it covers the surfaces of the articulating bones, the hyaline cartilage does not attach the bones together. Fourth, the inner surface of the joint capsule is lined with a thin synovial membrane. The synovial membrane's primary function is the secretion of synovial fluid, which represents the fifth and final unique characteristic of all synovial joints. Synovial fluid acts as a lubricant for the joint and provides nutrition to the articular (hyaline) cartilage. Normally, only a very small amount of synovial fluid (one or two teaspoons) is present in even the largest joints, such as the knee and shoulder. However, acute injury to, or overuse of, these synovial joints can stimulate the synovial membrane to secrete excessive fluid, typically producing pain, swelling, and decreased range of motion.

In addition to these five features, some synovial joints have fibrocartilage disks called menisci (singular = meniscus). An important weightbearing joint like the knee has two menisci. At large joints, such as the shoulder, hip, and knee, fibrocartilages help to absorb shock, increase joint stability, aid in joint nutrition by directing the flow of synovial fluid, and increase the joint contact area. By increasing the contact area between the bones of a joint, the fibrocartilages spread the load and reduce the pressure (force per unit area) on the weightbearing structures. Injury to a fibrocartilage changes the load-bearing pattern and shock-absorptive capabilities in that joint, and this change typically accelerates the wear and tear on the joint's load-bearing surfaces, leading to premature degeneration and osteoarthritis.

Types of Movement at Synovial Joints

The functional classification of synovial joints is based on the degree and type of movement they allow. Revisit the discussion of the anatomical planes of motion used to describe the actions of the body (see Figure 2.1). For a joint to move in a given plane, there must typically be an axis of rotation. An axis of rotation is an imaginary line perpendicular to the plane of movement about which a joint rotates. Due to their configuration, many joints have several axes of rotation, enabling bones to move in the various planes or directions.

Joints with one axis of rotation can only move in one plane and are known as uniplanar joints. These uniplanar joints are also known as hinge joints, in that hinges typically work only in one plane. The ankle (talocrural) and the elbow (ulnohumeral) joints are examples of uniplanar joints (Figure 2.12a).

Some joints have two axes of rotation, permitting motion in two planes that are at right angles to one another. These biplanar joints include a category of synovial joints known as condyloid joints, formed by the rounded, widened ends (condyles) of the two articulating bones. Condyloid joints allow full motion in one plane and have limited range of motion in a second plane. The knee (tibiofemoral), the joints of the hand and fingers (metacarpal-phalangeal), and the joints of the foot and toes (metatarsal-phalangeal joints) are all examples of condyloid joints (Figure 2.12b).

Triplanar joints have three axes of motion and permit movement in three planes. Examples include the hip joint and the shoulder (glenohumeral), both of which are ball-and-socket joints (Figure 2.12c), and the thumb (the first metacarpal-phalangeal), which is a saddle joint. A summary of the major joints in the body, classified by type and movements possible, is presented in Table 2.5.

Figure 2.12
Movement of synovial joints

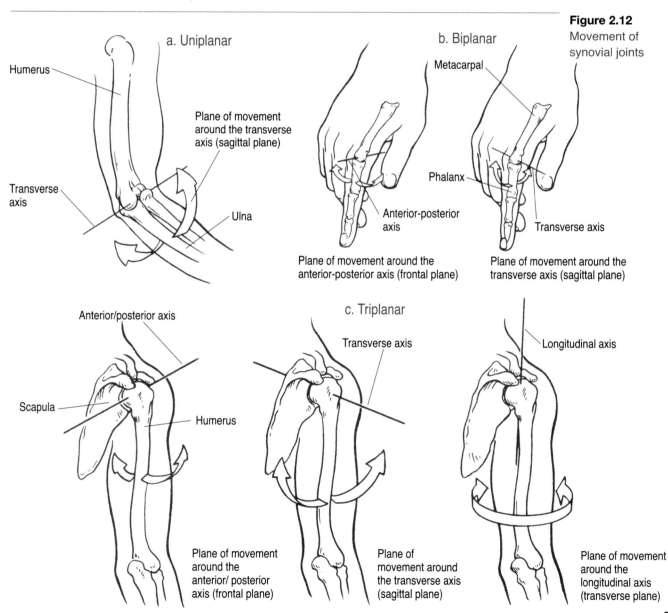

a. Uniplanar

Humerus

Plane of movement around the transverse axis (sagittal plane)

Transverse axis

Ulna

b. Biplanar

Metacarpal

Phalanx

Anterior-posterior axis

Transverse axis

Plane of movement around the anterior-posterior axis (frontal plane)

Plane of movement around the transverse axis (sagittal plane)

Anterior/posterior axis

Scapula

Humerus

Plane of movement around the anterior/ posterior axis (frontal plane)

c. Triplanar

Transverse axis

Plane of movement around the transverse axis (sagittal plane)

Longitudinal axis

Plane of movement around the longitudinal axis (transverse plane)

51

Fundamentals of Anatomy

Human Movement Terminology

Human motion occurs in three dimensions as body parts rotate about the joints. **Flexion** usually involves a decrease in the angle between the anterior surfaces of articulating bones, whereas **extension** most often describes an increase in this angle. Flexion and extension both occur in the **sagittal** plane and this fundamental movement occurs at most of the synovial joints (Figure 2.13). **Abduction** is a **lateral** movement away from the midline of the body. When the arm or leg is moved away from the midline of the body, abduction occurs. **Adduction** is the return motion from abduction and involves movement of the body part toward the midline of the body, to regain

anatomical position. Abduction and adduction movements occur in the **frontal plane** and are possible at many joints, some examples of which are presented in Figure 2.14. Movement at a joint that occurs in the transverse plane around a longitudinal axis is described as being either **internal rotation** or **external rotation** of the body segment involved. The hip, shoulder, and joints of the spine are among the joints most frequently requiring **rotation** for the performance of the activities of daily living (Figure 2.15).

At some synovial joints, the fundamental movements are given specialized names that clarify their action; these are summarized in Table 2.6. Forearm **supination** and **pronation** are motions that occur in the

Table 2.5
Major Joints in the Body

Region/Joint	Type	Number of Axes of Rotation	Movement(s) Possible
Lower Extremity			
Foot (metatarsal-phalangeal)	Synovial (condyloid)	2	Flexion and extension; abduction and adduction; circumduction
Ankle (talocrural)	Synovial (hinge)	1	Plantarflexion and dorsiflexion
Between distal tibia and fibula	Fibrous	0	Slight movement possible
Knee (tibia and femur)	Synovial (modified hinge)	2	Flexion and extension; internal and external rotation
Hip	Synovial (ball and socket)	3	Flexion and extension; abduction and adduction; circumduction; internal and external rotation
Upper Extremity			
Hand (metacarpal-phalangeal)	Synovial (condyloid)	2	Flexion and extension; abduction and adduction; circumduction
Thumb	Synovial (saddle)	3	Flexion and extension; abduction and adduction; circumduction; opposition
Wrist (radiocarpal)	Synovial	2	Flexion and extension; abduction and adduction; circumduction
Proximal radioulnar	Synovial (pivot)	1	Pronation and supination
Elbow (ulna and humerus)	Synovial (hinge)	1	Flexion and extension
Shoulder	Synovial (ball and socket)	3	Flexion and extension; abduction and adduction; circumduction; internal and external rotation
Ribs and sternum	Cartilaginous	0	Slight movement possible

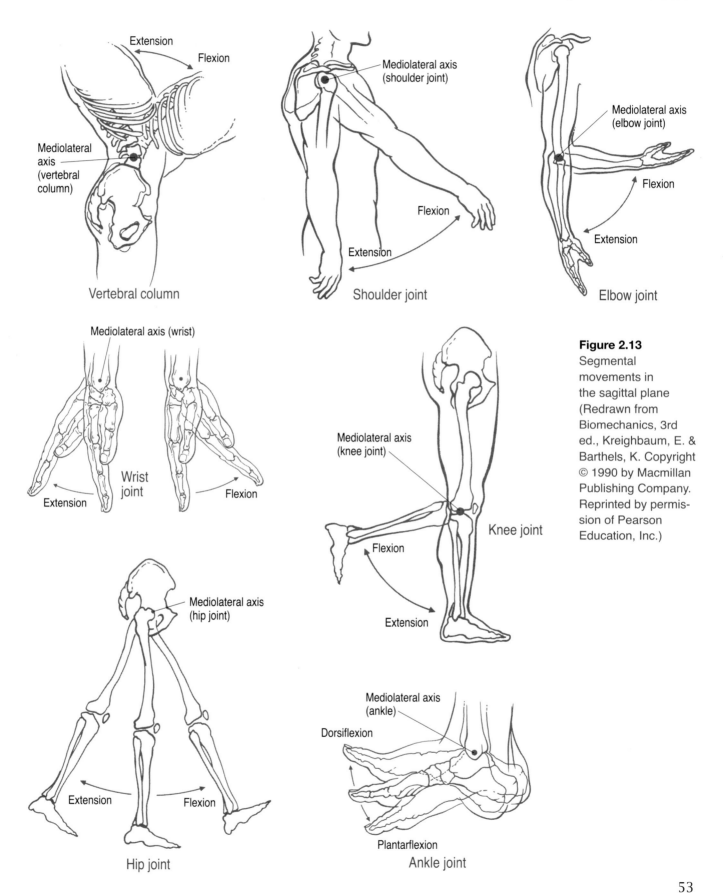

Vertebral column

Shoulder joint

Elbow joint

Wrist joint

Knee joint

Hip joint

Ankle joint

Figure 2.13
Segmental
movements in
the sagittal plane
(Redrawn from
Biomechanics, 3rd
ed., Kreighbaum, E. &
Barthels, K. Copyright
© 1990 by Macmillan
Publishing Company.
Reprinted by permission of Pearson
Education, Inc.)

Fundamentals of Anatomy

transverse plane. Supination is a term that specifically describes the external rotation of the forearm (radioulnar joint) that causes the palm to face anteriorly. The radius and the ulna are parallel in this position, which is the anatomical or reference position for the forearms (see Figure 2.1). Pronation describes the internal rotation of the fore-

arm that causes the radius to cross diagonally over the ulna and the palms to face posteriorly. **Circumduction** is a biplanar movement that involves the sequential combination of flexion, abduction, extension, and adduction. Circumduction is possible at the shoulder, hip, wrist, and spinal joints, among others.

Figure 2.14
Segmental movements in the frontal plane (Redrawn from *Biomechanics,* 3rd ed., Kreighbaum, E. & Barthels, K. Copyright © 1990 by Macmillan Publishing Company. Reprinted by permission of Pearson Education, Inc.)

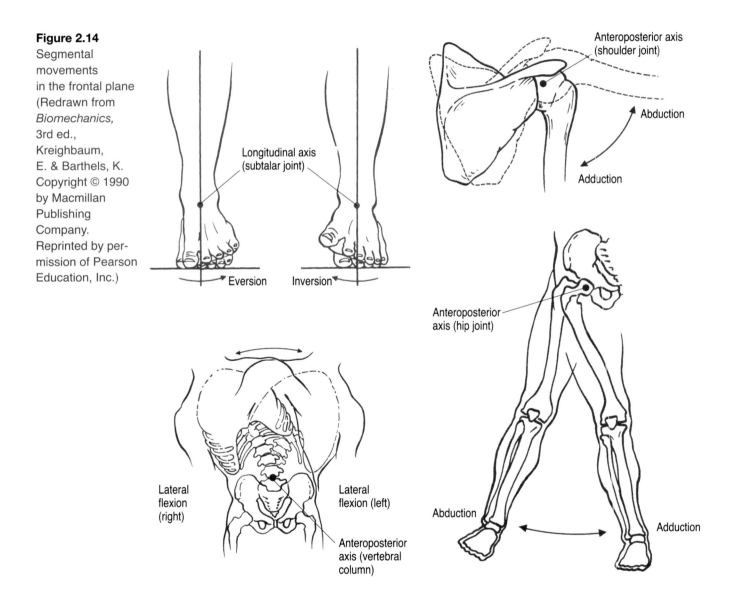

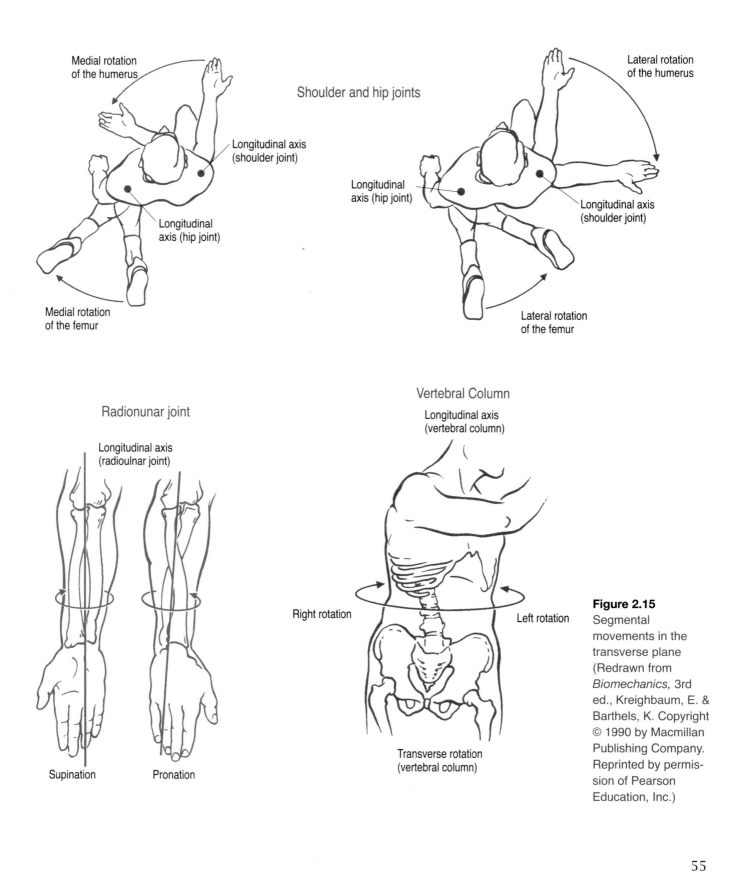

Shoulder and hip joints

Medial rotation
of the humerus

Longitudinal axis
(shoulder joint)

Longitudinal
axis (hip joint)

Medial rotation
of the femur

Lateral rotation
of the humerus

Longitudinal
axis (hip joint)

Longitudinal axis
(shoulder joint)

Lateral rotation
of the femur

Radionunar joint

Longitudinal axis
(radioulnar joint)

Supination

Pronation

Vertebral Column

Longitudinal axis
(vertebral column)

Right rotation

Left rotation

Transverse rotation
(vertebral column)

Figure 2.15
Segmental
movements in the
transverse plane
(Redrawn from
Biomechanics, 3rd
ed., Kreighbaum, E. &
Barthels, K. Copyright
© 1990 by Macmillan
Publishing Company.
Reprinted by permis-
sion of Pearson
Education, Inc.)

Fundamentals of Anatomy

Muscular System

While bones and joints provide the structural framework for the body, the system most directly affected by exercise is the muscular system, through the coordinated activation and relaxation of specific muscles that enable people to move. There are three types of human muscle tissue: cardiac, visceral, and skeletal. Cardiac muscle tissue forms the walls of the heart and its contractile activity is involuntary by nature. The second type, visceral (smooth) muscle, is found in the walls of internal organs like the stomach and intestines and in blood vessels. Visceral muscle activity is also involuntary, and thus it is not under conscious control. Skeletal muscle tissue is attached to bones by tendons and is typically named according to its location, function, or size. Skeletal muscle is voluntary muscle; that is, it can be made to act by conscious effort. While all three types of muscle have vital functions, the structure and function of skeletal muscles warrant fur-

Table 2.6
Fundamental Movements (From Anatomical Position)

Plane	Action	Definition
Sagittal	Flexion	Decreasing the angle between two bones
	Extension	Increasing the angle between two bones
	Dorsiflexion	Moving the top of the foot toward the shin (only at the ankle joint)
	Plantarflexion	Moving the sole of the foot downward; "pointing the toes" (only at the ankle)
Frontal	Abduction	Motion away from the midline of the body (or part)
	Adduction	Motion toward the midline of the body (or part)
	Elevation	Moving to a superior position (only at the scapula)
	Depression	Moving to an inferior position (only at the scapula)
	Inversion	Lifting the medial border of the foot (only at the subtalar joint)
	Eversion	Lifting the lateral border of the foot (only at the subtalar joint)
Transverse	Rotation	Internal (inward) or external (outward) turning about the vertical axis of bone
	Pronation	Rotating the hand and wrist medially from the elbow
	Supination	Rotating the hand and wrist laterally from the elbow
	Horizontal flexion	From a 90-degree abducted arm position, the humerus is flexed in, toward the midline of the body in the transverse plane
	Horizontal extension	The return of the humerus from horizontal flexion
Multiplanar	Circumduction	Motion that describes a "cone"; combines flexion, abduction, extension, and adduction in sequence
	Opposition	Thumb movement unique to humans and primates

ther discussion. Both ends of a skeletal muscle are attached to bone via tendons (cords of inelastic connective tissue). In some cases, skeletal muscles are attached to bone by an aponeurosis, a broad, flat type of tendon. The broad, flat insertion of the rectus abdominis is an example of an aponeurosis.

There are more than 650 muscles in the human body, but only the major muscles involved in human movement are discussed in this chapter. Muscles are named according to their location (anterior tibialis, posterior tibialis, subscapularis); shape (deltoid, trapezius, rhomboid); action (adductor magnus, pronator teres, erector spinae); number of divisions (biceps brachii, triceps brachii, quadriceps femoris); bony attachments (coracobrachialis, brachioradialis, iliocostalis); and size (gluteus maximus, gluteus medius, gluteus minimus). In addition, several muscles have the descriptive terms "longus" (long) or "brevis" (short) in their names.

When skeletal muscle is stimulated by an impulse from its motor nerve, it performs one function: it develops tension (**force**). There are three ways in which a muscle can develop tension: by shortening and producing joint movement (**concentric** muscle action), by lengthening and controlling the motion (**eccentric** muscle action), or by staying the same length and creating no joint motion (**isometric** muscle action). Generally speaking, concentric muscle actions occur when the muscle fibers contract and move toward the center ("concentric"), when the direction of movement is opposite the pull of gravity (e.g., the upward phase of a biceps curl with a dumbbell). In contrast, eccentric muscle actions occur when the muscle's fibers lengthen away from the center ("eccentric") to the anatomical or reference position, and the direction of body motion is

the same as the direction of gravity (e.g., the downward phase of the biceps curl).

From a functional perspective, most muscles are arranged in opposing pairs on the axial (trunk) or appendicular (extremities) skeleton. When one muscle is acting to achieve a desired movement, it is referred to as the **agonist;** the muscle that opposes the action of the agonist is known as the **antagonist.** For example, during the upward phase of a bent-knee curl-up, the abdominal muscles act concentrically as agonists to produce flexion of the trunk, while the erector spinae group of muscles of the back are elongated as antagonists. At most joints, several muscles work together to perform the same anatomical function; these muscles are functionally known as **synergists** (syn = together; erg = work). For the example just given, the synergistic actions of the rectus abdominis, external oblique, and internal oblique produce flexion of the trunk.

Perhaps the most difficult and often confusing aspect of functional anatomy is the fact that any given skeletal muscle can perform different, exactly opposite functions, depending on the circumstances and desired human movement. Most anatomy books only describe the concentric function(s) of a muscle, ignoring the motions produced when that same muscle acts eccentrically. To better understand this point, consider the functional roles played by the quadriceps femoris, the very large muscle located on the anterior thigh, during a mini-squat exercise. Focusing attention on the knee joint, the downward phase of a squat requires knee flexion, while the upward phase involves knee extension. The quadriceps, when acting concentrically, are the primary knee extensors and the hamstrings are the major knee flexors. However, since the direction of movement in the downward phase of the squat is the same direction as the pull of gravity, the observed knee flexion movement is controlled by an eccentric (lengthening) action of the quadriceps, not by the hamstrings. During the upward phase of the squat, the quadriceps act concentrically (shortening) to produce powerful extension of the knee, overcoming gravity and pushing the body upward in the direction opposite of gravity's pull. This one simple exercise illustrates how the quadriceps femoris acted as both a knee flexor and knee extensor, and how the only role the hamstrings had at the knee was that of the antagonist, rather than agonist. Every skeletal muscle has this same functional capability of producing opposite anatomical movements when it acts concentrically (shortens) versus when it acts eccentrically (lengthens).

The greatest amount of muscle force (tension) is generated during eccentric muscle actions, followed by isometric and then concentric muscle actions. Voluntary, coordinated maximal or submaximal efforts produce muscle actions that may or may not result in joint movement. Locomotion (walking, running) is the result of the complex, combined functioning of the bones, joints, nerves, and muscles. Isometric muscle actions enable the maintenance of posture in stationary positions (e.g., sitting and standing). As a by-product of performance of the activities of daily living, muscles produce heat, which is important in maintaining normal body temperature.

Muscles of the Lower Extremity

The major links of the lower extremity are (a) the ankle joint formed by the distal tibia, distal fibula, and talus; (b) the knee joint, which is composed of the tibiofemoral and patellofemoral joints; and (c) the hip joint,

which links the femur with the hip (coxal) bone. When compared to the muscles of the upper extremity, the muscles of the lower extremity tend to be larger and more powerful. Many of the muscles of the lower extremity cross two joints, either the hip and the knee or the knee and the ankle. The major muscles of the lower extremity that act at more than one joint are listed in Table 2.7.

Muscles That Act at the Ankle and the Foot

The muscles of the leg are grouped into four compartments that are divided by fibrous interosseous membranes (inter = between; os = bone) between the tibia and fibula (Figure 2.16). The anterior tibial compartment muscles act concentrically to extend the toes and dorsiflex the ankle. These muscles include the anterior tibialis, extensor digitorum longus, and extensor hallucis longus (Figure 2.17). The muscles of the lateral tibial compartment are known as the peroneals (peroneus longus and peroneus brevis) and act to cause **eversion** (movement outward, away from the middle) of the foot and assist in **plantarflexion** of the ankle (Figure 2.18). The posterior muscles of the leg are contained in two separate spaces—the superficial and deep posterior tibial compartments. The largest muscles of the calf (soleus and gastrocnemius), along with the much smaller plantaris, are located in the superficial posterior tibial compartment (Figure 2.19a & b). The deep posterior tibial compartment contains the posterior tibialis, flexor hallucis longus, flexor digitorum longus, and the popliteus (Figure 2.19c). The primary functions of these posterior muscles include plantarflexion of the ankle, flexion of the toes, and **inversion** (movement inward, toward the middle) of the foot. The popliteus has no function at the ankle or foot, but instead plays a vital role by con-

Table 2.7
Actions of Major Lower-extremity Multijoint Muscles

Muscle	Hip	Knee	Ankle
Rectus femoris	Flexion	Extension	—————
Biceps femoris	Extension (long head) External rotation	Flexion External rotation	—————
Semitendinosus	Extension Internal rotation	Flexion Internal rotation	—————
Semimembranosus	Extension Internal rotation	Flexion Internal rotation	—————
Gracilis	Adduction Internal rotation	Flexion Internal rotation	—————
Sartorius	Flexion External rotation	Flexion Internal rotation	—————
Gastrocnemius	—————	Flexion	Plantarflexion

tributing to knee flexion. The largest tendon in the body, the Achilles tendon, is found in the superficial posterior compartment and connects the gastrocnemius and soleus via one common tendon to the calcaneus (heel bone). The origins, insertions, primary functions, and examples of exercises to develop the muscles that act at the ankle and the foot are presented in Table 2.8.

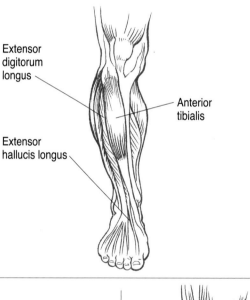

Extensor digitorum longus

Anterior tibialis

Extensor hallucis longus

Figure 2.17
Anterior tibial compartment muscles of the lower leg; primary muscles for dorsiflexion and inversion

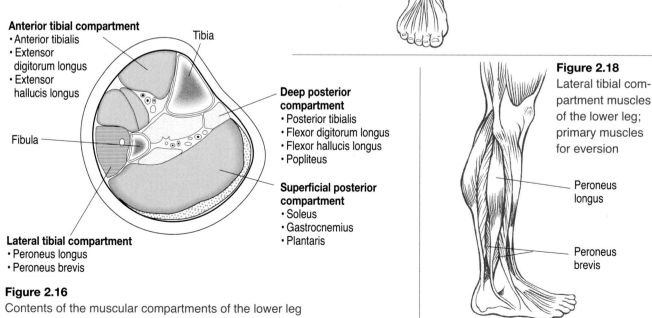

Anterior tibial compartment
• Anterior tibialis
• Extensor digitorum longus
• Extensor hallucis longus

Tibia

Fibula

Deep posterior compartment
• Posterior tibialis
• Flexor digitorum longus
• Flexor hallucis longus
• Popliteus

Superficial posterior compartment
• Soleus
• Gastrocnemius
• Plantaris

Lateral tibial compartment
• Peroneus longus
• Peroneus brevis

Figure 2.16
Contents of the muscular compartments of the lower leg

Figure 2.18
Lateral tibial compartment muscles of the lower leg; primary muscles for eversion

Peroneus longus

Peroneus brevis

Table 2.8
Major Muscles That Act at the Ankle and Foot

Muscle	Origin	Insertion	Primary Function(s)	Selected Exercises
Anterior tibialis	Proximal 2/3 of lateral tibia	Medial aspect of 1st cuneiform and 1st metatarsal	Dorsiflexion at ankle; inversion at foot	Cycling with toe clips; resisted inversion (with dorsiflexion)
Peroneus longus	Head of fibula and proximal 2/3 of lateral fibula	Inferior aspects of medial tarsal (1st cuneiform) and 1st metatarsal	Plantarflexion at ankle; eversion at foot	Resisted eversion of foot; walking on inside of foot
Peroneus brevis	Distal 2/3 of lateral fibula	Base of the 5th metatarsal	Plantarflexion at ankle; eversion at foot	Resisted eversion of foot with rubber tubing; walking on inside of foot
Gastrocnemius	Posterior surfaces of femoral condyles	Posterior surface of calcaneus via Achilles tendon	Plantarflexion at ankle	Hill running, jumping rope, calf raises with barbell on shoulder, cycling, stair-climber machine, in-line skating
Soleus	Proximal 2/3 of posterior surfaces of tibia and fibula	Posterior surface of calcaneus via Achilles tendon	Plantarflexion at ankle	Virtually the same as for gastrocnemius; bent-knee toe raises with resistance
Posterior tibialis	Posterior surface of tibia-fibular interosseous membrane	Lower medial surfaces of medial tarsals and metatarsals	Plantarflexion at ankle; inversion at foot	Resisted inversion of foot with surgical tubing (with plantarflexion)

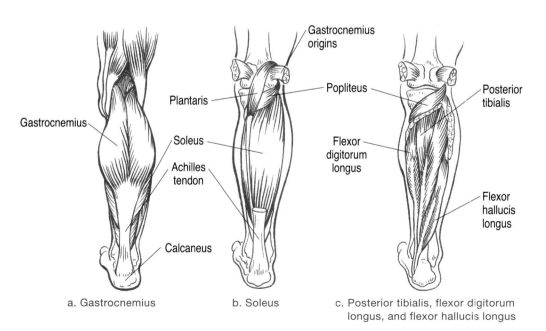

a. Gastrocnemius

b. Soleus

c. Posterior tibialis, flexor digitorum longus, and flexor hallucis longus

Figure 2.19
Posterior tibial compartment muscles primarily responsible for plantarflexion of the ankle

Muscles That Act at the Knee Joint

The muscles that cross the tibiofemoral (knee) joint can be divided into three functional groups based upon their location in one of the muscular compartments of the thigh. While the lower leg has four separate muscular compartments, the thigh has three distinct compartments, each innervated by a different peripheral nerve (Figure 2.20). The anterior compartment of the thigh is supplied by the femoral nerve, the **medial** compartment by the obturator nerve, and the posterior compartment is innervated by the sciatic nerve, the largest and longest peripheral nerve in the body.

The four major muscles on the front of the thigh are located in the anterior compartment. The primary function of these muscles is to extend the knee. These muscles are typically grouped together and referred to as the quadriceps femoris, although each muscle has its own individual name: rectus femoris, vastus medialis, vastus intermedius, and vastus lateralis. Of these four muscles, only the rectus femoris crosses the hip and functions as a hip flexor; the three vasti (medialis, intermedius, and lateralis) act only at the knee joint. The four muscles of the quadriceps femoris attach to the proximal tibia at the tibial tuberosity via one common tendon known as the patellar tendon (Figure 2.21).

The muscles found in the posterior compartment of the thigh are the biceps femoris, semitendinosus, and semimembranosus. These muscles, collectively known as the hamstrings, cross the knee joint and cause flexion of the leg. This large group of muscles has a common origin at the ischial tuberosity. Below the knee, the biceps femoris attaches laterally, while the semitendinosus and semimembranosus attach on the medial aspect of the tibia (Figure 2.22). Given these attachment sites, the biceps femoris is an external rotator of the knee, while

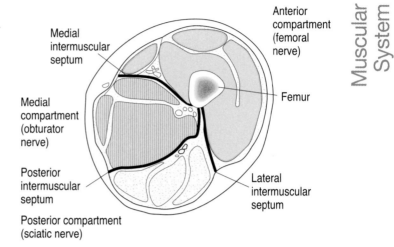

Figure 2.20
Muscular compartments of the thigh

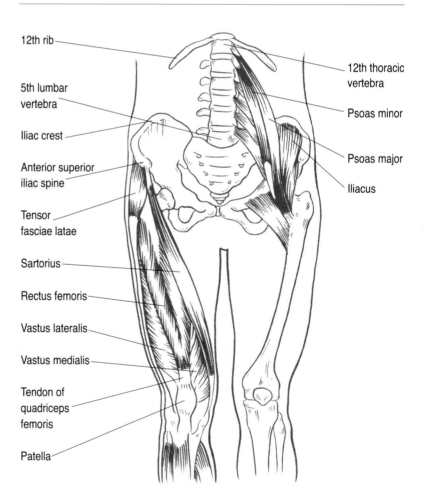

Figure 2.21
Anterior musculature of the hip and knee joints

61

Fundamentals of Anatomy

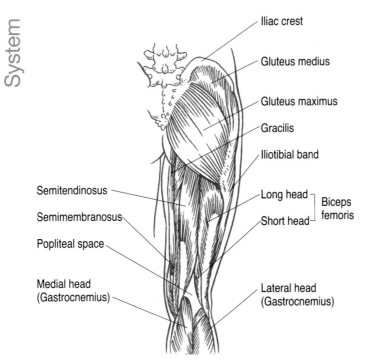

Figure 2.22
Posterior musculature of the hip and knee, prime movers for
hip extension (gluteus maximus and hamstrings) and knee flexion
(hamstrings and gastrocnemius)

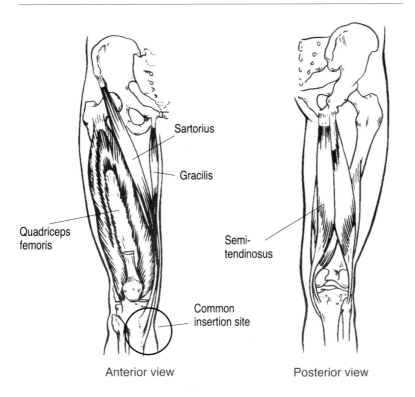

Figure 2.23
Pes anserine muscles: sartorius, gracilis, and semitendinosus

the semitendinosus and semimembranosus
are internal rotators (when flexed). In the area
between the hamstring tendons is the popliteal
space, a triangular area on the posterior-medial
aspect of the knee joint.

The third major group of muscles that act at
the knee is located in the medial compartment
of the thigh and includes two of the three muscles in the pes anserine (literally "goose's foot")
group (Figure 2.23). The pes anserine group got
its name from the flat, web-shaped common
tendon of attachment of the sartorius, the gracilis, and the semitendinosus. These muscles
are grouped together because of their common
site of insertion on the medial tibia, just below
the knee. The sartorius, the longest muscle in
the body, originates on the ilium and courses
diagonally across the anterior aspect of the
thigh to its insertion on the proximal tibia. Even
though the sartorius is an anterior thigh muscle,
its concentric action causes flexion of the knee,
functioning like the hamstrings. As a group, the
three pes anserine muscles internally rotate the
tibia when the knee is flexed. (Remember—no
rotation of the knee is possible when the
joint is fully extended.) The origins, insertions, primary functions, and examples of
exercises to develop the major muscles that
act on the leg are presented in Table 2.9.

Muscles That Act at the Hip Joint

Most of the muscles that act at the hip joint
have their origins on the pelvis and the bulk of
the muscle tissue is located on the thigh.
Recall the three muscular compartments of the
thigh presented in Figure 2.20. At the anterior
aspect of the hip, the psoas major and the
psoas minor muscles originate from the transverse processes of the five lumbar vertebrae.
These two muscles, along with the iliacus,
have a common attachment on the lesser
trochanter of the femur and work together as

Table 2.9
Major Muscles That Act at the Knee Joint

Muscle	Origin	Insertion	Primary Function(s)	Selected Exercises
Rectus femoris	Anterior-inferior spine of ilium	Superior aspect of patella and patellar tendon	Extension (most effective when the hip is extended)	Cycling, leg press machine, squat, vertical jumping, stair climbing, jumping rope, plyometrics
Vastus lateralis, intermedius, and medialis	Proximal 2/3 of anterior femur at midline	Patella and tibial tuberosity via the patellar tendon	Extension (particularly when the hip is flexed)	Same as for rectus femoris, resisted knee extension, in-line skating, cross-country skiing
Biceps femoris	Ischial tuberosity	Lateral condyle of tibia and head of fibula	Flexion and external rotation	Jumping rope, hamstring curls with knee in external rotation
Semitendinosus	Ischial tuberosity	Proximal anterior medial aspect of tibia	Flexion and internal rotation	Essentially the same as for biceps femoris; hamstring curls with knee in internal rotation
Semimembranosus	Ischial tuberosity	Posterior aspect of medial tibial condyle	Flexion and internal rotation	Same as semitendinosus

powerful flexors of the thigh. This group of three muscles is collectively known as the iliopsoas. The rectus femoris is the only muscle of the quadriceps femoris group that crosses the hip joint to cause hip flexion when acting concentrically (see Figure 2.21).

Posteriorly, several muscles combine to give shape to the buttocks and serve as very powerful movers of the hip joint. The largest and most superficial of the three is the gluteus maximus, which extends and externally rotates the hip. The gluteus maximus is a very large muscle that has fibers that pass both superiorly and inferiorly to the hip joint's axis of frontal plane motion. When the superior (upper) fibers of the gluteus maximus are stimulated to act concentrically, they produce hip abduction. Activation of the inferior (lower) fibers of the gluteus maximus pulls the hip toward the midline (adduction). Deep to the gluteus maximus are the gluteus medius and the gluteus minimus, which combine to abduct and internally rotate the hip. Also on the posterior aspect of the thigh are the hamstring muscles (biceps femoris, semitendinosus, semimembranosus), which function concentrically to extend the hip joint (see Figure 2.22).

The muscles located in the medial compartment of the thigh are named for both their function and their size. The adductor magnus, adductor longus, and adductor brevis work together to adduct the hip joint. In addition, the gracilis and pectineus muscles are synergists for adduction of the hip (Figure 2.24). The origins, insertions, primary

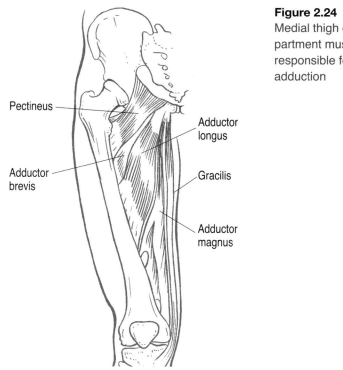

Figure 2.24
Medial thigh compartment muscles responsible for hip adduction

Pectineus

Adductor brevis

Adductor longus

Gracilis

Adductor magnus

Fundamentals of Anatomy

actions, and examples of exercises to develop the major muscles that act at the hip are presented in Table 2.10.

Muscles of the Trunk

The axial skeleton (trunk) forms the core of the human body, serving as the attachment site (origin or insertion) for nearly 30 muscles of the abdomen, low back, pelvis, and hips that combine to functionally link the upper and lower extremities. From an applied perspective, core stability is a widely used term that has numerous definitions. Hip and trunk muscle strength, abdominal muscle endurance, the ability to maintain a particular pelvic or vertebral alignment ("neutral spine"), and the absence of ligamentous laxity in the vertebral column have all been described as "core stability" (Willson et al., 2005)

Core stability, however defined, may provide significant direct benefits to a client's musculoskeletal system, including reduced low-back pain during, before, and after pregnancy (Berk, 2001); overuse-injury prevention in middle- and long-distance runners (Fredericson & Moore, 2005); and prevention of anterior cruciate ligament injuries to the knees of female athletes (Willson et al., 2005).

Generally speaking, the lumbo-pelvic-hip complex ("core") is composed of the five lumbar vertebrae, the pelvis, the hip joints, and the muscles, tendons, ligaments, and other connective tissues that either create or limit movement in any of these segments. Both static (the bony configuration of joints,

Table 2.10
Major Muscles That Act at the Hip Joint

Muscle	Origin	Insertion	Primary Function(s)	Selected Exercises
Iliacus	Inner surface of the ilium and base of sacrum	Lesser trochanter of femur	Flexion and external rotation	Straight-leg sit-ups, running with knees lifted up high, leg raises
Psoas major and minor	Transverse processes of all 5 lumbar vertebrae	Lesser trochanter of femur	Flexion and external rotation	Essentially same as iliacus
Rectus femoris	Anterior-inferior spine of ilium	Superior aspect of patella and patellar tendon	Flexion	Running, leg press, squat, jumping rope
Gluteus maximus	Posterior 1/4 of iliac crest and sacrum	Gluteal line of femur and iliotibial band	Extension and external rotation	Cycling, plyometrics, jumping rope, squat, stair-climbing machine
Biceps femoris	Ischial tuberosity	Lateral condyle of tibia and head of fibula	Extension	Cycling, hamstring curls with knee in external rotation
Semitendinosus	Ischial tuberosity	Proximal anterior-medial aspect of tibia	Extension	Essentially the same as for biceps femoris; hamstring curls with knee in internal rotation
Semimembranosus	Ischial tuberosity	Posterior aspect of medial tibial condyle	Extension	Same as semitendinosus
Gluteus medius and minimus	Lateral surface of ilium	Greater trochanter of femur	Abduction	Side-lying leg raises, walking, running
Adductor magnus	Pubic ramus and ischial tuberosity	Medial aspects of femur	Adduction	Side-lying bottom-leg raises; manual-resistance adduction exercises
Adductor brevis and longus	Pubic ramus and ischial tuberosity	Medial aspects of femur	Adduction	Side-lying bottom-leg raises, resisted adduction

fibrocartilages, and ligaments) and dynamic (active muscle-tendon units) structures contribute to core stability. When compared to the contributions to core stability made by the dynamic structures (muscles), the contributions of the static tissues to core stability are relatively small. There are three mechanisms by which the muscles that comprise the core contribute to the stability of the whole region (i.e., the capacity of these tissues to resist internal and external loads)— intra-abdominal pressure, spinal compressive forces, and hip and trunk muscle stiffness (Willson et al., 2005).

The discussion of the muscles of the trunk in this chapter includes the muscles associated with the spinal column and the walls of the abdomen. Current perspectives are changing with regard to the major muscles of the trunk, as there is a growing body of knowledge related to the contributions by muscles not previously thought to have highly significant roles in core stability (e.g., transverse abdominis, multifidus) (Hodges & Richardson, 1997). Chapter 3 includes specific examples of how to develop muscular strength, power, and endurance of the core.

Concentric actions of the largest muscles of the trunk result primarily in sagittal plane motion (i.e., flexion and extension). The three major muscles responsible for extension of the vertebral column, from lateral to medial, are the iliocostalis, the longissimus, and the spinalis. These are better known by their functional group name—erector spinae. Each of the three columns of muscles in this group has a subdivision name based on the particular portion of the spinal column to which it attaches. For example, the iliocostalis muscle has three divisions: iliocostalis lumborum (in the lumbar region of the spine), iliocostalis thoracis (in the tho-

racic region of the spine), and iliocostalis cervicis (in the cervical, or neck, region of the spine) (Figure 2.25). The anatomical function of the erector spinae muscle group is assisted by the multifidus and semispinalis (thoracis, cervicis, capitis) muscles. When these muscles act bilaterally (i.e., right and left side muscles stimulated at the same time), their concentric action produces extension of the spine. Unilateral concentric action of the erector spinae muscles will produce **lateral flexion** of the trunk to the same side that the muscles are active.

The rectus abdominis is a narrow, flat, superficial muscle on the anterior aspect of the abdominal wall that flexes the vertebral column; its fibers run vertically from the pubis to the rib cage. The rectus abdominis is crossed by three transverse fibrous bands

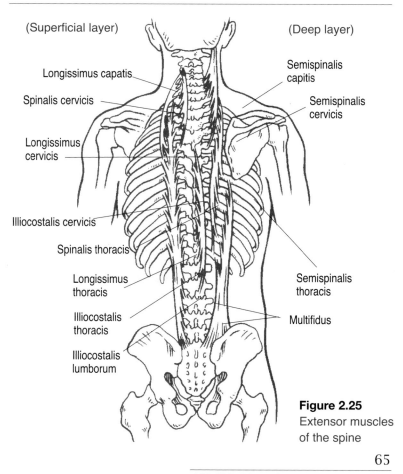

(Superficial layer)   (Deep layer)

Longissimus capatis

Spinalis cervicis

Longissimus cervicis

Illiocostalis cervicis

Spinalis thoracis

Longissimus thoracis

Illiocostalis thoracis

Illiocostalis lumborum

Semispinalis capitis

Semispinalis cervicis

Semispinalis thoracis

Multifidus

Figure 2.25
Extensor muscles
of the spine

65

Fundamentals of Anatomy

called tendinous inscriptions that, if combined with a well-developed rectus abdominis, form the "six-pack" appearance sought after by many exercisers (Figure 2.26).

The anterolateral walls of the abdominal cavity are supported entirely by the strength of the muscles located there, as there are no bones to support this region. To make up for the lack of a skeletal framework, the three layers of muscles in the abdominal wall run in different directions, providing additional support (see Figure 2.26). In the outermost (superficial) layer is the external oblique muscle, the fibers of which run anteriorly downward and toward the midline. In the second layer, the fibers of the internal oblique muscle run posteriorly and downward. An easy way to remember the orientation of these two muscles is to picture the fibers of the external oblique running into the front pockets of a pair of pants and the fibers of the internal oblique running diagonally into the back pockets. Unilateral (one-sided) activation of the lateral fibers of the obliques (external and internal) produces lateral flexion of the spinal column on that side. Trunk rotation to the right is produced by the simultaneous activation of

the left external oblique and the right internal oblique muscles; the opposite combination (right external oblique, left internal oblique) will produce left trunk rotation. Bilateral (both sides) concentric muscle action of the external and internal obliques will flex the trunk and compress the abdominal cavity.

The deepest of the three muscular layers of the abdominal wall contains the transverse abdominis muscle (see Figure 2.26). The fibers of this thin muscle run horizontally, encircling the abdominal cavity. Stimulation of this muscle compresses the abdomen, and the transverse abdominus is the first muscle recruited to initiate core stability (along with the multifidus) during voluntary movements of the lower extremity, regardless of the direction of the movement. Hodges and Richardson (1997) theorized that the central nervous system creates a stable foundation for movement of the lower extremities by first establishing core stability through isometric co-activation of the transverse abdominis and multifidus muscles.

The origins, insertions, primary functions, and examples of exercises to develop the

Figure 2.26
Muscles of the
abdominal wall

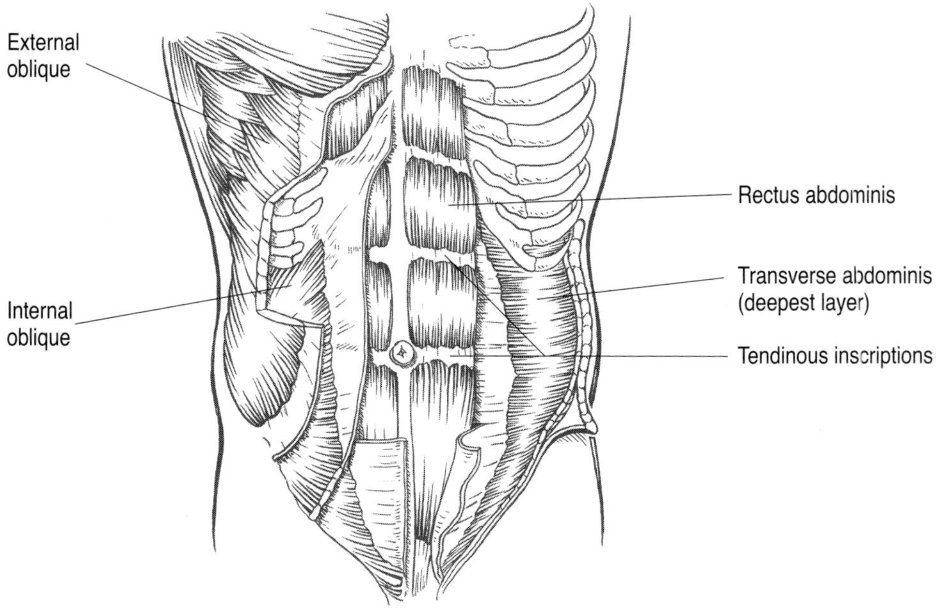

External oblique

Internal oblique

Rectus abdominis

Transverse abdominis (deepest layer)

Tendinous inscriptions

muscles that act on the trunk are presented in Table 2.11.

Muscles of the Upper Extremity

A group fitness instructor studying the musculature of the upper extremity must be familiar with the anatomical motions (and the muscles responsible for producing these movements) at the four major links in the upper body. Specifically, these four joints are the wrist joint, composed of the distal radius and adjacent carpal bones; the elbow joint, formed by the union of the olecranon process of the ulna and the distal humerus; the shoulder joint, consisting of the proximal humerus and the glenoid fossa of the scapula; and the **scapulothoracic articulation.** The connection between the scapula and the thorax is not a bony joint, per se, but more like an important functional, soft-tissue (muscle and fascia) link between the scapula and the trunk. Similar to the lower extremity, there are many muscles in the upper extremity that act at two joints; these muscles are identified in Table 2.12.

Muscles That Act at the Wrist

The muscles that act at the wrist joint can be grouped according to their origin and function. The flexor-pronator muscles originate on the medial epicondyle of the humerus and cause flexion of the wrist and pronation (palm facing down) of the forearm (radius and ulna). The primary wrist flexors are the flexor carpi radialis, palmaris longus, and flexor carpi ulnaris (Figure 2.27a). The palmaris longus muscle is absent in approximately 10% of the population. The major pronators of the forearm are the pronator teres at the elbow and the pronator quadratus at the wrist (Figure 2.27b).

The antagonist muscles to the flexor-pronators are the extensor-supinator muscles, which arise from a common tendon on the lateral humeral epicondyle and, as their group name indicates, produce extension of the wrist and supination of the forearm. The major wrist extensors are the extensor carpi radialis longus, extensor carpi radialis brevis, and the extensor carpi ulnaris (Figure 2.27c). Simply enough, the supinator muscle (with substantial synergistic help from

Table 2.11
Major Muscles That Act at the Trunk

Muscle	Origin	Insertion	Primary Function(s)	Sample Exercises
Rectus abdominis	Pubic crest	Cartilage of 5th through 7th ribs and xiphoid process	Flexion and lateral flexion of the trunk (unilateral action)	Bent-knee sit-ups, partial curl-ups, good posture, pelvic tilts
External oblique	Anteriolateral borders of lower 8 ribs	Anterior 1/2 of the ilium, pubic crest, and anterior fascia	Flexion, lateral flexion, and rotation of the trunk	Twisting bent-knee sit-ups (rotation opposite), side bridges, curl-ups
Internal oblique	Iliac crest	Cartilage of last 3–4 ribs	Flexion, lateral flexion, and rotation of the trunk	Twisting bent-knee sit-ups (rotation same side), side bridges, and curl-ups
Transverse abdominis	Iliac crest, lumbar fascia, and cartilages of last 6 ribs	Xiphoid process of sternum, anterior fascia, and pubis	Compression of abdomen	No motor function
Erector spinae	Posterior iliac crest	Angles of ribs, transverse and sacrum	Extension of trunk processes of all ribs	Squat, dead lift, prone back-extension exercises, good standing posture

Fundamentals of Anatomy

Table 2.12
Actions of Major Upper-extremity Multijoint Muscles

Muscle	Shoulder	Elbow	Forearm	Wrist
Biceps brachii	Flexion	Flexion	Supination	--------
Brachioradialis	--------	Flexion	Pronation, supination	--------
Triceps brachii	Extension (long head)	Extension	--------	--------
Flexor carpi radialis	--------	Flexion	--------	Flexion, abduction
Flexor carpi ulnaris	--------	Flexion	--------	Flexion, adduction
Extensor carpi radialis longus and brevis	--------	Extension	--------	Extension
Extensor carpi ulnaris	--------	Extension	--------	Extension, adduction

Figure 2.27
Muscles of
the forearm
and wrist

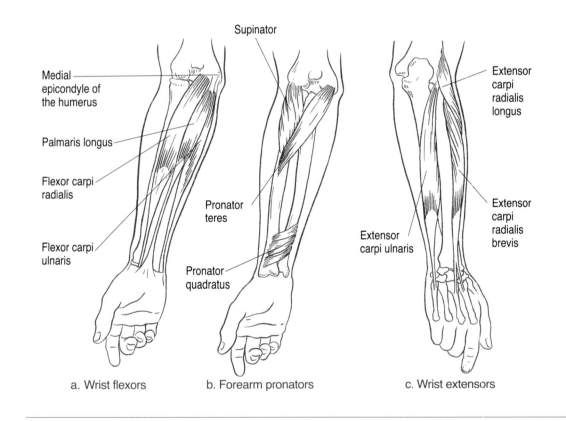

a. Wrist flexors   b. Forearm pronators   c. Wrist extensors

the biceps brachii) is responsible for supination of the forearm (see Figure 2.27b). The origins, insertions, primary functions, and examples of exercises to develop the muscles that act at the wrist and forearm are presented in Table 2.13.

Muscles That Act at the Elbow Joint

The elbow (ulnohumeral) joint is a hinge joint, and as such, permits motion in only one plane. In the case of the elbow, that one plane is the sagittal plane, and the only motions that occur in the sagittal plane are flexion and extension.

Table 2.13
Major Muscles That Act at the Wrist

Muscle	Origin	Insertion	Primary Function(s)	Sample Exercises
Flexor carpi radialis	Medial epicondyle of humerus	2nd and 3rd metacarpals	Flexion	Wrist curls against resistance; grip-strengthening exercises; baseball and softball; racquet sports, particularly racquetball and badminton
Flexor carpi ulnaris	Medial epicondyle of humerus	5th metacarpal	Flexion	Same as flexor carpi radialis
Extensor carpi radialis longus	Lateral epicondyle of humerus	2nd metacarpal	Extension	"Reverse" wrist curls, racquet sports, particularly tennis
Extensor carpi ulnaris	Lateral epicondyle of humerus	5th metacarpal	Extension	Same as extensor carpi radialis longus

The flexors of the elbow—the biceps brachii, brachialis, and brachioradialis—are located on the anterior aspect of the arm (humerus) (Figure 2.28). The brachialis is commonly referred to as the "workhorse" of the elbow, as it is active throughout the entire range of elbow flexion. While not wholly visible because it lies deep to the biceps brachii, the brachialis is the largest of the elbow flexors and generates the greatest

amount of force of any muscle crossing the anterior aspect of the joint—nearly twice that of the biceps brachii (Neumann, 2002).

The triceps brachii is the major extensor of the elbow joint and is located on the posterior aspect of the arm. As its name suggests, the triceps brachii has three heads, or origins—one on the scapula and two on the proximal humerus. All three heads converge and insert via a common tendon into the olecranon process of the ulna (Figure 2.29). The origins, insertions, primary functions, and examples of

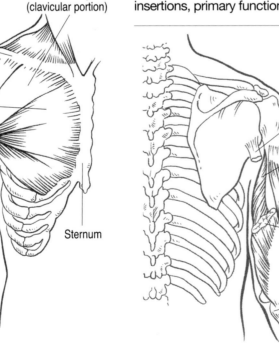

Pectoralis major (clavicular portion)

Clavicle

Deltoid

Pectoralis major (sternal portion)

Biceps brachii

Brachialis

Brachioradialis

Sternum

Figure 2.28
Superficial musculature of the anterior chest, shoulder, and arm (humerus)

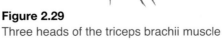

Long head

Medial head

Lateral head

Long head

Olecranon process

Figure 2.29
Three heads of the triceps brachii muscle

Fundamentals of Anatomy

exercises to develop the muscles that act at the elbow joint are presented in Table 2.14.

Muscles That Act at the Shoulder Joint

The shoulder (glenohumeral) joint is the most mobile joint in the body. Only the 10 major muscles that cross the shoulder joint and act on the arm are covered in this chapter. The two muscles with the largest physiological cross-sectional area, the pectoralis major and the latissimus dorsi, have their origins on the thorax. The pectoralis major has several important functions at the shoulder: When acting concentrically, the clavicular portion of the pectoralis major causes flexion, while its sternal fibers produce shoulder extension in the sagittal plane, adduction in the frontal plane, and internal rotation in the **transverse plane** (see Figure 2.28). The latissimus dorsi arises posteriorly from the pelvis and lumbar and lower thoracic vertebrae. Interestingly, due to its medial insertion on the arm, the latissimus dorsi shares two functions with the pectoralis major. While the latissimus dorsi is a prime extensor of the

shoulder joint, it complements the pectoralis as an adductor and internal rotator of the arm (Figure 2.30). The smaller teres major, often referred to as the "little lat," has a similar point of attachment on the proximal

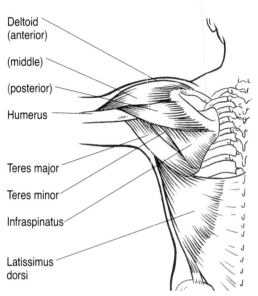

Deltoid
(anterior)

(middle)

(posterior)

Humerus

Teres major

Teres minor

Infraspinatus

Latissimus
dorsi

Figure 2.30
Superficial musculature of the superior and inferior shoulder joint (Redrawn from *Biomechanics,* 3rd ed., Kreighbaum, E. & Barthels, K. Copyright © 1990 by Macmillan Publishing Company. Reprinted by permission of Pearson Education, Inc.)

Table 2.14
Major Muscles That Act on the Elbow

Muscle	Origin	Insertion	Primary Function(s)	Sample Exercises
Biceps brachii	Long head from tubercle above glenoid cavity; short head from coracoid process of scapula	Radial tuberosity and bicipital aponeurosis	Flexion at elbow; supation at forearm	Curling with barbell, rowing machine, chin-ups, rock climbing, upright rows with barbell
Brachialis	Anterior humerus	Ulnar tuberosity and coronoid process of ulna	Flexion at elbow	Same as for biceps brachii
Brachioradialis	Distal 2/3 of lateral condyloid ridge of humerus	Radial styloid process	Flexion at elbow	Same as for biceps brachii
Triceps brachii	Long head from lower edge of glenoid cavity of scapula; lateral head from posterior humerus; short head from distal 2/3 of posterior humerus	Olecranon process of ulna	Extension at elbow	Push-ups, dips on parallel bars, bench press, military press, triceps kickbacks
Pronator teres	Distal end of medial humerus and medial aspect of ulna	Middle 1/3 of lateral radius	Flexion at elbow; pronation at forearm	Pronation of forearm with dumbbell

humerus and thus has the same anatomical functions as the latissimus dorsi.

The remaining muscles that act at the shoulder joint have their origins on the scapula itself. The superficial deltoid muscle is located on the superior aspect of the shoulder joint and resembles its name in several ways. The deltoid muscle is shaped like a triangle (Greek letter delta = Δ) and is divided into three functional sections. The anterior deltoid fibers flex and internally rotate the shoulder. The fibers of the middle deltoid lie parallel to the frontal plane, and, as such, this muscle is ideally situated to be the primary abductor of the glenohumeral joint. The posterior deltoid fibers extend the shoulder as well as produce external rotation when activated concentrically (see Figures 2.28 and 2.30).

The rotator cuff muscles, a group of four relatively small muscles, are functionally very important to the shoulder joint (Figure 2.31). These muscles act to oppose the constant force of gravity to dislocate the joint and stabilize the humeral head by pulling it inward and slightly downward into the glenohumeral joint. For this reason, the rotator cuff muscles are

sometimes referred to as the compressor cuff, in that they compress the humeral head in against the glenoid fossa of the scapula. The four rotator cuff muscles are easily remembered with the acronym SITS: the supraspinatus, which abducts the arm; the infraspinatus and teres minor, which externally rotate the arm; and the subscapularis. As its name describes, the subscapularis is located on the inferior surface of the scapula, and internally rotates the arm. The origins, insertions, primary functions, and examples of exercises designed to develop the muscles that cross the shoulder joint are presented in Table 2.15.

The rotator cuff muscles are frequently injured due to errors in training (e.g., general overuse, improper or insufficient warm-up, and excessive repetitions of shoulder abduction with internal rotation). Inflammation of the rotator cuff commonly results in a painful condition known as impingement syndrome in which the irritated rotator cuff muscles, their tendons, and the nearby bursa sacs are compressed between the humeral head and the acromion process of the scapula when the arm is abducted. A group fitness instructor

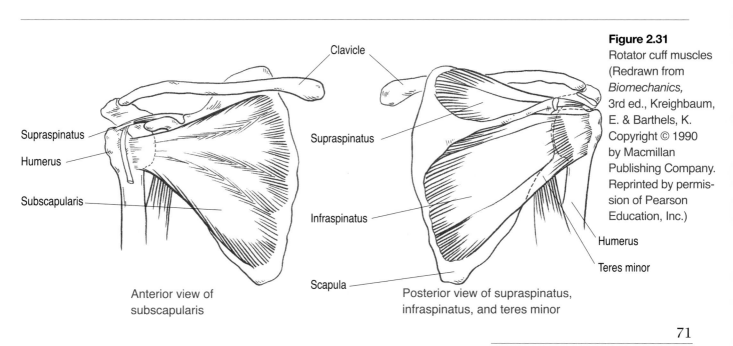

Clavicle

Supraspinatus
Humerus
Subscapularis

Anterior view of
subscapularis

Supraspinatus

Infraspinatus

Scapula

Posterior view of supraspinatus,
infraspinatus, and teres minor

Humerus

Teres minor

Figure 2.31
Rotator cuff muscles (Redrawn from *Biomechanics,* 3rd ed., Kreighbaum, E. & Barthels, K. Copyright © 1990 by Macmillan Publishing Company. Reprinted by permission of Pearson Education, Inc.)

Fundamentals of Anatomy

Table 2.15
Major Muscles That Act at the Shoulder

Muscle	Origin	Insertion	Primary Function(s)	Sample Exercises
Pectoralis major	Clavicle, sternum, and first six costal cartilages	Greater tubercle of humerus	Flexion, adduction, internal rotation	Push-ups, dips on parallel bars, incline bench press, regular bench press, climbing a rope, all types of throwing, tennis serve
Deltoid	Anterolateral clavicle, border of the acromion, and lower edge of the spine of the scapula	Deltoid tubercle of humerus on midlateral surface	Entire muscle: abduction Anterior fibers: flexion, internal rotation Posterior fibers: extension, external rotation Note: anterior deltoid has similar functions as the pectoralis major	Lateral "butterfly" (abduction) exercises with dumbbells
Latissimus dorsi	Lower six thoracic vertebrae, all lumbar vertebrae, crests of ilium and sacrum, lower four ribs	Medial side of intertubercular groove of humerus	Extension, adduction, internal rotation	Pull-ups, chin-ups, rope climbing, rowing, any exercise that involves pulling the arms downward against resistance (e.g., lat pull-downs on exercise machine)
Rotator cuff	Various aspects of scapula	All insert on greater tubercle of humerus except for the subscapularis, which inserts on the lesser tubercle of humerus	Infraspinatus and teres minor: external rotation Subscapularis: internal rotation Supraspinatus: abduction	Exercises that involve internal and external rotation (e.g., tennis serve, throwing a baseball, internal and external rotation exercises from prone/supine position with dumbbells)

who recommends exercise regimens that include repeated overhead arm motions, such as swimming, resistance training, and racquet sports, should closely monitor participant performance to avoid inducing shoulder-impingement syndrome.

Muscles That Act at the Scapulothoracic Articulation

The primary function of the muscles and fascia that make up the soft-tissue connection between the scapula and the trunk is to stabilize the scapula during movement of the arm (humerus). A commonly used analogy likens the relationship between the glenoid fossa of the scapula and the rounded head of the humerus to a circus seal balancing a beach ball on its nose. The seal, like the scapula, must be constantly moving to keep the ball (head of the humerus) in the proper position on its nose (the glenoid fossa). The critical functional relationship between the scapula and the humerus is termed **scapulohumeral rhythm.**

The four major muscles that anchor the scapula to the thorax are named according to their shape (trapezius, rhomboid major, and rhomboid minor) and function (levator scapulae) (Figure 2.32). The trapezius is one of the largest muscles in the body, originating at the external occipital protuberance of the skull and terminating distally at the 12th thoracic vertebra. Due to its shape and the varied directions of pull of its fibers, the superficial trapezius

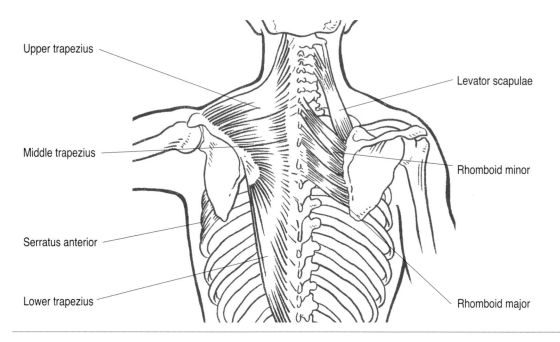

Figure 2.32
Superficial and deep muscles that act at the scapulothoracic articulation

Upper trapezius

Middle trapezius

Serratus anterior

Lower trapezius

Levator scapulae

Rhomboid minor

Rhomboid major

muscle has several different functions. The upper portion of the trapezius is responsible for **elevation** of the scapula (i.e., shrugging the shoulders). The middle section of the trapezius has horizontally directed fibers, resulting in adduction of the scapula when acting concentrically. The fibers of the lower portion of the trapezius are angled downward toward their attachment on the thoracic vertebrae. Isolated concentric action of the lower trapezius primarily results in adduction and **depression** of the scapula. Simultaneous concentric activation of the upper and lower trapezius, along with the serratus anterior, results in upward rotation of the scapula.

Deep to the trapezius are the rhomboids (major and minor), which work in unison to produce adduction and slight elevation of the scapula (see Figure 2.32). Good muscle tone in the rhomboids will help maintain good upper-back posture, and thereby help avoid the "rounded shoulders" posture. The levator scapulae runs from the upper cervical vertebrae to the medial border of the scapula and, together with the upper part of the trapezius, elevates the scapula. The origins, insertions, primary functions, and examples of exercises to develop the muscles of the scapulothoracic articulation are presented in Table 2.16.

Table 2.16
Major Muscles That Act at the Scapulothoracic Articulation

Muscle	Origin	Insertion	Primary Function(s)	Sample Exercises
Trapezius	Occipital bone, spines of cervical and thoracic vertebrae	Acromion process and spine of scapula	Upper: elevation of scapula Middle: adduction of scapula Lower: depression of scapula	Upright rowing, shoulder shrugs with resistance
Levator scapulae	Upper four or five cervical vertebrae	Vertebral border of scapula	Elevation of scapula	Shoulder shrugs with resistance
Rhomboid major and minor	Spines of 7th cervical through 5th thoracic vertebrae	Vertebral border of scapula	Adduction and elevation of scapula	Chin-ups, supported dumbbell bent-over row

Fundamentals of Anatomy

Summary

Group fitness instructors are required to design exercise programs that are safe and effective and that accomplish the desired fitness and/or personal goals of their class participants. Without a fundamental understanding of human anatomy, this task is nearly impossible. Anatomical terminology and the five major anatomical systems— cardiovascular, respiratory, nervous, skeletal, and muscular—were presented in this chapter. Chapter 3 focuses on the musculoskeletal aspects discussed in this chapter, with specific emphasis on functional anatomy and **kinesiology.** Chapter 3 also provides sufficient information to identify specific exercises and physical activities that will safely and efficiently accomplish the fitness goals of participants.

References

Berk, B. (2001). Yoga for moms—Building core stability before, during and after pregnancy. *Midwifery Today,* 59, 27.

Fredericson, M. & Moore, T. (2005). Muscular balance, core stability, and injury prevention for middle- and long-distance runners. *Physical Medicine and Rehabilitation Clinics of North America*, 16, 3, 669–689.

Hodges, P.W. & Richardson, C.A. (1997). Contraction of the abdominal muscles associated with movement of the lower limb. *Physical Therapy,* 77, 132–142.

Kandel, E.R., Schwartz, J.H., & Jessell, T.M. (2000). *Principles of Neural Science* (4th ed). New York: McGraw-Hill.

Neumann, D.A. (2002). *Kinesiology of the Musculoskeletal System.* St. Louis: Mosby.

Willson, J.D. et al. (2005). Core stability and its relationship to lower extremity function and injury. *Journal of the American Academy of Orthopaedic Surgeons,* 13, 5, 316–325.

Suggested Reading

Golding, L.A. & Golding, S.M. (2003). *Musculoskeletal Anatomy and Human Movement.* Monterey, Calif.: Healthy Learning.

Hamilton, N. & Luttgens, K. (2002). *Kinesiology: Scientific Basis of Human Motion* (10th ed.). Boston: McGraw-Hill.

Marieb, E.N., Mallatt, J., & Wilhelm, P.B. (2005). *Human Anatomy and Physiology* (4th ed.). Redwood City, Calif.: Benjamin-Cummings.

Moore, K.L. & Dalley, A.F. (1999). *Clinically Oriented Anatomy* (4th ed) Philadelphia: Lippincott Williams & Wilkins.

Oates, C.A. (2004). *Kinesiology: The Mechanics and Pathomechanics of Human Movement.* Philadelphia: Lippincott Williams & Wilkins.

Watkins, J. (1999). *Structure and Function of the Musculoskeletal System.* Champaign, Ill.: Human Kinetics.

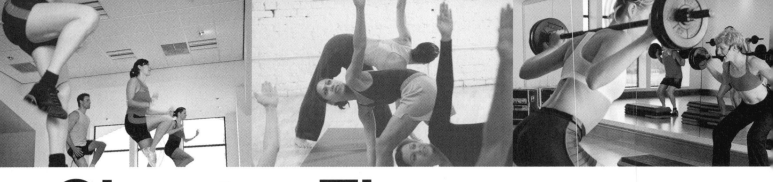

Chapter Three

Rod A. Harter, Ph.D., A.T.C., F.A.C.S.M., is an associate professor in the Department of Nutrition and Exercise Sciences at Oregon State University in Corvallis. Dr. Harter is a certified athletic trainer and a fellow of the American College of Sports Medicine. His areas of specialization include kinesiology, biomechanics, and sports medicine.

IN THIS CHAPTER:

Fundamentals of Applied Kinesiology

By Rod A. Harter

Kinesiology, as it is known to teachers and students of exercise science, involves the study of human movement from biological and physical science perspectives. A common way for professors to describe kinesiology to their students is to have them imagine the human body as a living machine designed for the performance of work. To accomplish this work, there must be meaningful and purposeful integration of the anatomical, neurological, and physiological systems in accordance with the physical laws of nature. Understanding the principles and concepts of kinesiology will provide a framework with which to analyze the vast multitude of human movements, and to make decisions and judgments regarding the safety and effectiveness of a particular movement sequence or sport skill and its role in the accomplishment of a specific fitness or personal goal of a participant.

In this context, expertise in kinesiology will provide the tools to analyze common activities of daily living (ADL), as well as the specialized movements associated with group fitness classes. To use these tools, consider the body's daily activities, postures, and the mechanical stresses that it undergoes in these positions. Next, identify possible areas of weakness or tightness caused by those habitual positions and activities. Then, design activities to improve the body's function under those specific conditions. The result will be balanced fitness programs for participants that not only include cardiovascular endurance, but also proper body mechanics, neutral postural alignment, and muscular balance.

Biomechanical Principles Applied to Human Movement

As an area of study, biomechanics involves the application of mechanics to living organisms (chiefly human beings) and the study of the effects of the forces applied. Within the study of mechanics, there are two major areas of interest to the group fitness instructor: kinematics and kinetics. **Kinematics** involves the study of the form, pattern, or sequence of movement without regard for the forces that may produce that motion. **Kinetics** is the branch of mechanics that describes the effects of forces on the body—from a kinesiology viewpoint, a force can be either internal (e.g., produced by

muscles) or external (e.g., produced by gravity's pull on a barbell), to cause, modify, or oppose motion.

The analytical process within kinesiology can either be quantitative (mathematically derived) or qualitative (subjective). Biomechanics research laboratories at major universities, medical schools, and hospitals use state-of-the art equipment costing hundreds of thousands of dollars to perform precise quantitative analyses of movement. In contrast, current digital camera technology is relatively inexpensive and will allow an instructor to create a record of a participant's movement pattern at the beginning and later stages of learning a new skill or task (e.g., exercising on a stability ball). Sharing this visual record with the participant, along with a critique of the movement, allows for self-analysis and improvement. A more common example of a "low-tech" kinesiological qualitative analysis is the real-time use of a mastery of kinesiological principles when teaching in an exercise facility with mirrored walls to give participants verbal cues for immediate self-correction when necessary.

While an instructor will use the naked eye rather than expensive digital cameras and computers to analyze human movement, he or she will still need to understand the physical laws that apply to the motion of all objects. While Sir Isaac Newton, a 17th century English mathematician, is perhaps best known for his conceptualization of the **law of gravity** after observing an apple falling from a tree to the ground, his formulation of three important natural laws that govern motion represents his greatest contribution to science. When taken together, Newton's laws of motion provide a better understanding of the interrelationships among forces, mass, and human movement—at individual joints or of the body as a whole.

Law of Inertia

Newton's first law of motion, known as the **law of inertia**, states that a body at rest will stay at rest and that a body in motion will stay in motion (with the same direction and velocity) unless acted upon by an external force. A body's inertial characteristics are proportional to its mass. Therefore, it is more difficult to start moving a heavy object than a light one. Similarly, if two objects are moving at the same velocity, it requires more effort to stop or slow the heavier object than the lighter one. For group fitness instructors, resistance-training programs probably have the greatest association with Newton's first law. For example, the "sticking point" at the beginning of a biceps curl occurs in part due to the difficulty of overcoming the dumbbell's inertial property of being at rest, and in part due to the mechanical disadvantage of the human body to generate internal forces when the elbow is fully extended.

Law of Acceleration

The **law of acceleration,** Newton's second law, states that the force (F) acting on a body in a given direction is equal to the body's mass (m) multiplied by the body's acceleration (a) in that direction (F = ma). Newton's second law also relates to a moving body's momentum (M), in that a body's linear momentum is equal to its mass multiplied by its velocity (M = mv). For a given mass, the application of additional force will accelerate the body to a higher velocity, thus creating greater momentum. For a given velocity, linear momentum will be increased if the mass of the body is increased. Angular momentum is governed by similar principles, but the motion performed is about an axis. If a participant is

using a 10-pound dumbbell to perform biceps curls to slow-tempo music, there will be less momentum produced than when moving that same weight at a faster tempo. If the tempo of movement to the music (velocity = v) is held constant, but the participant switches to a 15-pound dumbbell (greater mass, m), then momentum (M = mv) will increase proportionally.

Law of Reaction

Newton's third law, commonly referred to as the **law of reaction,** states that every **applied force** is accompanied by an equal and opposite reaction force. Said differently, for every action there is an equal and opposite reaction. This law has bearing on the ground-reaction forces (impact forces) that the body must absorb during activities such as step training, plyometrics, and jogging. According to Newton's principles, the ground exerts a force against the body equal to the force that the body applies to the ground as a person walks, jogs, or sprints. Step training and martial arts–derived exercise programs remain popular group fitness activities even though the magnitude of the ground-reaction forces associated with each puts participants at risk for a variety of overuse injuries. Athletic shoes designed specifically for step training have additional cushioning in the metatarsal region of the foot for injury prevention, as the forefoot is where much of the vertically directed ground-reaction force is concentrated. A biomechanical analysis of step aerobic exercise reported that significantly smaller-magnitude ground-reaction forces occurred with a 6-inch step when compared to 8-inch and 10-inch step heights (Maybury & Waterfield, 1997). Little difference in ground-reaction forces existed between the 8-inch and 10-inch step heights; these findings suggest that participants should use a lower step height to reduce the risk of an overuse injury to the lower limb.

An understanding of the anatomical and biomechanical factors that affect muscles and create movement is crucial for effective exercise design and program implementation. The next step in this process is to apply these principles to identify the individual and collective contributions of muscles through an analytical process. Leonardo da Vinci, perhaps the premier anatomist in all of history, simplified the study of functional anatomy when he likened human tendons to "cords attached to skeletons." Remembering a muscle's location, the attachment sites of its tendons, and its lines of action (i.e., the orientation of the muscle fibers in relation to a particular joint) will provide a clear understanding of the anatomical motions that muscle produces.

A helpful analogy is to view the production of human movement similar to how a puppeteer manipulates the strings of a puppet to make it move; the "strings" that produce motion are the tendons connected to the muscles that have been activated by the central nervous system (CNS). The following sections contain numerous examples of common movements produced during exercise by the muscles of the lower and upper extremities.

Kinesiology of the Lower Extremity

In this chapter, movements of the lower extremity are defined as those that occur at the hip, knee, and ankle joints. The normal ranges of motion for these joints are presented in Figure 3.1. The subsequent sections provide details regarding the functions of the primary muscles in the lower extremity and examples of exercises to develop strength and improve flexibility.

Anterior Hip Muscles: Hip Flexors

The most important muscles, or **prime movers**, for hip flexion are the iliopsoas, rectus femoris, sartorius, and tensor fasciae latae. These muscles act synergistically to cause hip flexion, as in a straight-leg raise or knee lift. They also act eccentrically to control hip extension, such as in the downward phases of a straight-leg raise or knee lift.

The iliopsoas is actually three muscles—the iliacus, psoas major, and psoas minor (absent in about 40% of people)—that function together as one unit. The iliacus gets its name from the Latin root ilium, meaning groin or flank. The iliacus has its origin on the inner surface of the ilium bone of the hip (near the sacroiliac joint) and inserts into the lesser trochanter of the femur. The psoas major and psoas minor originate on the transverse processes of the five lumbar vertebrae and attach to the femur at the lesser trochanter. Given the origin of the psoas muscles in the low back and attachment to the proximal femur, they have poor mechanical efficiency (leverage) when recruited to raise or lower the mass of a straight leg. In most people, the abdominals are not strong enough to balance the large force created by the psoas to keep the spine in neutral position during a straight-leg lift. This is one reason why straight-leg sit-ups and leg-lowering exercises are not recommended. Because of its origin at the lumbar spine, psoas tightness (inflexibility) or hypertrophy can result in passive hyperextension of the lumbar spine, a condition known as **lordosis.** Tightness in the iliopsoas can also be attributed to a lack of stretching exercises and poor standing and sitting postures.

To stretch the iliopsoas, have participants stand in a forward lunge position with one

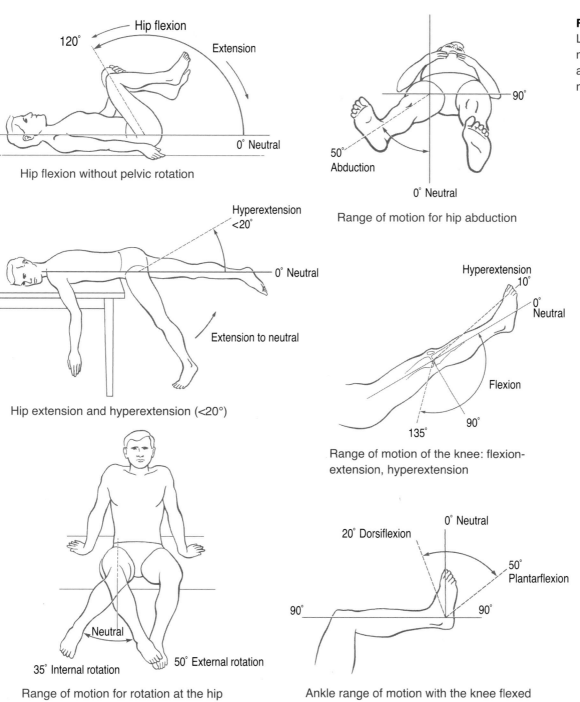

Figure 3.1
Lower-extremity
movements and
active range of
motion

Hip flexion without pelvic rotation

Range of motion for hip abduction

Hip extension and hyperextension (<20°)

Range of motion of the knee: flexion-
extension, hyperextension

Range of motion for rotation at the hip

Ankle range of motion with the knee flexed

knee flexed and foot flat, and the heel of the other leg off the floor (Figure 3.2). Instruct them to activate their abdominal muscles to slightly flex the lumbar spine and hold this position for at least 15 seconds. Careful supervision of this activity is important, as the tendency is to hyperextend the lumbar spine during this stretch, putting unwanted compressive loads on the joints of the lumbar spine. To strengthen the iliopsoas, use the abdominals to tilt the pelvis posteriorly from a supine position to stabilize the low back (Figure 3.3). Most healthy active people have adequate strength in their hip flexors

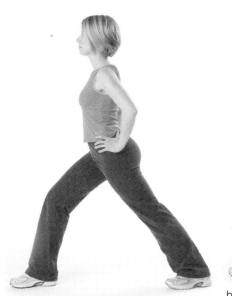

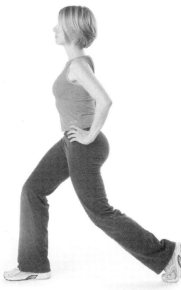

a. Straight leg hip flexor

b. Bend the back leg at the knee (lift the heel off the floor) for a deeper stretch of the left iliopsoas and rectus femoris muscles.

Figure 3.2
Hip flexor stretch

knee and hip; concentric action of the rectus femoris results in hip flexion, knee extension, or both simultaneously. An effective exercise to strengthen this muscle is the standing straight-leg raise, producing an overload in both hip flexion and knee extension. To stretch the rectus femoris, perform the iliopsoas lunge stretch, then lower the body so that the back knee bends (see Figure 3.2b).

The sartorius is the longest muscle in the body, originating from the anterior superior iliac spine (ASIS) and inserting onto the medial tibia, just below the knee. This multijoint muscle flexes, abducts, and externally rotates the hip while flexing and internally rotating the knee. Just lateral to the sartorius is the tensor fasciae latae (TFL), a short muscle with a very long tendon that combines with tendon fibers from the lower fibers of the gluteus maximus to form the **iliotibial band**. The TFL originates on the ASIS and inserts on the lateral tibia just below the knee. Sprinters typically have highly developed TFL muscles from the explosive hip flexion action required when coming out the starting blocks at the beginning of a race.

through ADL such as walking and stair climbing. As people age, there is a tendency to become less active, and the decreased stride length and hip flexion range of motion observed in many elders during walking is the direct result of the loss of hip flexor muscular strength.

The rectus femoris is the only one of the four muscles of the quadriceps femoris that crosses the hip joint. This muscle works at both the

Posterior Hip Muscles: Hip Extensors

The primary hip extensors are the hamstrings (biceps femoris, semitendinosus,

Figure 3.3
Hip flexor (iliopsoas) strengthening exercise; may be performed with one knee extended for greater resistance

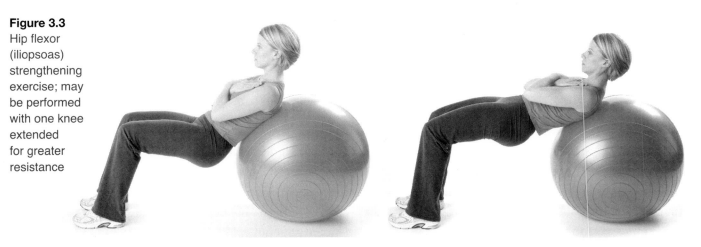

and semimembranosus) and the gluteus maximus. Working concentrically, these muscles extend the hip joint against gravity, such as during a prone leg lift. They are also activated eccentrically to control hip flexion (e.g., motion during the downward phase of a squat or lunge) (Figure 3.4).

Figure 3.4
Eccentric action of the gluteus maximus and hamstrings controls the downward phase of the squat into hip flexion.

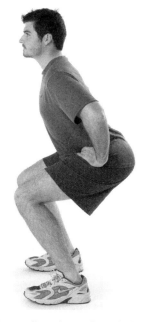

Electromyographic studies show that during normal walking and other low-intensity movements, the hamstrings act as prime movers for hip extension. There also is some electrical activity in the gluteus maximus muscle. During higher-intensity activities such as stationary cycling, stair climbing, and sprinting, in which greater hip ranges of motion and more powerful hip extension are required, the gluteus maximus plays the primary role. Most of the activities in a step-training class recruit the gluteus maximus for hip extension in addition to the always-active hamstrings, but other group activities, such as indoor cycling classes, jumping rope, and power walking on hilly terrain, also recruit the gluteus. If a participant has "buns of steel" as a fitness goal, be sure to include moderate- to higher-intensity activities that extend and hyperextend the hip. One

guideline for choosing activities that involve the gluteus maximus is to select exercises that require at least 90 degrees of hip flexion. These activities tend to be more vigorous and require firing of the gluteus maximus to provide the extra force needed to help the hamstrings accomplish the task of extending the hip through such a large range of motion.

Lateral Hip Muscles: Hip Abductors and External Rotators

The abductors and external rotators of the hip are found posterior and lateral to the hip joint in an area commonly referred to as the buttocks. The three gluteal muscles—gluteus medius, gluteus minimus, and the superior fibers of the gluteus maximus—are the primary hip abductors and are assisted by the tensor fasciae latae (TFL) (Figures 3.5 and 3.6). The gluteus medius is the largest of the hip abductor muscles, two times larger than the gluteus minimus; the TFL is the smallest (Clark & Haynor, 1987).

The origins of these muscles are superior to the joint; therefore, when these muscles act concentrically (remember da Vinci's analogy of "cords attached to skeletons"),

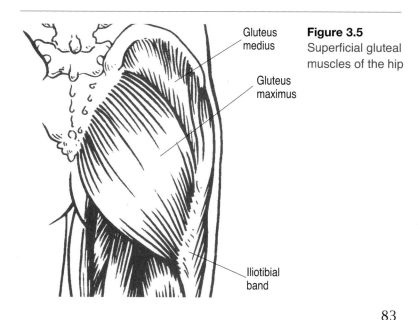

Gluteus medius

Gluteus maximus

Iliotibial band

Figure 3.5
Superficial gluteal muscles of the hip

Fundamentals of Applied Kinesiology

the hip is pulled away from the midline of the body into abduction. Recall that the function of a muscle depends on the orientation (line of pull) of its fibers in relation to the joint at which it is acting. The primary function of the gluteus maximus is hip extension, while the main action of the gluteus medius is hip abduction. However, about one-third of the fibers of the gluteus maximus cross the hip superior to the functional axis of the joint, while the other two-thirds of the muscle fibers cross inferior to the joint axis for abduction and adduction. This means that concentric activation of those fibers of the gluteus maximus superior to the joint axis will produce abduction, while the inferior fibers will cause adduction. In a similar anatomical paradigm, the anterior fibers of the gluteus medius attach medial to the hip joint axis for rotation, and produce internal rotation when acting concentrically. The posterior fibers of the gluteus medius insert lateral to the hip's axis for rotation and thus will create external rotation when activated concentrically.

There are six external rotators of the hip located deep to the gluteus maximus. From superior to inferior, these muscles are the piriformis, superior gemellus, obturator internus, obturator externus, inferior gemellus, and the quadratus femoris (see Figure 3.6). The orientation of the muscle fibers in this group is horizontal and this, coupled with their position posterior to the joint, makes them highly efficient external rotators of the hip. When the hip is extended, the gluteus maximus also functions as an external rotator.

The optimal arc of motion for the gluteus medius to produce hip abduction is between 0 and 40 degrees of hip flexion, as its mechanical efficiency as an abductor diminishes beyond that range. When abduction exercises are performed with the hip flexed

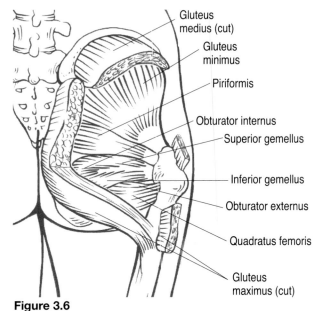

Figure 3.6
Six external rotators of the hip

more than 40 degrees, the six small external rotators of the hip take on the role of prime movers (Lundy, 2006).

To stretch the external rotator muscles, have the participant lie flat on his or her back and pull the flexed knee and hip diagonally across the body (Figure 3.7). This position involves adduction and internal rotation, which effectively stretches these muscles.

An understanding of concentric and eccentric muscle actions is critical for the proper design of exercise programs. Recall the discussion in Chapter 2 of the general

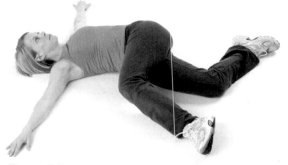

Figure 3.7
Stretching of the deep external rotators of the left hip. Keep the shoulders and back flat; pull the flexed hip and knee across the torso.

rules for determining what type of muscle action is occurring. If the movement direction is opposite the pull of gravity, the active muscle is working concentrically; if the direction of movement is the same as the pull of gravity, then the muscle is working eccentrically. However, when gravity is "eliminated" during movements that occur parallel to the mat, each muscle group acts concentrically to produce the desired motion. When resistance is added through the use of elastic bands or stability balls, the same principles apply in all planes of motion; concentric muscle actions occur if the movement increases the resistance in the elastic tubing, and eccentric muscle actions occur if the motion decreases the resistance offered by the stability ball.

Figure 3.8 employs a series of hip abduction and adduction exercises to provide four examples of how body position can modify the influence of gravity. In Figure 3.8a, side-lying leg lifts are depicted. The initial action is hip abduction upward against gravity's downward pull. No motion will occur until sufficient internal muscle forces are created. Therefore, the hip abductors are acting concentrically as agonists. In the downward phase of the leg lift, the hip joint action is adduction. This joint motion occurs slowly in the same direction as gravity's pull; therefore, the hip abductors are working eccentrically as agonists to control hip adduction. The hip abductors are the prime movers for the hip abduction and adduction motions seen in this activity.

Figure 3.8b shows a supine hip abduction/adduction exercise with the hips flexed, knees extended, and feet in the air; the initial action that occurs is abduction of the hip joints as the legs move farther apart. Since the movement occurs in the same direction as the force of gravity, the hip

adductors control the motion via eccentric muscle action. To bring the legs back together again in a vertical position, the hip adductor muscles work concentrically against the pull of gravity. The hip adductors are the prime movers for the hip abduction and adduction motions observed in this exercise.

In the third example (Figure 3.8c), hip abduction and adduction are performed from a supine position, effectively eliminating the force of gravity as a source of resistance. From this position, the motions occur neither against nor in the same direction as gravity, but perpendicular to the pull of gravity. There is a concentric action of the hip abductors when the extended legs are moved away from midline and a concentric action of the hip adductors when the legs are moved back to anatomical position.

In the final example (Figure 3.8d), elastic tubing is added to the exercise pictured in Figure 3.8c. Concentric muscle actions of the hip abductors occur when the participant moves her legs away from midline, increasing the resistance in the elastic tubing. Conversely, eccentric muscle actions occur in the hip abductors during the return to the starting position (adduction), against the force supplied by the elastic band at the lower leg.

Medial Hip Muscles: Hip Adductors and Internal Rotators

The muscles that produce adduction and internal rotation are located anterior, inferior, and medial to the hip joint. In this case, the muscle names clearly indicate their function—the primary adductors are the adductor magnus, adductor longus, and adductor brevis. Figure 3.8 provided several good examples of exercises that recruit the adductors of the hip.

Fundamentals of Applied Kinesiology

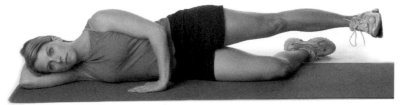

a. Side-lying leg lifts; abductors work concentrically in the upward phase
and eccentrically in the downward phase

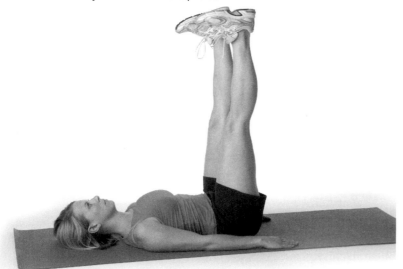

b. Supine with feet toward ceiling; legs are abducted (spread apart) and
lowered slowly, resisting gravity's downward pull in the eccentric phase, and
brought back together in the concentric phase

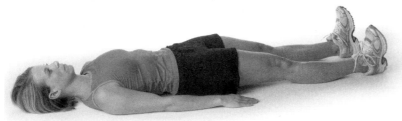

c. Moving apart involves concentric action of hip abductors; moving together
involves concentric activation of hip adductors

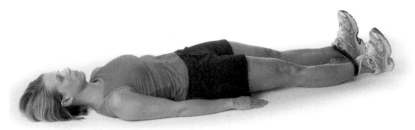

d. Concentric (legs apart) and eccentric (legs together) actions of the hip
abductors with elastic resistance

Figure 3.8a-d
Concentric and eccentric hip muscle actions

Because of the anatomical configuration of the hip, there are no true primary internal rotators of the hip for movements starting from the anatomical position because no single muscle has a superior mechanical advantage over another to produce internal rotation torque (Neumann, 2002). As the hip joint is increasingly flexed toward 90 degrees, the most important internal rotators of the hip are the adductor longus and brevis muscles, gluteus medius and minimus, pectineus, and tensor fasciae latae. Lindsay et al. (1992) point out that the changes in the mechanical advantage (leverage) of the internal rotators improves dramatically when strength is tested in a flexed-hip versus an extended-hip position, increasing maximum internal rotation torque by as much as 50%.

The inner thigh is an area of concern for many participants. Many people want to lose the fat that has accumulated along the medial thigh and improve both the muscle tone and strength of their adductors. It is important to educate participants that spot reduction of fat does not work, regardless of what they see on television infomercials. To decrease body-fat stores along the inner thigh or anywhere else in the body, daily caloric expenditure must consistently exceed daily caloric intake. Irrespective of gender, participation in physical activity for 30 minutes a day on most days of the week will most effectively help with weight loss and help decrease body-fat percentage.

Anterior Knee Muscles:
Knee Extensors

The large muscle on the front of the thigh, the quadriceps femoris, is the prime mover for knee extension when acting concentrically. As the Latin roots of its name implies,

Fundamentals of Applied Kinesiology

the quadriceps femoris is composed of four different muscles located on the femur that work together to extend the knee. Three of the four muscles—the vastus lateralis, vastus medialis, and vastus intermedius—originate on the proximal femur. The rectus femoris is the only one of the quadriceps that crosses the hip joint and produces hip flexion when acting concentrically, a function made possible by its origin on the anterior inferior iliac spine. The quadriceps muscles combine distally to form the patellar tendon, the second largest tendon in the body. The patella, the largest sesamoid ("seed-like") bone in the body, is found within the patellar tendon and acts like a pulley to increase the mechanical advantage of the quadriceps by as much as 30% at some knee-joint angles.

During relaxed standing there is little activity in the quadriceps to keep the knees extended, as most of the body weight is borne statically on the joint surfaces of the lower extremity. When moving from a standing position to a seated position, the quadriceps act eccentrically to allow knee flexion, thereby permitting a controlled (safe) descent of the body into the chair. When getting up from a chair, the quadriceps muscles act concentrically as prime movers to extend the knee. In the varied activities of daily living, strong quadriceps femoris muscles are needed for lifting heavy objects, walking, and climbing stairs. Squats, lunges, and stepping are important exercises in preparing the quadriceps for most ADL. Many experts agree that the safest approach in a group fitness class is to limit knee flexion to no more than 90 degrees during weightbearing exercises.

Posterior Knee Muscles: Knee Flexors and Rotators

The primary knee flexors are the hamstrings muscle group: semitendinosus, semimembranosus, and biceps femoris. The hamstrings are referred to as a bi-articular group of muscles, producing knee flexion as well as hip extension when acting concentrically. Additionally, the two medial hamstrings—semimembranosus and semitendinosus—are internal rotators of the knee. The lateral hamstring, the biceps femoris, is an external rotator of the knee. Knee-joint rotation is only possible in flexed-joint positions, as a phenomenon known as the **screw-home mechanism** increases knee-joint stability by locking the femur on the tibia (or vice-versa) when the knee is fully extended.

The sartorius, popliteus, gastrocnemius, and gracilis are secondary knee flexors (see Figures 2.19 and 2.23). The popliteus plays a very unique role in that it is responsible for initiating knee flexion and "unlocking" the knee from its extended position.

To stretch the hamstrings effectively, have participants assume a position that places the targeted limb in hip flexion and knee extension (Figure 3.9). From a standing position, put

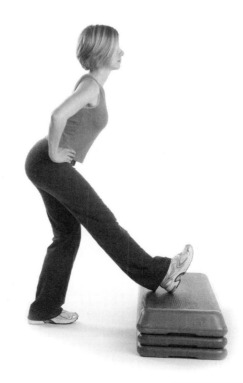

Figure 3.9
Standing hamstring stretch; hands should be used for balance—do not apply pressure on the knee

Fundamentals of Applied Kinesiology

the foot of the leg to be stretched on a step and slowly bend forward at the waist, keeping a flat back **(neutral spine position).** This stretch can also be performed while sitting on a stability ball. Both of these positions isolate the stretch to the hamstrings group and avoid overstressing the erector spinae muscles. To increase the intensity of this stretch, have the participant flex the knee and hip of the limb not being stretched.

Anterior Leg Muscles: Dorsiflexors

Recall from Chapter 2 that the muscles below the knee are organized into four finite compartments. The muscles in the anterior compartment of the lower leg (see Figures 2.16 and 2.17) are the anterior tibialis, extensor hallucis longus, and extensor digitorum longus. When acting concentrically, these muscles produce dorsiflexion of the ankle. These muscles also work together during locomotor activities, such as walking and running, to eccentrically lower the foot to the ground with control. Without the vital eccentric action of the dorsiflexor muscles as dynamic shock absorbers, the foot would slap the ground with each stride or impact. Given that the ground-reaction forces during running are three to five times one's body weight with each stride and that there are approximately 1,500 to 1,800 strides (ground impacts) per mile (1.6 km), the importance of the shock-absorption role of these muscles cannot be overstated.

The anterior tibialis inserts on the medial aspect of the foot and combines with the posterior tibialis to serve as the prime movers for inversion of the foot. A common method of warming these muscles prior to impact activities is to perform toe tapping, stepping either straight ahead or side-to-side. Having participants walk for short dis-tances with only their heels touching the ground is also a good warm-up activity for these anterior-compartment muscles.

Posterior Leg Muscles: Plantarflexors

The large muscles of the superficial posterior tibial compartment (see Figures 2.16 and 2.19) are the primary plantarflexors of the ankle joint. While more easily palpated and more visible than the underlying soleus muscle, the gastrocnemius is actually the smaller of the two. These muscles combine distally to form the Achilles tendon, the largest tendon in the body, which attaches posteriorly to the calcaneus. The gastrocnemius, as mentioned previously, acts at both the knee and the ankle; the soleus only works at the ankle joint. Indeed, there are eight muscles that act as synergists for plantarflexion, evidence of the adaptive importance of plantarflexion force production (e.g., "fight or flight" mechanism). The remaining six muscles—the posterior tibialis, flexor hallucis longus, flexor digitorum longus, plantaris, peroneus longus, and peroneus brevis—play secondary functional roles in producing the propulsion force required for human locomotion.

The gastrocnemius and soleus muscles are often inflexible, particularly among participants who regularly wear high-heeled shoes. To stretch the two-joint gastrocnemius, the hip and knee should be extended and the ankle should be in a dorsiflexed position while the heel remains on the ground. To stretch the soleus, a similar posture is assumed, except that the knee is flexed to about 20 degrees to isolate the soleus. These stretches can be performed while seated or lying down, but more commonly are performed against a real or imagined wall or by utilizing a step aerobics bench (Figure 3.10).

Figure 3.10
Stretching of the
gastrocnemius
(rear leg) and
soleus (front leg)
muscles

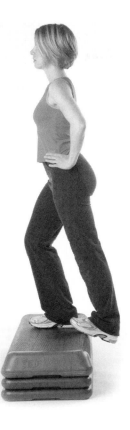

Lateral Leg Muscles: Evertors

The peroneus longus and peroneus brevis are muscles found in the lateral tibial compartment (see Figures 2.16 and 2.18) that are responsible for eversion of the foot (i.e., pulling the foot laterally in the frontal plane). The tendons of these muscles curve around behind the lateral malleolus and attach on the foot. Both muscles play secondary roles as plantarflexors at the ankle due to their posterior location relative to the axis of motion of the talocrural (ankle) joint. These muscles are active during virtually all locomotor activities to provide dynamic stability at the subtalar joint, acting eccentrically to prevent the joint from rolling too far into inversion and overloading the lateral ankle ligaments, possibly causing a sprain.

Medial Leg Muscles: Invertors

There are two muscles that are primarily responsible for concentric inversion (i.e., pulling the foot toward the midline in

the frontal plane): the tibialis anterior and tibialis posterior. A key anatomical point is to focus on the insertion sites of the distal tendons of these muscles. As their names suggest, the tibialis anterior muscle is located on the front of the tibia and is a key muscle for dorsiflexion in the sagittal plane. Its antagonist muscle in the sagittal plane is the tibialis posterior, found on the posterior aspect of the tibia and acting as a plantarflexor. While the functions of these muscles are opposite in the sagittal plane, they function as synergists in the frontal plane to produce inversion when they act concentrically. Similar to the evertors, these muscles are active during most weightbearing activities as dynamic stabilizers of the ankle joint.

Kinesiology of the Spine and Pelvis

Posture and the Neutral Spine

Given the wide variation of human body shapes, sizes, and types, there are few people who actually have what can be called an "ideal" posture. Muscularity, flexibility, and pattern of fat deposition are just three of many factors that influence real (versus idealized) posture (Neumann, 2002). The spine of a fully grown healthy adult has 24 movable vertebrae and three normal curves: the cervical and lumbar regions are naturally convex anteriorly and concave posteriorly, referred to as a **lordotic** curvature. In contrast, the thoracic region possesses a curve that first develops in utero from the fetal position—concave anteriorly and convex posteriorly—known as a **kyphotic** curve (Figure 3.11).

This idealized neutral spine position requires the mathematical balance of 12 vertebrae that are curved in an anterior direction (7 cervical vertebrae plus 5 lumbar vertebrae) with the 12 thoracic region vertebrae that are

Fundamentals of Applied Kinesiology

curved in a posterior direction. The normal active ranges of motion of the thoracic and lumbar regions of the spine are presented in Figure 3.12.

An instructor can assess muscular balance by having a participant stand in the anatomical position and observing him or her from the back and from the side. If a person stands in this neutral alignment and is viewed from the rear, the line of gravity (envision a plumb bob suspended from above) would pass through the midline of the skull, the center of the vertebral column over the spinous processes, the

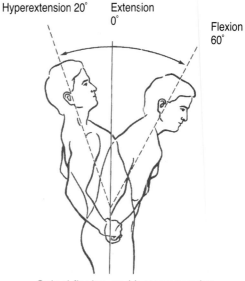

Spinal flexion and hyperextension

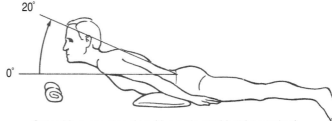

Spinal hyperextension (thoracic and lumbar spine)

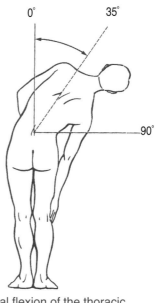

Lateral flexion of the thoracic and lumbar spine

Figure 3.11
Neutral spine alignment with slight anterior (lordotic) curves at neck and low back and a posterior (kyphotic) curve in the thoracic region

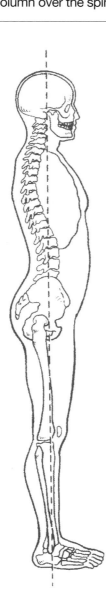

Figure 3.12
Active range of motion of the thoracic and lumbar spine

vertical crease between the buttocks, and
touch the ground midway between the feet.
Group fitness classes can promote good
posture and muscular balance by having
participants perform all activities with as
close to a neutral spine alignment as possible. Effective cueing and correction techniques, combined with verbal and visual
feedback, will help participants become
more aware of their posture. Good posture is
a neuromuscular skill that can be achieved or
reacquired through repetition and practice.

The position of the pelvis plays a major role
in the determination of the forces applied at
the lumbar spine. If the lumbar spine is correctly aligned with regard to the pelvis, and the
pelvis is properly balanced in relation to the
legs, then the forces applied to the low back
can be reduced. To achieve this balance
requires excellent muscle strength and flexibility on both sides of the trunk—the trunk and
hip flexors anteriorly and the trunk and spine
extensors posteriorly (Figure 3.13).

Abnormal and Fatigue-related Postures

Deviations from neutral spine position can
be temporary or permanent; muscle spasm
and pain following a soft-tissue injury to the
back, fatigue, or muscular imbalance may
cause these deviations. When applied at the
appropriate time with the correct dosage
(frequency, intensity, and duration), exercise
can help alleviate each of these conditions.
Some postural deviations are structural
(bony) in nature, and typically do not
respond to corrective exercise. The three
most common abnormal postures are lordosis, kyphosis, and scoliosis.

Lordosis is an excessive anterior curvature of the spine that typically occurs at the
low back, but may also occur at the neck

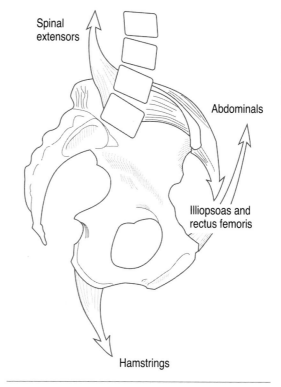

Spinal extensors

Abdominals

Illiopsoas and rectus femoris

Hamstrings

Figure 3.13
Muscular control of the pelvis by the ab-dominals and hip flexors (iliopsoas) anteriorly and the spinal extensors (erector spinae) and hamstrings posteriorly

(Figure 3.14a). The lay term for lordosis of the
lumbar spine is "swayback," a condition
marked by protruding buttocks and weak
abdominal muscles. This lordotic or swayback
posture has been associated with low-back
pain, a condition commonly experienced by
late-term pregnant women and individuals with
large concentrations of abdominal fat. Lordotic
posture will cause an anterior tilting of the
pelvis, placing tension on the anterior longitudinal ligaments of the spine and compression
on the posterior part of the intervertebral discs.
If this posture is maintained over weeks and
months, the back extensor and hip flexor muscles will adapt by losing their extensibility
and adaptively shorten. In contrast, the
hamstring and abdominal muscles will
lengthen under these constant loads,
becoming more lax and further decreasing
their control of the pelvis. Unlike obesity,
pregnancy has a finite beginning and end,
and most back pain and changes in posture
associated with pregnancy are resolved

Fundamentals of Applied Kinesiology

postpartum. The overweight or obese participant with lordosis presents a significant challenge to the group fitness instructor. To correct the anterior pelvic tilt position associated with lumbar lordosis, focus on strengthening the participant's abdominal and hip extensor (hamstring) muscles, while stretching the hip flexors (iliopsoas) and spine extensors (erector spinae).

Kyphosis is defined as an excessive posterior curvature of the spine, typically seen in the thoracic region (Figure 3.14b). The presence of kyphosis will give the individual a characteristic "humpback," with associated rounded shoulders, sunken chest, and head-forward posture with neck hyperextension. Kyphosis is a common postural abnormality among older adults with osteoporosis. In some instances, their rounded-shoulders posture is caused by weakness or disuse atrophy of the muscles that control scapular movement—the rhomboids and trapezius. Strengthening programs intended to correct this postural deformity have had varying levels of success.

Scoliosis is an excessive lateral curvature of the spine and is more prevalent among women than men (Figure 3.14c). With scoliosis, the pelvis and shoulders often appear uneven and the vertebrae may rotate, causing a posterior shift of the rib cage on one side.

If a participant has one of these three postural abnormalities and cannot actively assume a neutral spine posture, refer him or her to a physician.

Figure 3.14
Postural deviations

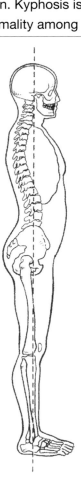

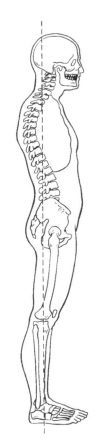

a. Lordosis: increased anterior lumbar curve from neutral

b. Kyphosis: increased posterior thoracic curve from neutral

c. Scoliosis: lateral spinal curvature often accompanied by vertebral rotation

Temporary lordotic (in standing position) or kyphotic (in sitting position) postures may occur every day when participants are tired— so-called fatigue postures. Fatigue postures may cause, or be the result of, physical stress, muscle imbalance, and/or pain. If these postures are continued for extended periods of time (e.g., months or years), the bones of the spine may adapt these postures, causing skeletal (rather than soft tissue) deviations that become irreversible.

Muscular Balance and Imbalance

When muscular balance is present on all sides of the cylindrical trunk, the neutral spine position can occur. However, a problem in one muscle group often creates problems in the opposing muscle group. If one muscle group is too tight (inflexible), it may pull the body out of the neutral position, causing increased stress and a tendency toward imbalance on the opposite side of the body. Conversely, if a particular muscle group is weakened from injury or fatigue, the body will fall out of alignment in the opposite direction.

The term **muscular balance** refers to the symmetry of the interconnected components of muscle and connective tissue. Specifically, muscular balance involves (a) equal strength and flexibility on the right and left sides of the body (bilateral symmetry); (b) proportional strength ratios in opposing (agonist/antagonist) muscle groups, although they may not be exactly equal; and (c) a balance in flexibility, in that normal ranges of motion are achieved but not exceeded.

One example of agonist/antagonist muscle imbalance is the relationship between the erector spinae and the abdominal muscles. Very commonly, the abdominals are overmatched by the muscles that extend the trunk and neutral spine is lost. Persons with localized low-

back pain from mechanical causes (no intervertebral disk or spinal nerve root involvement) are typically given abdominal-strengthening rehabilitation exercises to regain muscular control of the pelvis and balance with the erector spinae.

While not directly affecting the spine, a frequent muscular imbalance affects the function of the quadriceps and hamstrings. In untrained individuals, the naturally occurring size of the quadriceps is about twice that of the hamstrings, resulting in a significant imbalance in the agonist/antagonist relationship. With regular training, the ratio of hamstrings-to-quadriceps size and strength will improve, but hamstring strains unfortunately remain an all-too-frequent result of this muscular imbalance. Similarly, strength differences are often present between the dominant and nondominant limbs, particularly in the upper extremity. One method to counteract this is to have participants perform unilateral resistance exercises with dumbbells, isolating the right and left sides, rather than using a barbell to perform the same activity.

Core Stability

As introduced in Chapter 2, the axial skeleton (trunk) forms the "core" of the body, serving as the origin or insertion site for nearly 30 muscles in the abdomen, low back, pelvis, and hips. Biomechanically, the muscles that attach to the axial skeleton work to transfer forces to and from the upper and lower extremities. For example, a baseball pitch begins with generation of muscular force in the lower extremity (i.e., the forward stride toward home plate). These internal forces are transferred upward through a kinetic link system to the axial skeleton and into the throwing arm, concluding with the transfer of momentum to the ball via the fingers.

Fundamentals of Applied Kinesiology

While pitching coaches and athletic trainers go to great lengths to care for the shoulder muscles of professional pitchers, they, along with strength and conditioning specialists, also understand the need to develop trunk and lower-extremity muscular strength and endurance.

While not a particularly new concept, **core stability** is currently a popular topic of debate among group fitness instructors, personal trainers, clinicians, coaches, and athletes. There is an increasing body of knowledge that suggests that core stability is a key component necessary for successful performance of most gross motor activities (Willson et al., 2005). Hip and trunk muscle strength, abdominal muscle endurance, the ability to maintain a particular spinal or pelvic alignment, and the absence of ligamentous laxity in the vertebral column have all been identified as "core stability."

The lumbo-pelvic-hip "core" is formed by the lumbar vertebrae, the pelvis, the hip joints, and the muscles, tendons, ligaments, and other connective tissues that either create or limit movement in any of these segments. **Static stabilizers** (the bony configuration of joints, fibrocartilages, and ligaments) and **dynamic stabilizers** (the muscles) contribute to the creation of core stability. When compared to the contributions to core stability made by the dynamic structures (muscles), the contributions of the static tissues are relatively small. There are three mechanisms by which the muscles that comprise the core contribute to the stability of the trunk: intra-abdominal pressure, spinal compressive forces, and hip and trunk **muscle stiffness**, which is the capacity of these tissues to resist internal and external loads (Willson et al, 2005).

Trunk Flexors: Abdominal Muscles

The abdominal muscles are found on the anterior and lateral surfaces of the trunk, and they flex, laterally flex, and rotate the trunk. Trunk flexion occurs in the sagittal plane, right and left lateral flexion occurs in the frontal plane of motion, and right and left trunk rotation occurs in the transverse plane. The abdominal muscle group is composed of the rectus abdominis, the external oblique, the internal oblique, and the transverse abdominis (see Figure 2.26).

The fibers of the rectus abdominis are superficial and run longitudinally from the lower part of the chest to the pubic bone. Synergistic concentric actions of the right and left rectus abdominis muscles produce flexion of the trunk, as in the upward phase of an abdominal curl or crunch. While the anatomical movement during the return (downward) phase of the crunch is trunk extension, it is the eccentric muscle actions of the right and left rectus abdominis muscles (trunk flexors) that control the slow return to the mat. Unilateral concentric activation of the right or left rectus abdominis will result in lateral flexion of the trunk. Highly effective exercises to develop this muscle are posterior pelvic tilts, supine abdominal curls, straight reverse abdominal curls (eccentric action emphasized), and abdominal crunches (Figure 3.15a).

Also in the superficial layer of trunk muscles are the external obliques. These muscles originate on the ribs and attach to the iliac crest and the aponeurosis of the rectus abdominis; their fibers run diagonally downward and forward, as if into the front pockets of a pair of pants. When the right and left external obliques act together concentrically, they produce trunk flexion. The right and left sides can be activated independently to cause lateral flexion and, when combined with concentric action of the opposite internal oblique, produce trunk rotation to the opposite side. An example is the oblique (twisting) abdominal curl with the shoulder moved toward the opposite hip. Effective exercises to develop the external obliques are supine pelvic tilts, straight abdominal curls with the hips and knees partially extended to create more resistance, oblique abdominal curls, side-lying torso raises, and straight and oblique reverse abdominal curls (i.e., lifting the feet toward the ceiling until the buttocks leave the floor).

The internal oblique muscles are found deep to the external obliques, and their fibers run diagonally downward and posteriorly, as if into the back pockets of a pair of pants. Their functions include flexion, lateral flexion, and rotation of the trunk to the same side. Helpful exercises to develop and strengthen the internal obliques are supine pelvic tilts, straight and oblique reverse abdominal curls, and side-lying torso raises (Figure 3.15b).

Until the last decade, the transverse abdominis, found in the deepest layer of the abdominal wall, was thought to have no voluntary motor function; its only known anatomical contributions were to compress the viscera and support the spine. A series of studies (Hodges, 1999; Hodges & Richardson, 1997; 1999) have shown that the transverse abdominis, together with the multifidi muscles of the spine, play a critical role in core stability. These authors demonstrated that co-activation of the transverse abdominis and multifidi muscles occurred before any movements of the limbs. Specifically, these two muscles were activated an average of 30 milliseconds before shoulder movement and 110 milliseconds before leg movement. What is the impor-

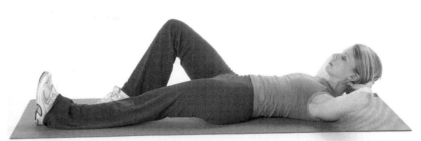

a. Abdominal curl for rectus abdominis

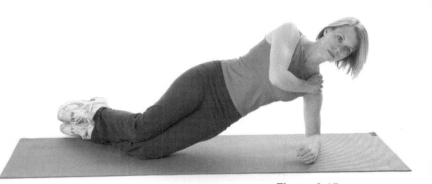

b. Side-lying torso raise for internal and external obliques

Figure 3.15
Abdominal strength and endurance exercises

tance of this temporal pattern of trunk muscle recruitment? The transverse abdominis and multifidi muscles are thought to play a vital role in providing feedback about spinal joint position, and thus forewarn the central nervous system about impending dynamic forces to be created in the extremities that may destabilize the spine (Fredericson & Moore, 2005).

Knowing how to activate the transverse abdominis muscles is an important aspect of core stability. Have participants lie on their backs with their knees flexed and feet flat on the floor. While they are relaxed and breathing normally, have them visualize pulling their navel inward toward the spine. They should hold this position for several seconds, relax, and then repeat several times. There are several different floor and standing exercises that will help participants activate their transverse abdominis

95

Fundamentals of Applied Kinesiology

and multifidi muscles. If a participant has a history of low-back pain or injury, he or she may have difficulty recruiting the transverse abdominis and multifidi muscles early enough to stabilize the spine (Hides, Richardson, & Jull, 1996). An instructor may need to refer these participants to a certified athletic trainer or physical therapist to assist them in learning these exercises. Figure 3.16

provides examples of static core stability exercises (prone plank, side plank) and dynamic core stability exercises (abdominal rollout on a stability ball, alternate leg bridges with shoulders on a stability ball).

There are several effective methods of increasing the resistance and loading pattern during abdominal exercises; one such variation is to change body positions relative

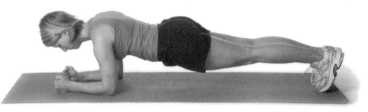

Prone plank with forearms on mat, elbows at 90°

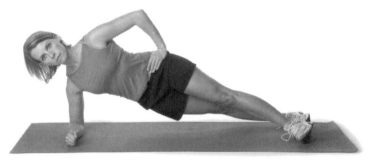

Side plank for abdominals and quadratus lumborum

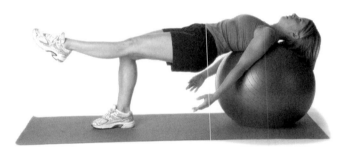

Alternate leg bridge with shoulders and head fully supported on a stability ball

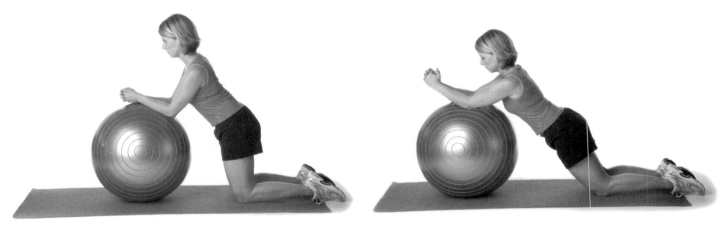

Abdominal rollout with stability ball; the farther the rollout, the more this exercise targets the latissimus dorsi

Figure 3.16
Core stability exercises (Adapted from Fredericson & Moore, 2005)

to gravity (e.g., partial abdominal curl on an incline bench with the head down rather than on a flat mat). Another variation is to change the end of the muscle that is stabilized and the one that is moved (e.g., perform abdominal curls with the shoulders lifted, and then change to a reverse curl with the hips elevated). Emphasize endurance training for the abdominals by having the participant hold an abdominal curl at various points in the arc of motion while performing exercises for the hip adductors or flexors.

Trunk Extensors:
Erector Spinae Group

When acting bilaterally and concentrically, the erector spinae group of muscles, formed by the iliocostalis, longissimus, and spinalis, will produce trunk extension and hyperextension. These muscles also act eccentrically to control flexion of the spine from a standing position, as in bending over to pick up the morning newspaper. When the erector spinae muscles are stimulated unilaterally, they cause lateral flexion to that same side. In normal standing posture, the level of activity in these muscles is quite low.

Exercises that are effective for strengthening this muscle group include the prone trunk hyperextension lift (Figure 3.17a), and, from a kneeling (all-fours) position, simultaneous lifting of the opposite arm and leg (Figure 3.17b). The latter exercise causes the erector spinae muscles to function as stabilizers of the spine to maintain a neutral position. For participants seeking more advanced challenges, incorporate a BOSU™ into the exercise program to develop balance and proprioception along with trunk extensor strength (Figure 3.18).

To stretch the erector spinae group, have participants lie on a mat in a supine position

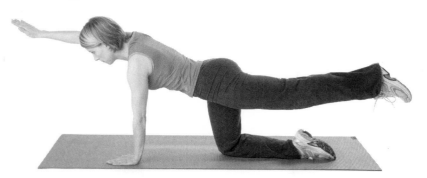

a. Prone hyperextension

b. Birddog: lift the opposite arm and leg simultaneously while keeping the spine in neutral position

Figure 3.17
Basic and intermediate difficulty strength exercises for the trunk extensors

with a posterior pelvic tilt and gently pull either one or both knees to the chest with the arms; hold this position for at least 15 seconds (Figure 3.19). The posterior pelvic tilt position flattens the anterior (lordotic) curve in the lumbar region of the spine and places the erector spinae in a stretched position.

Kinesiology of the Upper Extremity

Upper-extremity segments include the head and neck, shoulder girdle (scapulothoracic articulation), shoulders, elbows, wrists, and hands. Tables 2.13 through 2.16 summarize the muscles in each of these regions, their origins and insertions, primary function(s), and specific examples of exercises involving these muscles. Prior to discussion of the functional relationships of the muscles in the upper extremity, the terms shoulder joint complex, glenohumeral joint, and shoulder girdle must be differentiated. The term **shoulder joint complex** describes the coordinated functioning of four separate

Fundamentals of Applied Kinesiology

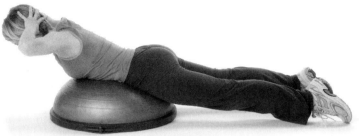

Starting position using both arms for balance

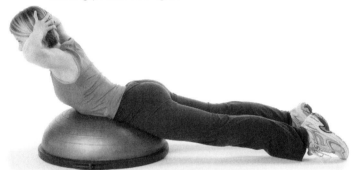

Trunk extension exercise (modified "Superman")

Figure 3.18
Advanced trunk extension exercise with a BOSU.

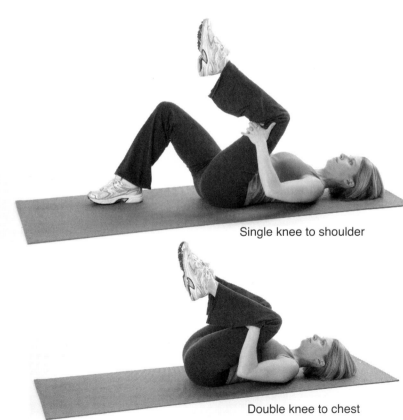

Single knee to shoulder

Double knee to chest

Figure 3.19
Flexibility exercises for the erector spinae muscles in a supine position with posterior pelvic tilt

upper-extremity segments: the **sternoclavicular (S/C) joint,** the junction of the sternum and the proximal clavicle; the **acromioclavicular (A/C) joint,** the junction of the acromion process of the scapula with the distal clavicle; the **glenohumeral (G/H) joint,** the ball-and-socket joint composed of the glenoid fossa of the scapula and the humeral head; and the **scapulothoracic (S/T) articulation,** the muscles and fascia connecting the scapulae to the thorax (Figure 3.20). The more general term, **shoulder girdle,** is synonymous with the formal anatomical term, scapulothoracic articulation.

The glenohumeral (G/H) joint is the most mobile joint in the body, the beneficiary of contributions to range of motion by the other components of the shoulder complex (S/C, A/C, and S/T). Voluntary movement at the G/H joint is possible in all three anatomical planes: flexion and extension in the sagittal plane, abduction and adduction in the frontal plane, circumduction in a combination of the sagittal and frontal planes, and internal and external rota-

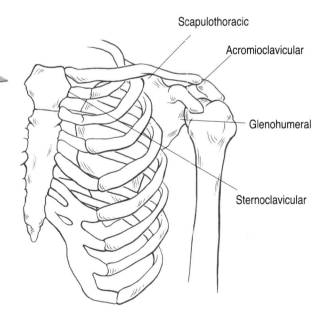

Scapulothoracic

Acromioclavicular

Glenohumeral

Sternoclavicular

Figure 3.20
The four articulations of the shoulder joint complex

tion and horizontal flexion and extension in the transverse plane (Figure 3.21).

The glenohumeral joint and the scapulothoracic articulation work together to produce coordinated flexion and extension in the sagittal plane and abduction and adduction in the frontal plane. This relationship is referred to as **scapulohumeral rhythm** and, throughout the available range of motion for flexion/extension and abduction/adduction, approximately 2 degrees of humeral motion occurs for every 1 degree of scapular motion. Translated to absolute terms, to achieve 180 degrees of flexion or abduction,

Figure 3.21
Shoulder joint range of motion

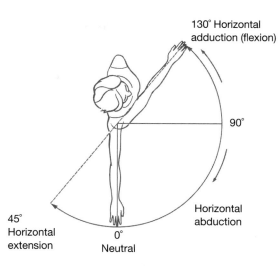

Shoulder range of motion in the transverse plane: horizontal adduction (flexion) 130°; horizontal abduction to 0°; horizontal extension 45° past neutral

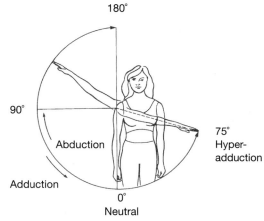
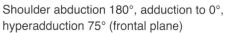

Shoulder abduction 180°, adduction to 0°, hyperadduction 75° (frontal plane)

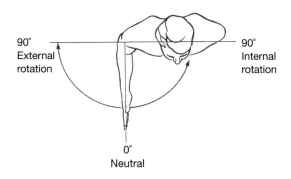

Shoulder rotation range of motion in the transverse plane (shoulder is adducted to 0°): external rotation 90°, internal rotation 90°

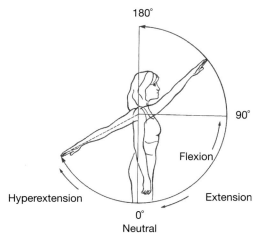
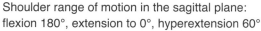

Shoulder range of motion in the sagittal plane: flexion 180°, extension to 0°, hyperextension 60°

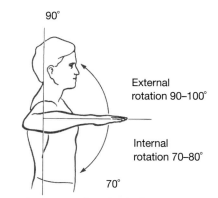

Shoulder rotation range of motion in the transverse plane, viewed from the sagittal plane: external rotation 90–100°, internal rotation 70–80°

approximately 120 degrees of that motion occurs at the glenohumeral joint and 60 degrees of the motion occurs as the result of movement of the scapula on the thorax (Figure 3.22).

In common activities of daily living, the scapular muscles function primarily as stabilizers, but they also are powerful muscles involved in upper-extremity movements. Anatomical movements of the scapulae on the thorax include elevation and depression, abduction (also termed "protraction") and adduction ("retraction"), and upward and downward rotation (Figure 3.23). Scapular muscles are typically divided into two groups based on their location and function. Anterior shoulder girdle muscles connect the scapulae to the front of the trunk, while the posterior shoulder girdle muscles hold the scapulae to the back of the trunk.

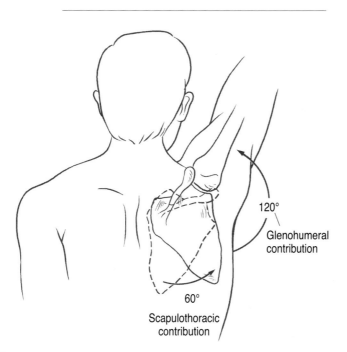

Figure 3.22

The movement of the arm is accompanied by movement of the scapula—a ratio of approximately 2° of arm movement for every 1° of scapular movement occurs during shoulder abduction and flexion; this relationship is known as scapulohumeral rhythm.

There are many anatomical movements possible throughout the upper extremity. However, within the scope of this chapter, only the kinesiology of the scapulothoracic articulation and glenohumeral joint are addressed.

Anterior Shoulder Girdle Muscles

The major anterior shoulder girdle muscles—the pectoralis minor and serratus anterior—attach the scapula to the front of the thorax (Figure 3.24). Concentric and eccentric activity in these muscles results in scapular movement on the thorax; these muscles have no attachment to the humerus and thus do not directly cause glenohumeral motion. The pectoralis minor originates on the coracoid process of the scapula and inserts on the third, fourth, and fifth ribs. The pectoralis minor can have a positive or negative effect on posture, depending on the amount of muscular tone in the scapular adductors, specifically the middle trapezius and rhomboids. Concentric activity of the pectoralis minor results in abduction, depression, and downward rotation of the scapula. However, if the scapular adductors are weak, fatigued, or injured, the muscular tension created by the pectoralis minor will tilt the scapulae forward and down, worsening a rounded-shoulders posture (kyphosis).

The serratus anterior is a broad, knife-edged muscle that originates along the underside of the entire length of the medial border of the scapula and inserts onto the front parts of the first through ninth ribs. The serratus anterior abducts the scapula and works as a synergist with the upper trapezius to produce upward rotation of the scapula. A key function of the serratus is to hold the medial border of the scapula firmly

100

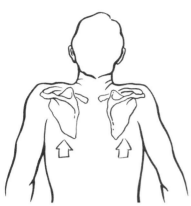

Figure 3.23
Scapular
movements

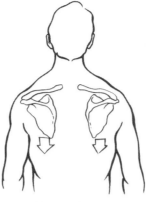

Elevation

Depression

Adduction (retraction)

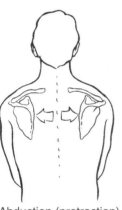

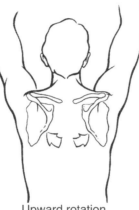

Abduction (protraction)

Upward rotation

Downward rotation (return to anatomical position)

against the rib cage, preventing "winging" of the scapula posteriorly away from the thorax. Concentric action of the serratus anterior enables powerful forward motion of the arm, as in the overhead throwing motion. Strengthening of the serratus can be done from a supine position with the shoulder flexed to 90 degrees and the elbow extended, by pushing a dumbbell or medicine ball held in the hand toward the ceiling in a "punching" motion without bending the elbow. The shoulder blade(s) should lift off the floor slightly when performing this exercise (Figure 3.25). Another effective method of working the serratus anterior is to have participants perform push-ups with a "plus"—the addition of scapular abduction at the end of the upward phase of a regular push-up.

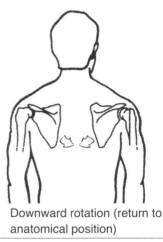

Figure 3.24
Anterior muscles of the shoulder girdle

Coracoid process

Serratus anterior

Pectoralis minor

Figure 3.25
Exercise to
strengthen
the serratus
anterior muscle

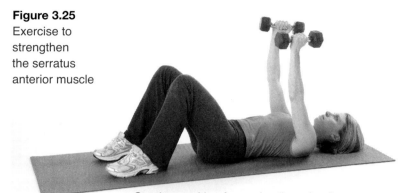

Starting position for supine "punches"

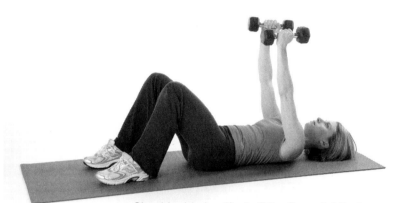

Shoulder blades lifted off the floor slightly; keep
elbows fully extended

Posterior Shoulder Girdle Muscles

The posterior shoulder girdle muscles—the
trapezius, rhomboids, and levator scapulae—
attach the scapula to the back of the thorax.
Since these muscles have no attachment to
the humerus, their action does not directly
result in glenohumeral motion.

The trapezius is the largest and most superficial of the posterior shoulder girdle muscles; it
originates at the base of the skull and has
attachments to all 19 vertebrae in the cervical
and thoracic regions of the spine. Resembling
the shape of a trapezoid, the muscle attaches
laterally to the spine of the scapula and the lateral aspect of the clavicle. Recalling da Vinci's
perspective of functional human anatomy as
"cords attached to skeletons," it is easy to
understand why the different sections of the
trapezius have three different names. The

trapezius is divided into three distinct units—
upper, middle, and lower—because of the different directions and line of action of its fibers.
The fibers of the upper trapezius are angled
upward and obliquely, the muscle fibers of the
middle trapezius are purely horizontal in their
direction and pull, and the fibers of the lower
trapezius are angled obliquely downward.
Therefore, if the upper fibers are activated concentrically, they will produce elevation and
adduction of the scapula. Stimulation of the
fibers of the middle trapezius will cause pure
adduction of the scapula, while concentric
activity of the lower trapezius fibers will both
depress and adduct the scapula.

The different fibers of the trapezius are
alternately activated and relaxed to cause
scapular rotation. If the arms are lifted in front
(G/H flexion) or out to the side (G/H abduction), the shoulder blades rotate upward and
away from the spine. This critical anatomical
motion, upward rotation, occurs as the result
of the upper and middle trapezius, rhomboids, and serratus anterior pulling on different aspects of the scapula. Concentric action
of the lower trapezius, together with eccentric
activity in the rhomboids and levator scapulae, will return the shoulder blades to their
original (anatomical) position.

To design effective exercises to strengthen
each of the sections of the trapezius, consider
the stresses and loads that the muscle encounters regularly. In typical sitting and standing
postures, the upper trapezius acts isometrically
to support the arms and head. The upper
trapezius is also active when a heavy weight or
object is held at arm's length. This portion of
the trapezius needs stretching and strengthening throughout the full range of motion and
does not require long-duration, isometric-resis-
tance activities. The upper trapezius and the
levator scapulae are strengthened in an upright

standing or a sitting position by performing shoulder shrugs with dumbbells or tubing with the arms extended behind (Figure 3.26).

The middle trapezius is commonly weak or fatigued in a participant who has rounded shoulders (kyphotic) in a standing or sitting posture. Typically, the middle trapezius does not need to be stretched, but rather strengthened in an "antigravity" position; that is, the muscle must be used to lift some resistance against gravity. Simply adducting the scapulae in a standing position does not overload the middle trapezius because there is no resistance (other than gravity) to overcome. Examples of antigravity positions include a fully prone or a simulated-prone position (e.g., forward lunge, half-kneeling with the torso supported on the front thigh). Using dumbbells, the desired movement in the modified forward-lunge position is to "squeeze" the shoulder blades together, causing the arms to lift in the direction opposite the pull of gravity (Figure 3.27a). To isolate the middle trapezius in a standing position, use elastic bands or surgical tubing to provide resistance. Instruct participants to abduct their G/H joints to 90 degrees, maintain a neutral spine, and then "pull" their scapulae together with no movement at the elbows or wrists (Figure 3.27b).

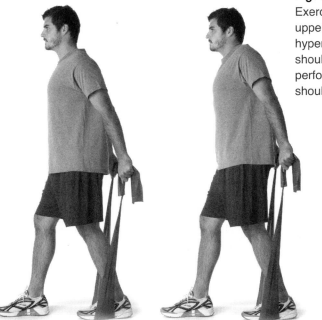

Figure 3.26
Exercise for the upper trapezius–hyperextend the shoulders, then perform a full shoulder shrug

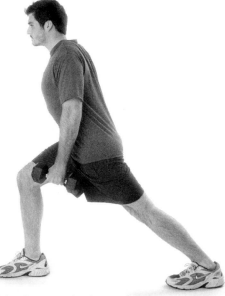

a. Maintain neutral spine and pull the scapulae toward the spine, keeping the elbows straight and arms hanging down

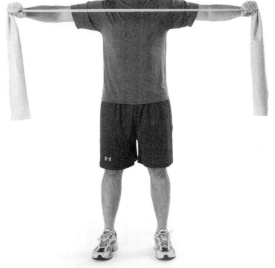

b. Maintain neutral spine and pull the scapulae together with the elbows slightly bent and the wrists neutral

Figure 3.27
Exercises for the middle trapezius

103

Fundamentals of Applied Kinesiology

The rhomboid major and minor work together as one functional unit; the fibers of these muscles run upward and obliquely from the spine to the vertebral border of the scapulae. These muscles act primarily to adduct and elevate the scapulae and assist with downward rotation of the scapulae. When the rhomboids are weak or overstressed, the shoulder blades may tilt and pull away from the thorax due to the unopposed tension exerted by the serratus anterior and pectoralis minor. Bent-over rows with a weighted bar or pulley machine weights or the use of a rowing ergometer are effective in strengthening the rhomboids (Figure 3.28).

Glenohumeral Joint Muscles

The final muscles discussed in this section are those that directly produce movement at the glenohumeral joint. These prime movers include the pectoralis major, deltoid, rotator cuff, latissimus dorsi, and teres major (Figure 3.29). Due to the complexity of the anatomical functions of the major muscles acting at the G/H joint, they are not listed in groups as adductors, extensors, and so on.

The pectoralis major is a very large muscle that makes up the majority of the muscle mass on the anterior chest wall. The pectoralis major is divided into three sections, with each portion named for its attachment point to the axial skeleton: (a) clavicular, (b) sternal, and (c) costal portions. The clavicular portion of the pectoralis major, originating on the anterior aspect of the clavicle, is located slightly superior to the G/H joint and acts concentrically as a flexor. The similar downward-oblique angles of the fibers of the sternal and costal portions of the pectoralis major allow them to be considered as one functional unit. The inferior location of these muscles relative to the shoulder joint makes the sternal and costal portions powerful shoulder extensors. When considered as a whole unit, the pectoralis major is a prime mover in glenohumeral adduction, internal rotation, and horizontal flexion.

To strengthen the pectoralis major using hand-held weights, have participants lie supine on a mat or on top of a step bench. From this position, a pectoral flye exercise involving horizontal flexion will overload the pectoralis major. The push-up is also an effective exercise for the pectoral muscles. The pectoralis major, serratus anterior, and triceps brachii act eccentrically to slowly lower the body in the downward phase (same direction of movement as the force of gravity) of the push-up. These same muscles act concentrically during the upward phase of the push-up. As an added challenge for an advanced class, utilize a step-bench as the starting position for the hands to increase the level of difficulty of the push-up, or have participants place two benches close together, positioning one hand

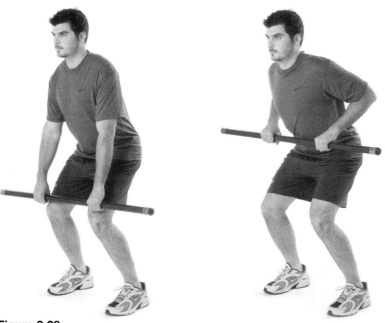

Figure 3.28
Bent-over row to strengthen scapular retractors (rhomboids and middle trapezius muscles)

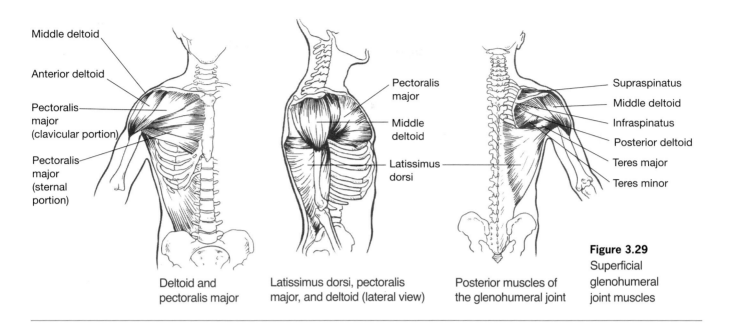

Middle deltoid

Anterior deltoid

Pectoralis major (clavicular portion)

Pectoralis major (sternal portion)

Deltoid and pectoralis major

Pectoralis major

Middle deltoid

Latissimus dorsi

Latissimus dorsi, pectoralis major, and deltoid (lateral view)

Supraspinatus

Middle deltoid

Infraspinatus

Posterior deltoid

Teres major

Teres minor

Posterior muscles of the glenohumeral joint

Figure 3.29
Superficial glenohumeral joint muscles

on each and performing the push-up between the benches. The increased height off the ground will permit a larger range of motion during the eccentric and concentric phases of the push-up, creating a greater overload of these muscles. A study of 12 different types of push-up exercises reported that ballistic (plyometric) push-ups (e.g., those involving a hand-clap) elicited significantly higher levels of muscle activation in upper-extremity and core musculature than did push-ups performed with the hands on unstable surfaces (e.g., using standard-size basketballs) (Freeman et al., 2006).

The deltoid has a configuration similar to the trapezius in that it has fibers running in three different directions and three names, according to location. As a whole, the deltoid muscle lies superior to the glenohumeral joint and collectively functions as the primary abductor of the shoulder joint. The anterior deltoid is easily palpated in the front of the shoulder, attaching to the lateral one-third of the clavicle. Since the anterior deltoid crosses the shoulder joint anteriorly, it flexes, internally rotates, and horizontally flexes the arm at the shoulder. The most

effective positions to strengthen the anterior deltoid are sitting and standing. Using free weights or elastic tubing, participants can flex the arms forward from 0 degrees (anatomical position) to full flexion (180 degrees), in sets of eight to 12 repetitions.

The fibers of the middle deltoid are aligned perfectly with the frontal plane, and thus this muscle is the prime mover in concentric abduction of the shoulder joint (e.g., upward phase of a seated military press). During the downward phase of a seated military press, the middle deltoid acts eccentrically to control the lowering of the weight via adduction (Figure 3.30). When performing overhead resistance training, such as a shoulder press, it is important to maintain the glenohumeral joint in neutral or external rotation.

Shoulder abduction combined with internal rotation, particularly in participants over 40 years of age, will commonly irritate the rotator cuff muscles, impinging their tendons between the acromion process of the scapula, the subacromial bursa, and the head of the humerus. For those participants who have existing shoulder pain or those who develop impingement symptoms, avoid recommending resistance exercises that combine shoulder abduction with internal rotation.

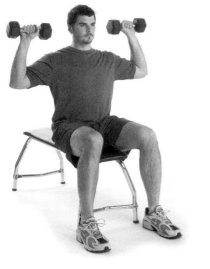

Figure 3.30
Seated military press for the deltoid muscle group

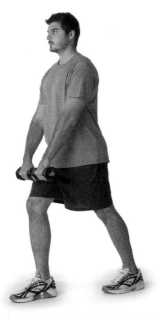

Starting position: maintain a neutral spine—shoulder blades flexed and internally rotated (hands together)

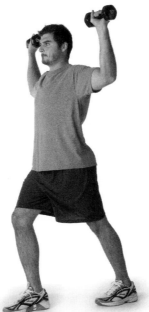

Finishing position: shoulders extended, adducted, and externally rotated

Figure 3.31
Strengthening exercise for the posterior deltoid

The posterior deltoid is located on the back side of the G/H joint and acts as an antagonist to the anterior deltoid. The posterior deltoid has the exact opposite functions as the anterior deltoid; it extends, externally rotates, and horizontally extends the arm at the shoulder. To strengthen the posterior deltoid, have participants stand in a forward lunge position with a neutral spine. Using hand weights, begin with the shoulder flexed, adducted, and internally rotated, and move into extension, abduction, and external rotation (Figure 3.31).

A group of four relatively small muscles comprise the rotator cuff (Figure 3.32). These muscles act synergistically to pull the head of the humerus down and into the glenoid fossa, thus helping to stabilize the G/H joint against the constant downward pull of gravity acting to dislocate the joint. The rotator cuff muscles are sometimes referred to as the "compressor cuff" because they stabilize the humeral head within the joint. The tendons of these muscles cover the head of humerus, while the muscles themselves are mostly named for their location in relation to the scapula. The acronym "SITS" is used as a memory device to recall the names of the muscles in this group. The supraspinatus, located superior to the spine of the scapula, initiates abduction and is a prime mover through the early abduction range of motion. The infraspinatus, found inferior to (below) the spine of the scapula, and the teres minor are synergists for external rotation of the G/H joint. The subscapularis, located on the anterior undersurface of the scapula, is not easily palpated and attaches to the anterior aspect of the joint. Since it is located anterior and medial, the subscapularis functions as an internal rotator of the humerus.

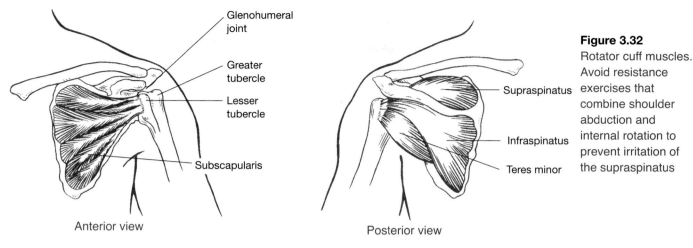

Glenohumeral joint

Greater tubercle

Lesser tubercle

Subscapularis

Anterior view

Supraspinatus

Infraspinatus

Teres minor

Posterior view

Figure 3.32
Rotator cuff muscles. Avoid resistance exercises that combine shoulder abduction and internal rotation to prevent irritation of the supraspinatus

Caution must be used when working the rotator cuff in isolation; the four tendons (primarily the supraspinatus) can become inflamed by performing many repetitions of movements that involve abduction, flexion, and rotation. For injury prevention, make sure that participants' shoulders are in neutral or external rotation any time the arms are abducted or flexed.

The latissimus dorsi and the teres major are similar muscles from a functional perspective (see Figure 2.30). Kinesiology instructors often nickname the teres major the "little lat" because its functions are identical to the much larger latissimus dorsi. The latissimus dorsi originates over a wide area in the lower thoracic and all of the lumbar regions of the spine, while the teres major arises from the inferior portion of the scapula. What makes these two muscles so functionally similar is the close proximity of their insertion sites on the medial aspect of the proximal humerus. Both muscles act concentrically to produce adduction, extension, and internal rotation of the glenohumeral joint. In the class setting, these muscles are strengthened with elastic resistance, starting with the arms overhead (elbows extended) and adducting and extending the G/H joint against the resistance

provided by the tubing. Performing this same exercise with dumbbells will not involve the latissimus and teres major in adduction, but rather recruit the abductors (deltoids) eccentrically to lower the weights. Regardless of the muscle targeted for strengthening, when working with hand-held weights, be sure that the initial effort is in a direction opposite the pull of gravity.

Summary

Group fitness instructors are required to design exercise programs that are safe and effective, and that accomplish the desired fitness and/or personal goals of participants. Without a fundamental understanding of biomechanical principles and kinesiology, this task is nearly impossible. This chapter has provided a detailed region-by-region summary of the functional relationships of skeletal muscles in the upper and lower extremities, as well as a review of the most current information available related to core stability. With this information, an instructor has at his or her disposal sufficient information to identify specific exercises and physical activities that will safely and efficiently accomplish the fitness goals of participants.

References and Suggested Reading

References

Clark, J.M. & Haynor, D. R. (1987). Anatomy of the abductor muscles of the hip as studied by computed tomography. *Journal of Bone and Joint Surgery,* 69A,1021–1031.

Fredericson, M. & Moore, T. (2005). Muscular balance, core stability, and injury prevention for middle- and long-distance runners. *Physical Medicine and Rehabilitation Clinics of North America,* 16, 3, 669–689.

Freeman, S. et al., (2006). Quantifying muscle patterns and spine load during various forms of the push-up. *Medicine & Science in Sports & Exercise,* 38, 570–577.

Hides, J.A., Richardson, C.A., & Jull, G.A. (1996). Multifidus muscle recovery is not automatic after resolution of acute, first-episode low-back pain. *Spine,* 21, 2763–2769.

Hodges, P.W. (1999). Is there a role for transverse abdominis in lumbo-pelvic stability? *Manual Therapy,* 4, 74–86.

Hodges, P.W. & Richardson, C.A. (1999). Altered trunk muscle recruitment in people with low back pain with upper limb movement at different speeds. *Archives of Physical Medicine and Rehabilitation,* 80, 1005–1012.

Hodges, P.W. & Richardson, C.A. (1997). Contraction of the abdominal muscles associated with movement of the lower limb. *Physical Therapy,* 77, 132–142.

Lindsay, D.M. et al. (1992). Comparison of isokinetic internal and external hip rotation torques using different testing positions. *Journal of Orthopedic and Sports Physical Therapy,* 16, 43–50.

Lundy, J. (2006). Gluteus medius stimulates lower extremity movement. *Biomechanics,* 13, 41–52.

Maybury, M.C. & Waterfield, J. (1997). An investigation into the relation between step height and ground reaction forces in step exercise: A pilot study. *British Journal of Sports Medicine,* 31, 109.

Neumann, D.A. (2002). *Kinesiology of the Musculoskeletal System.* St. Louis, Mo.: Mosby.

Willson, J.D. et al. (2005). Core stability and its relationship to lower extremity function and injury. *Journal of the American Academy of Orthopaedic Surgeons,* 13, 316–325.

Suggested Reading

Golding, L.A. & Golding, S.M. (2003). *Musculoskeletal Anatomy and Human Movement.* Monterey, Calif.: Healthy Learning.

Hamilton, N. & Luttgens, K. (2002). *Kinesiology: Scientific Basis of Human Motion* (10th ed.). Boston, Mass.: McGraw-Hill.

Marieb, E.N., Mallatt, J., & Wilhelm, P.B. (2005). *Human Anatomy and Physiology* (4th ed.). Redwood City, Calif.: Benjamin-Cummings.

Mayo Clinic (2005). Core strengthening: Improve your balance and stability. *Mayo Clinic Women's HealthSource,* 9, 7.

Mow, V.C. & Huiskes, R. (Eds). (2005). *Basic Orthopaedic Biomechanics and Mechano-Biology* (3rd ed.). Philadelphia, Pa.: Lippincott Williams & Wilkins.

Oates, C.A. (2004). *Kinesiology: The Mechanics and Pathomechanics of Human Movement.* Philadelphia: Lippincott Williams & Wilkins.

Watkins, J. (1999). *Structure and Function of the Musculoskeletal System.* Champaign, Ill.: Human Kinetics.

Chapter Four

Claudia S. Plaisted Fernandez, Dr.P.H., M.S., R.D., L.D.N., earned her doctorate in public health from the University of North Carolina at Chapel Hill, where she directs leadership institutes for public health, healthcare, university deans, and other professionals. She earned her master's degree in clinical nutrition at Boston University and her baccalaureate in home economics and nutrition from Miami University of Ohio. At UNC, she has taught a graduate course in nutrition called "The Psychology of Eating," taught in the UNC medical school, and served as director of *Nutrition in Medicine,* a series of interactive CD-ROMs that teach nutrition to medical students. She also teaches in the executive education program at the Duke Fuqua School of Business. Clinically, she specializes in eating disorders and disordered eating, weight cycling and obesity, and wellness.

Kelly M. Adams, M.P.H., R.D., L.D.N., earned her B.A. in biology from the University of Virginia and her master's degree in public health nutrition from the University of North Carolina at Chapel Hill, where she now works on the *Nutrition in Medicine* project. This CD-ROM and Web-based curriculum is used to teach nutrition at many medical schools across the U.S. and abroad. She has held positions in public health nutrition at a county health department and in the wellness program at Duke University.

IN THIS CHAPTER:

Introduction to Nutrition

By Claudia S. Plaisted Fernandez and Kelly M. Adams

Group fitness instructors are in a position to both teach and demonstrate healthy habits to their participants. This responsibility includes not only fitness habits, but nutritional habits as well. Since many participants will see the instructor as an authority on basic issues of health, it is important to be able to instruct them on appropriate nutritional guidelines, identify individuals at risk, and know when it is appropriate to make referrals.

Introduction to Nutrition

An understanding of **nutrition** is fundamental to providing sound guidance to participants. There are two basic sets of dietary recommendations with which an instructor should be very familiar: the USDA Dietary Guidelines 2005 and the MyPyramid Food Guidance System (www.MyPyramid.gov) (Figure 4.1, Table 4.1).

This chapter is designed to provide the basics of nutrition so that an instructor can serve as a guide in improving participants' health, based on these sets of public health guidelines. Some participants may have more complex health issues, such as chronic diseases or eating disorders. In these cases, it will be important to give sound nutritional guidance and to refer the participant for the appropriate medical intervention, such as a medical doctor or a registered dietitian. Although an instructor should have an understanding of basic nutrition after mastering this chapter, it is not a substitute for a degree or a license in nutrition. In some states, nutrition assessment and prescription is a legally protected area of practice. An instructor must be aware of the laws governing the practice of

nutrition in his or her state. Regardless of the state's licensure laws, advanced training in nutrition (such as a bachelor's or master's degree in nutrition and passing a national competency exam) is required before a person is competent to make assessments or give specific dietary recommendations. However, all allied health professionals should be able to give sound advice based on the two sets of guidelines mentioned above. Studying this chapter will help an instructor guide participants to better health and answer some of their most common questions about nutrition.

Human Metabolism

Energy is a word with many meanings, but when it comes to the human body, it refers exclusively to the capacity to do work. The ultimate source of **energy** is the sun, which plants turn into chemical energy through a process called **photosynthesis.** Animals, such as humans, eat plants (and some animals eat other animals) to gain this energy. The energy in food is chemical energy. The human body can convert chemical energy from foods into mechanical energy (muscle activity), electrical energy (nerve conduction), and heat energy (metabolism). Energy is found in two forms: active (kinetic) energy and stored (potential) energy. Active energy is ready for the body's immediate use (e.g., **ATP** in muscles), while stored energy is in the body's reserves (body fat and **glycogen** stores).

Energy is measured in units called **kilocalories,** often written as "kcal," "Cal," or **"Calories"** (note the capital C). A kilocalorie is the amount of energy needed to raise the temperature of 1 kilogram of **water** by 1° C. Although many people simply call these "calories," the correct scientific terminology is kilocalories. One kilocalorie equals 1,000 calories

Figure 4.1
MyPyramid Food
Guidance System

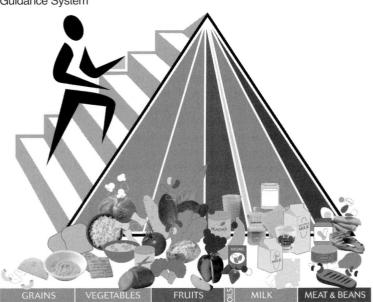

| GRAINS | VEGETABLES | FRUITS | OILS | MILK | MEAT & BEANS |

Table 4.1
USDA Dietary Guidelines for Americans 2005

Key Recommendations for the General Population

ADEQUATE NUTRIENTS WITHIN CALORIE NEEDS

• Consume a variety of nutrient-dense foods and beverages within and among the basic food groups while choosing foods that limit the intake of saturated and trans fats, cholesterol, added sugars, salt, and alcohol.

• Meet recommended intakes within energy needs by adopting a balanced eating pattern, such as the U.S. Department of Agriculture (USDA) Food Guide or the Dietary Approaches to Stop Hypertension (DASH) Eating Plan.

WEIGHT MANAGEMENT

• To maintain body weight in a healthy range, balance calories from foods and beverages with calories expended.

• To prevent gradual weight gain over time, make small decreases in food and beverage calories and increase physical activity.

PHYSICAL ACTIVITY

• Engage in regular physical activity and reduce sedentary activities to promote health, psychological well-being, and a healthy body weight.

• To reduce the risk of chronic disease in adulthood: Engage in at least 30 minutes of moderate-intensity physical activity, above usual activity, at work or home on most days of the week.

• For most people, greater health benefits can be obtained by engaging in physical activity of more vigorous intensity or longer duration.

• To help manage body weight and prevent gradual, unhealthy body-weight gain in adulthood: Engage in approximately 60 minutes of moderate- to vigorous-intensity activity on most days of the week while not exceeding caloric-intake requirements.

• To sustain weight loss in adulthood: Participate in at least 60 to 90 minutes of daily moderate-intensity physical activity while not exceeding caloric-intake requirements. Some people may need to consult with a healthcare provider before participating in this level of activity.

• Achieve physical fitness by including cardiovascular conditioning, stretching exercises for flexibility, and resistance exercises or calisthenics for muscle strength and endurance.

FOOD GROUPS TO ENCOURAGE

• Consume a sufficient amount of fruits and vegetables while staying within energy needs. Two cups of fruit and 2½ cups of vegetables per day are recommended for a reference 2,000-calorie intake, with higher or lower amounts depending on the calorie level.

• Choose a variety of fruits and vegetables each day. In particular, select from all five vegetable subgroups (dark green, orange, legumes, starchy vegetables, and other vegetables) several times a week.

• Consume three or more ounce-equivalents of whole-grain products per day, with the rest of the recommended grains coming from enriched or whole-grain products. In general, at least half of the grains should come from whole grains.

• Consume 3 cups per day of fat-free or low-fat milk or equivalent milk products.

FATS

• Consume less than 10% of calories from saturated fatty acids and less than 300 mg/day of cholesterol, and keep trans fatty acid consumption as low as possible.

• Keep total fat intake between 20 and 35% of calories, with most fats coming from sources of polyunsaturated and monounsaturated fatty acids, such as fish, nuts, and vegetable oils.

• When selecting and preparing meat, poultry, dry beans, and milk or milk products, make choices that are lean, low-fat, or fat-free.

• Limit intake of fats and oils high in saturated and/or trans fatty acids, and choose products low in such fats and oils.

CARBOHYDRATES

• Choose fiber-rich fruits, vegetables, and whole grains often.

• Choose and prepare foods and beverages with little added sugars or caloric sweeteners, such as amounts suggested by the USDA Food Guide and the DASH Eating Plan.

• Reduce the incidence of dental caries by practicing good oral hygiene and consuming sugar- and starch-containing foods and beverages less frequently.

SODIUM AND POTASSIUM

• Consume less than 2,300 mg (approximately 1 teaspoon of salt) of sodium per day.

• Choose and prepare foods with little salt. At the same time, consume potassium-rich foods, such as fruits and vegetables.

ALCOHOLIC BEVERAGES

• Those who choose to drink alcoholic beverages should do so sensibly and in moderation—defined as the consumption of up to one drink per day for women and up to two drinks per day for men.

• Alcoholic beverages should not be consumed by some individuals, including those who cannot restrict their alcohol intake, women of childbearing age who may become pregnant, pregnant and lactating women, children and adolescents, individuals taking medications that can interact with alcohol, and those with specific medical conditions.

• Alcoholic beverages should be avoided by individuals engaging in activities that require attention, skill, or coordination, such as driving or operating machinery.

FOOD SAFETY

• To avoid microbial foodborne illness:
  – Clean hands, food-contact surfaces, and fruits and vegetables. Meat and poultry should not be washed or rinsed.
  – Separate raw, cooked, and ready-to-eat foods while shopping, preparing, and storing foods.
  – Cook foods to a safe temperature to kill microorganisms.
  – Chill (refrigerate) perishable food promptly and defrost foods properly.
  – Avoid raw (unpasteurized) milk or any products made from unpasteurized milk, raw or partially cooked eggs or foods containing raw eggs, raw or undercooked meat and poultry, unpasteurized juices, and raw sprouts.

Introduction to Nutrition

(note the lowercase c) or one Calorie. The energy-burned units measured by exercise machines or the calories displayed on a food label are actually kilocalories, although they are often displayed as "calories."

The body requires energy—or calories—to function properly. **Total energy expenditure** is made up of basal metabolism (60–70%), **physical activity** (20–30%), and **dietary-induced thermogenesis** (10%). Metabolism describes the chemical processes that happen in your body every day. Your **basal metabolic rate (BMR)** is the energy required to complete the sum total of these processes—including ion transport (about 40% of BMR), protein synthesis (about 20% of BMR), and daily functioning like breathing, circulation, and nutrient processing (also about 40% of BMR).

Physical activity requires energy as well. The amount of kilocalories needed depends on the duration and type of activity as well as the size of the individual (larger people burn more calories). Energy expenditure also increases after eating, which is called the "thermic (heat-producing) effect of food" or sometimes "dietary-induced thermogenesis." This energy is spent on digesting the carbohydrates, proteins, and fats into other substances and for some storage of energy in the form of body fat and glycogen. This body fat is called adipose tissue.

How Much Energy?

Just how much energy does the human body need on a daily basis? General guidelines have been developed by the United States Department of Agriculture and the United States Department of Health and Human Services (summarized in Table 4.2). The Web site www.MyPyramid.gov allows individuals to estimate their own energy needs based on age, sex, and activity level.

Table 4.2
Sample Energy Needs at Different Activity Levels (kcal)

Age–Gender	Activity Level	
	Sedentary	Active
Age–Females		
19–30	2,000	2,400
31–50	1,800	2,200
51+	1,600	2,200
Age–Males		
19–30	2,400	3,000
31–50	2,200	3,000
51+	2,000	2,800

How energy needs translate into food choices is discussed later in this chapter. To get a general understanding of how much energy is needed by the human body, anticipate that about 10 kcal for every pound (0.45 kg) of body weight will be used to meet the body's energy needs at rest, which include tissue growth and repair. For a 160-pound (72 kg) male, that means his resting energy expenditure will be about 1,600 kcal/day. In addition, the body has energy needs for daily activities (general movement creates a need, often estimated at 300 to 500 kcal/day) and exercise, which varies with the individual. Growth, such as in children, pregnant women, and teenagers, requires extra energy. (Clearly, energy needs can add up quickly in active individuals.)

Since people generally eat several times a day rather than continuously, their bodies must store some of the energy they eat for later use, maybe minutes, hours, or even days away. The body ultimately converts all energy from food into ATP molecules—the energy currency of the body. Overall, only about 25% of ATP energy ends up being used for work, and the other 75% is lost as heat. ATP is always present in small amounts in all body tissues. Its purpose is to deliver energy instantaneously. When a person sprints for just a few seconds, he or she is drawing primarily on muscular ATP stores and another compound called **phosphocreatine,** or **creatine phosphate (CP).** As the person uses up immediate energy stores, he or she must continually provide more for the muscles to function.

Of course, many people perform activities for longer than just a few seconds, whether it is running, walking, or even standing. Food energy must be converted to meet these demands as well. This energy is directly related to the foods eaten: the type and the amount of **carbohydrates, proteins,** and **fats.** Not only does this food supply energy to the body, it also supplies the chemicals needed to process and use this energy. These chemicals are commonly called "vitamins" and "minerals." A diet high in carbohydrates helps the body to perform better during endurance activities, since a high-carbohydrate diet promotes glycogen storage. The other main energy source for the body is stored fat, called **fatty acids,** which are stored in adipose tissue in the form of **triglycerides.** Although a mix of fuel is consistently being used, during physical activity the body initially draws on ATP and CP, then primarily on glycogen, and eventually on fatty acids from fat stores. A well-trained athlete stores more glycogen and can mobilize fat faster and more efficiently than a poorly trained individual.

The chemistry and biology of health and physical fitness boils down to one major starting point: food. The energy to move, live, and grow comes from the foods people eat and the **nutrients** those foods contain. Helping participants make healthy food choices is an important role an instructor can play—a role that can have a positive impact not only on athletic performance, but also on life expectancy. To provide this guidance, an instructor must understand some of the basics of nutrition.

Macronutrients

The foods people eat supply energy. Energy only comes from four classes of nutrients: carbohydrates, protein, fat, and alcohol (Table 4.3). Fat is by far the most energy-dense of the substances, with 9 kcal/g. Carbohydrate and protein both contain only 4 kcal/g, less than half of that found in fat. Alcohol is very energy-dense at 7 kcal/g but, unlike carbohydrate, protein, and fat, is very nutrient-poor. It contributes mostly calories to the diet with little to no nutritional benefit. Any energy eaten in excess of needs is converted to body fat for storage, thus no one category is more "fattening" than another. However, it must be noted that because fat and alcohol are more calorically dense than carbohydrate and protein, they make it easier for a person to exceed his or her energy needs.

**Table 4.3
Energy Content**

Carbohydrate	4 kcal/g
Protein	4 kcal/g
Fat	9 kcal/g
Alcohol	7 kcal/g

Carbohydrate

Carbohydrate, protein, and fat are referred to as the **macronutrients,** while alcohol is not usually referred to as a macronutrient because it cannot be a large contributor to a healthy diet. Carbohydrate, protein, and fat are the "energy nutrients" because they provide the body with kilocalories. For example, they contain or carry vitamins, minerals, and other non-nutritive substances (e.g., dietary fiber, fluid, phytochemicals) that are critical for health.

Carbohydrates are compounds of carbon, oxygen, and hydrogen atoms. They are consumed either as **simple carbohydrates** or as **complex carbohydrates** (Table 4.4). The simple carbohydrates are also called sugars, which fall into the category of **monosaccharides**

Introduction to Nutrition

Table 4.4
Carbohydrates (sugars)

Simple

Monosaccharides	Disaccharides
Glucose	Sucrose
Fructose	Lactose
Galactose	Maltose

Complex

Starch (polysaccharides)	Fibers (viscous, incompletely fermented)

(single sugars) or **disaccharides** (double sugars). Regardless of the category into which they fall, all of these carbohydrates provide 4 kcal/g.

Simple carbohydrates contain naturally occurring sugars like those in fruit (fructose) and milk (lactose), and refined sugars (often sucrose or high-fructose corn syrup), such as table sugar, brown sugar, honey, and corn syrup. Since refined sugars provide little more than calories, excess consumption of foods high in refined sugars can cause health problems, particularly if sweetened, nutrient-poor foods replace more nutritious choices. The naturally occurring sugars in fruits and milk are found in combination with vitamins, minerals, proteins, and other non-nutritive but beneficial compounds (e.g., fiber and phytochemicals).

In contrast to the mono- and disaccharides, polysacchrides are complex carbohydrates, such as starch and dietary fiber, that contain longer chains of carbon atoms. Complex carbohydrates have different tastes, textures, and health effects than their simple, shorter-chain counterparts. Examples of complex carbohydrates are whole-grain breads and cereals, legumes (beans and peas), and vegetables. Similar to the naturally occurring simple carbohydrates, the com-

plex ones are good choices because they are packed with vitamins, minerals, some protein, and other non-nutritive but beneficial compounds.

Regardless of whether the carbohydrate eaten is in a simple or complex form, the processes of digestion, absorption, and metabolism turn all carbohydrates into **glucose,** the form of sugar in the blood and the main energy fuel for the body, brain, and central nervous system. Although muscle tissue can use fat as an energy source, the brain and central nervous system are dependent on glucose as their primary source of fuel. Glucose is one of the body's major energy sources and, after it is eaten, is stored as glycogen to be used later. The muscles contain some glycogen to meet their short-term energy needs while the liver stores up to approximately a 12-hour supply to meet the needs of the brain between meals or during an overnight fast (during sleep). Very active individuals must make sure they are getting enough carbohydrates to fuel their activities and to replenish depleted glycogen stores following exercise.

Many foods rich in carbohydrates actually contain a mix of simple and complex carbohydrates. There is some evidence that the body transforms this mix into blood glucose at slightly different rates. The speed of the relative rise in blood glucose is reflected in the **glycemic index**. The blood glucose response of foods eaten is compared to either the response to glucose or white bread (set at a reference standard of 100). Foods with higher glycemic index scores raise blood glucose more quickly than those with lower scores (Table 4.5).

It is this type of provocative research that has shown that people with diabetes can have food containing sugar—or any other kind of

Table 4.5
Glycemic Index Values of Sample High- and Low-index Foods

Sample High-glycemic Foods	Glycemic Index (food consumed alone)	Sample Low-glycemic Foods	Glycemic Index (food consumed alone)
Carrots	92	Bananas	53
Instant rice	91	Oranges	43
Corn flakes	84	Apples	36
Table sugar	65	Chocolate milk	34
Raisins	64	Yogurt	33
Potatoes	62	Nonfat milk	32
Orange juice	57	Whole milk	27
		Grapefruit	25

carbohydrates—just like anybody else. Research into the glycemic index provides evidence that foods cannot be classified into "good" or "bad" categories. It is important to remember that the glycemic index only applies when these foods are eaten alone; when they are eaten as part of a mixed meal, the values change in complex and unpredictable ways. Carrots eaten by themselves as a snack do not react the same way as those in a salad, on a sandwich, or cooked. The glycemic index is sometimes used by people with a poor understanding of nutrition to label foods inappropriately, such as "provokes a strong insulin response," "promotes fat storage," and "provokes high blood sugars." The science just does not give evidence to draw those kinds of conclusions.

Guiding participants to base their diet in complex carbohydrates and the naturally occurring simple carbohydrates can help them maximize their muscle glycogen stores, extend their endurance, and improve their athletic performance. However, even more importantly, it can help lower their risk for chronic diseases, such as cancer and heart disease, in part because of the **fiber, vitamins, minerals,** and **phytochemicals** they contain. The relationship between diet and disease is discussed later in this chapter, as is the definition and role of dietary fiber. See Table 4.6 for recommended daily carbohydrate intakes for several different calorie levels.

Protein

Proteins are large nitrogen-containing molecules made up of amino acids that play a variety of roles in the body. They make up the major part of the body's structural components like muscles, skin, tendons, organs, and bones. They also work in the form of enzymes to catalyze chemical reactions and they serve as neurotransmitters in the brain and are involved with thinking and emotions. Some hormones are made of protein and transmit messages throughout the body. Proteins help balance fluid and electrolytes in the body and help regulate acid–base balance. Also, they work as a veritable taxi service in the blood,

Table 4.6
Recommended Healthy Intakes/Day for Carbohydrate, Protein, and Fat for Several Calorie Levels

Energy Intake (kcal)	Carbohydrate	Protein	Fat
Goal % total kcal	45–65%	10–35%	20–35%
1,600	180–260 g/day	40–140 g/day	36–62 g/day
2,000	225–325 g/day	50–175 g/day	44–78 g/day
2,200	248–358 g/day	55–193 g/day	49–86 g/day
2,600	293–423 g/day	65–228 g/day	58–101 g/day
2,800	315–455 g/day	70–245 g/day	62–109 g/day

Macronutrients

serving as transport proteins for many nutrients, particularly fats. Proteins can provide energy as well (4 kcal/gram), but in light of all the other important functions they provide, it is best if carbohydrate and fat supply the majority of energy needs. In illness, severe injury, or poorly constructed diets (such as some fad diets), protein is sacrificed to meet energy demands instead of fulfilling its important biological roles. Protein is crucial in keeping the Krebs cycle functioning, which helps ensure that the body is able to use the energy contained in carbohydrates.

How do proteins accomplish this incredible variety of vital tasks? They do so by taking on a virtually infinite variety of shapes, most of them looking like long, twisted chains or balls of string. In fact, that is exactly what they are: Long chains of **amino acids** are the building blocks of proteins. There are approximately 20 amino acids, all but eight to 10 of which can be manufactured by the body if the basic metabolic parts are available. Those the body cannot make are called "essential amino acids" and must be provided in the diet. Complete proteins contain all of the essential amino acids and are found in animal products like seafood, poultry, dairy products, and red meats. Although grains and legumes do not contain all of the amino acids, they can be combined to provide complete protein sources. For example, serving black beans with rice, peanut butter on wheat bread, or tofu and stir-fried vegetables with brown rice will provide the complete array of essential amino acids.

In the 1970s, vegetarians were instructed to eat complementary proteins at every meal. Subsequent research has found that it is sufficient to consume a mixture of amino acids in the same day for adequate health. Agricultural research is also producing genetically modified grain products that contain complete proteins, although the primary beneficiaries of these products will be poor populations and those in developing countries.

Contrary to some beliefs, protein or amino-acid supplements are not necessary for either health or athletic performance. For most people living in industrialized societies, protein deficiency is not a health issue. Most individuals in these societies eat too much protein, rather than too little. Instead, excess protein intake is ultimately turned into fat and stored in the body.

Fat

Dietary fats, called **lipids,** are a group of organic compounds that are water-insoluble and include triglycerides, **cholesterol,** and **lecithin.** Triglycerides make up 95% of the fat people eat. This is also the major form of fat stored in the body's fat tissues, called adipose tissues. In the body, fat does more than store energy; it cushions vital organs, provides insulation, and is involved in basic functions, such as nerve conduction and tissue structure (e.g., brain tissue). As phospholipids, fats are present in the membranes surrounding every cell in the body. Fats are also important for the absorption and transport of **fat-soluble vitamins** and **essential fatty acids.**

Fat is the most efficient source of energy, since it contains 9 kcal/g. Even if 70 g sounds like a lot of fat (see Table 4.6), it is quite easy to consume when eating the typical American diet. Consider that a popular fast-food hamburger contains 35 g of fat and a "bloomin' onion" (a popular breaded and deep fried onion) contains nearly 120 g of fat.

Fats, or triglycerides, are organized into two groups: saturated and unsaturated (also referred to as fatty acids). Regardless of the type of fat, all fats contain 9 kcal/g. Like carbohydrates, fatty acids are made up of long chains of carbon molecules connected to hydrogen atoms. What determines whether a fat is saturated or unsaturated is how many carbons are bonded to each other (called a carbon–carbon double bond) and not just to hydrogen. **Saturated fats** have *no* double bonds, which makes them typically solid at room temperature. Examples include butter, lard, milk and meat fats, eggs, and tropical fats like coconut oil. Liquid oils that are turned into stick margarines or solid hydrogenated vegetable shortening undergo a process called **hydrogenation,** in which the carbon–carbon double bonds are destroyed and replaced with more hydrogen atoms. This process creates a new type of fat, the **trans fatty acid.** While trans fatty acids are not commonly found in unprocessed foods, they are found in high-fat baked goods, fried foods, and snacks, in addition to shortening and other partially hydrogenated oils and margarine. Now that food manufacturers in the U.S. are required to declare the trans-fat content on the food label, many are seeking alternatives to the use of trans fats in foods. The health implications of saturated fats are addressed later in this chapter.

Unsaturated fats, which have at least one carbon–carbon double bond, also fall into two categories: **polyunsaturated** and **monounsaturated.** The polyunsaturated fats have more than one double bond and are liquid at room temperature. Examples include corn, sunflower, and safflower oils. The monounsaturated fatty acids have only one double bond and are also liquid at room temperature. Examples of these include olive, sesame, canola, avocado, and nut oils. Most naturally occurring fats in foods are actually a mix of all three types of fat: saturated, monounsaturated, and polyunsaturated. The category is determined by the proportion of the fatty-acid types present. The health implications of these types of fats are addressed later in this chapter.

Cholesterol is not actually a fat, but rather a waxy, fat-like substance. People cannot derive calories from cholesterol because the body cannot break it down; it is absorbed relatively intact. Cholesterol is commonly found in foods of animal origin rich in saturated fats (primarily meat and milk fats). Cholesterol is also manufactured by the liver. For a food to contain cholesterol, it must come from an animal-based food, such as beef, pork, dairy, or poultry. Organ meats are particularly rich in cholesterol and saturated fat and, therefore, should be consumed only in moderation. Some foods, such as peanut butter made with hydrogenated fat, are rich in saturated fat but contain no cholesterol. It is recommended that people keep their average daily cholesterol intake to 300 mg or less.

Lecithin is a type of fat called a **phospholipid,** meaning that it has a water-soluble and a fat-soluble portion. It is manufactured by the body and does not contain calories. Although it is not needed as a supplement, it is sold in many health-food stores. The body can convert fatty acids to meet its needs for all fats except for **linoleic acid,** which is called an essential fatty acid. This fat is found in vegetable oils, nuts, seeds, wheat germ, and other foods that contain polyunsaturated fat. Supplements of essential fatty acids are not necessary because adequate amounts are supplied by even an extremely low-fat diet.

Micronutrients

The body needs more than just carbohydrate, protein, and fat to function; it needs the special chemicals it cannot manufacture on its own. These chemicals, among a multitude of other tasks, help the body create tissues, release energy, regulate metabolic processes, and make DNA. Unlike the macronutrients, these special chemicals are needed only in minute amounts and are found widely in the foods people eat. Most people know these special chemicals as vitamins and minerals.

Vitamins are organic (carbon-containing) compounds that the body cannot manufacture on its own and, therefore, must be consumed. If a vitamin is not supplied in the diet, a deficiency symptom occurs. For example, lack of vitamin C causes scurvy, a condition particularly prevalent among sailors before the nineteenth century. By definition, when the vitamin is returned to the diet the deficiency symptoms go away. If lack of a substance does not cause deficiency symptoms, it cannot be a vitamin. Vitamins provide no calories and therefore cannot be used as fuel. Some vitamins, such as the B-vitamins, help the body liberate the energy from foods, but they do not themselves provide energy.

The 13 vitamins identified fall into two groups: water soluble and fat soluble. The **water-soluble vitamins** include the B-vitamins and vitamin C. Most water-soluble vitamins need to be supplied on a daily basis because the body has a limited ability to store them and excretes excesses in the urine daily. Vitamins A, D, E, and K are the **fat-soluble vitamins.** Unlike their water-soluble counterparts, most fat-soluble vitamins are stored in the body, particularly in the liver and body-fat tissues. It is challenging to meet all of the nutrient needs when eating fewer than 1,600 kcal/day. Group fitness instructors should be aware that participants who are restricting their calorie intake might be depriving themselves of essential nutrition as well. They will need to make careful decisions about the foods they eat to protect their health. This chapter will soon address for whom supplements are appropriate.

Like vitamins, the minerals necessary for health are needed in tiny amounts. Minerals are inorganic compounds that enter the food chain as plants absorb them from soil and water. Humans eat either the plants or the animals that consumed the plants, and thus get minerals in their diets. There are several minerals that have been recognized as essential. However, excess intake of minerals can be dangerous. Since such small amounts are required for health, it is important to keep mineral intake well-balanced. Many minerals compete for absorption in the gut, such as iron, copper, and zinc. Supplementing with large doses of iron can cause a deficiency in copper or zinc, even if dietary intake meets the **recommended dietary allowances (RDA).** Similarly, the proper balance between minerals enhances their use. For example, magnesium and zinc affect how **calcium** is absorbed and used in the body.

Nutrient recommendations, called Dietary Reference Intakes, or DRIs, are set by a national panel of scientists for the Food and Nutrition Board of the Institute of Medicine, a subgroup of the National Academy of Sciences. DRIs have been established for energy, the macronutrients, fiber, vitamins, minerals, electrolytes, and water. While nutritional needs vary somewhat from person to person, the RDAs are set to meet the needs of 98% of the population.

When not enough scientific information was available to establish an RDA, the DRI panel set an Adequate Intake (AI) level for that particular nutrient. The needs of most people will be met adequately if they make good food choices. For those individuals who wish to "hedge their nutritional bet," a general purpose multivitamin/mineral supplement should be sufficient. Under no circumstances should an instructor ever suggest a participant take a supplement with more than 100 to 150% of the RDA. While most nutrients are safe even in large doses, some, particularly the minerals and certain fat-soluble vitamins, can have toxic side effects at just a few times the RDA level.

When vitamins and minerals are obtained through foods, it is difficult to upset the proportional balances that nature intended. However, when an individual starts taking large doses (called **megadoses**) of the micronutrients, he or she risks imbalances that could affect long-term health outcomes, particularly for diseases such as osteoporosis (via an upset in calcium absorption or use) or blood sugar control (via aberrations in zinc or chromium absorption and use). Some minerals (and some vitamins) are toxic in large amounts, so megadoses should be avoided. Some minerals are referred to as major minerals, which indicates their relative quantity, not their importance. The major minerals include calcium and phosphorus (used in bones and teeth), sodium, potassium, chloride (found in body fluids), sulfur, and magnesium.

The **trace minerals,** found in much smaller quantities, include iron, zinc, copper, manganese, iodine, and selenium, among many others. Despite the fact that the entire human body has less than 5 g in total of each of these minerals, they are far more likely to be consumed in nutritional supplements. Tables 4.7 and 4.8 provide an overview of these important vitamins and minerals: their function, how much is needed each day, and what foods contain these nutrients. Use these tables as references to steer participants to healthy food choices and away from pills.

Other Important Dietary Components

There is more to the story of good nutrition than just macro- and micronutrients. There are substances important to health that are not nutritive at all. Non-nutritive substances include water, fiber, and phytochemicals.

Fluid and Hydration

Fitness professionals know the value of adequate **hydration.** Water is the most commonly overlooked endurance aid. It is literally the fluid in which all life processes occur in every cell. The body uses fluids to help regulate body temperature via sweat (to dissipate heat); to maintain blood pressure, thus influencing how substances move between the bloodstream and the body cells; to deliver nutrients to cells; and to carry off waste products. A human can survive without water for only a few days. Sudden **dehydration** from heat or excessive exercise can be life-threatening.

Thirst guides most individual's water intake. Changes in the mouth, hypothalamus, and nerves help signal the need for increased fluid intake. Although thirst may drive a person to seek water, it lags behind the body's fluid needs. A fluid deficiency that develops quickly, such as during strenuous exercise, may not alert the body's fluid sensors in time to prevent dehydration. The adult body must excrete a minimum of about 500 mL (almost 17 oz) of urine per day to carry away the waste products generated by the day's metabolic activities.

Table 4.7
Vitamin Facts

Vitamin	RDA/AI*		Best Sources	Functions
	Men†	Women†		
A (carotene)	**900 µg**	**700 µg**	Yellow or orange fruits and vegetables, green leafy vegetables, fortified oatmeal, liver, dairy products	Formation and maintenance of skin, hair, and mucous membranes; helps people see in dim light; bone and tooth growth
B1 (thiamine)	**1.2 mg**	**1.1 mg**	Fortified cereals and oatmeals, meats, rice and pasta, whole grains, liver	Helps the body release energy from carbohydrates during metabolism; growth and muscle tone
B2 (riboflavin)	**1.3 mg**	**1.1 mg**	Whole grains, green leafy vegetables, organ meats, milk, eggs	Helps the body release energy from protein, fat, and carbohydrates during metabolism
B6 (pyridoxine)	**1.3 mg**	**1.3 mg**	Fish, poultry, lean meats, bananas, prunes, dried beans, whole grains, avocados	Helps build body tissue and aids in metabolism of protein
B12 (cobalamin)	**2.4 µg**	**2.4 µg**	Meats, milk products, seafood	Aids cell development, functioning of the nervous system, and the metabolism of protein and fat
Biotin	30 µg	30 µg	Cereal/grain products, yeast, legumes, liver	Involved in metabolism of protein, fats, and carbohydrates
Choline	550 mg	425 mg	Milk, liver, eggs, peanuts	A precursor of acetylcholine; essential for liver function
Folate (folacin, folic acid)	**400 µg**	**400 µg‡**	Green leafy vegetables, organ meats, dried peas, beans, lentils	Aids in genetic material development; involved in red blood cell production
Niacin	**16 mg**	**14 mg**	Meat, poultry, fish, enriched cereals, peanuts, potatoes, dairy products, eggs	Involved in carbohydrate, protein, and fat metabolism
Pantothenic Acid	5 mg	5 mg	Lean meats, whole grains, legumes, vegetables, fruits	Helps release energy from fats and carbohydrates
C (ascorbic acid)	**90 mg**	**75 mg**	Citrus fruits, berries, and vegetables— especially peppers	Essential for structure of bones, cartilage, muscle, and blood vessels; helps maintain capillaries and gums and aids in absorption of iron
D	5 µg	5 µg	Fortified milk, sunlight, fish, eggs, butter, fortified margarine	Aids in bone and tooth formation; helps maintain heart action and nervous system
E	**15 mg**	**15 mg**	Fortified and multigrain cereals, nuts, wheat germ, vegetable oils, green leafy vegetables	Protects blood cells, body tissue, and essential fatty acids from harmful destruction in the body
K	120 µg	90 µg	Green leafy vegetables, fruit, dairy, and grain products	Essential for blood-clotting functions

* Recommended Dietary Allowances are presented in bold type; Adequate Intakes are presented in non-bolded type.

† RDAs and AIs given are for men aged 31–50 and nonpregnant, nonbreastfeeding women aged 31–50; mg = milligrams; µg = micrograms

‡ This is the amount women of childbearing age should obtain from supplements or fortified foods.

Reprinted with permission from *Dietary Reference Intakes* (various volumes). Copyright 1997, 1998, 2000, 2001 by the National Academy of Sciences. Courtesy of the National Academies Press, Washington, D.C.

Table 4.8
Mineral Facts

Mineral	RDA/AI*		Best Sources	Functions
	Men†	Women†		
Calcium	1,000 mg	1,000 mg	Milk and milk products	Strong bones, teeth, muscle tissue; regulates heart beat, muscle action, and nerve function; blood clotting
Chromium	35 μg	25 μg	Corn oil, clams, whole-grain cereals, brewer's yeast	Glucose metabolism (energy); increases effectiveness of insulin
Copper	**900 μg**	**900 μg**	Oysters, nuts, organ meats, legumes	Formation of red blood cells; bone growth and health; works with vitamin C to form elastin
Fluoride	4 mg	3 mg	Fluorinated water, teas, marine fish	Stimulates bone formation; inhibits or even reverses dental caries
Iodine	**150 μg**	**150 μg**	Seafood, iodized salt	Component of hormone thyroxine, which controls metabolism
Iron	**8 mg**	**18 mg**	Meats, especially organ meats, legumes	Hemoglobin formation; improves blood quality; increases resistance to stress and disease
Magnesium	**420 mg**	**320 mg**	Nuts, green vegetables, whole grains	Acid/alkaline balance; important in metabolism of carbohydrates, minerals, and sugar (glucose)
Manganese	2.3 mg	1.8 mg	Nuts, whole grains, vegetables, fruits	Enzyme activation; carbohydrate and fat production; sex hormone production; skeletal development
Molybdenum	**45 μg**	**45 μg**	Legumes, grain products, nuts	Functions as a cofactor for a limited number of enzymes in humans
Phosphorus	**700 mg**	**700 mg**	Fish, meat, poultry, eggs, grains	Bone development; important in protein, fat, and carbohydrate utilization
Potassium	4700 mg	4700 mg	Lean meat, vegetables, fruits	Fluid balance; controls activity of heart muscle, nervous system, and kidneys
Selenium	**55 μg**	**55 μg**	Seafood, organ meats, lean meats, grains	Protects body tissues against oxidative damage from radiation, pollution, and normal metabolic processing
Zinc	**11 mg**	**8 mg**	Lean meats, liver, eggs, seafood, whole grains	Involved in digestion and metabolism; important in development of reproductive system; aids in healing

*Recommended Dietary Allowances are presented in bold type; Adequate Intakes are presented in non-bolded type.

† RDAs and AIs given are for men aged 31–50 and nonpregnant, nonbreastfeeding women aged 31–50; mg = milligrams; μg = micrograms

Reprinted with permission from *Dietary Reference Intakes* (various volumes). Copyright 1997, 1998, 2000, 2001 by the National Academy of Sciences. Courtesy of the National Academies Press, Washington, D.C.

Introduction to Nutrition

Under normal conditions, the kidneys can adjust to a high fluid intake to keep a person in a normal fluid balance. How much fluid does a person need in a day? Most people have probably heard the recommendation to consume eight 8-oz glasses of water, but the true amount varies with age, gender, activity, and environment.

Not all fluid intake must be in the form of water; fluid comes from other beverages as well as foods. The average adult consumes 75–80% of fluid via beverages and approximately 20–25% via foods. Although fluid needs are best met by water, particularly in an exercising adult, low-fat milk and juice are excellent choices to round out the day's liquid intake, since they contain the minerals involved in fluid balance: potassium, sodium, chloride, and, to some extent, calcium. Poor choices for rehydration include alcohol- and caffeine-containing beverages (sodas, coffees, and teas), since both of these substances act as diuretics.

The Adequate Intake for water from beverages and foods is 3.7 L/day for adult males and 2.7 L/day for adult females, although physically active individuals will need more and should take care to follow the recommendations of the National Athletic Trainers' Association (Table 4.9). It should be noted that while the recommendations provided in Table 4.9 provide good general guidelines, the best practice is to replace fluids lost in sweat.

Beverage choice for proper hydration during exercise depends on the duration of the activity. For exercise that lasts less than one hour, water is perfectly acceptable. However, for exercise of one hour or more, a sports drink containing 4 to 8% carbohydrate (4 to 8 g per 100 mL) and sodium is the best choice.

Dehydration is a serious risk to health and performance, but overhydration, though rare, is also a real risk. Overconsuming water can result in **hyponatremia** (low blood sodium levels), which can occur in otherwise healthy individuals. Hyponatremia can lead to convulsions, coma, and even death. It is most common in ultra-distance events such as a marathon. Females, especially slower athletes, are more prone to this condition, as they tend to have more time to overconsume beverages during the event.

Fiber

For many years, specific types of fiber were classified as either soluble or insoluble, depending on their functions. Soluble fibers, such as the type found in oat bran, are known to reduce blood cholesterol levels and help normalize blood sugar levels. On the other hand, insoluble fibers, such as the type found in wheat bran, are known to promote bowel regularity. Many commonly used plant sources of fiber contain both soluble and insoluble fibers. For example, psyllium husks contain a mixture of soluble and insoluble fibers.

Despite the widespread use of the terms "soluble" and "insoluble" to describe the health benefits of **dietary fiber,** many medical and nutrition experts contend that these terms do not adequately describe the physiological effects of the many different types of fiber. These experts advocate the use of the terms "viscous" and "incompletely fermented" in place of soluble and insoluble to describe the functions and associated health benefits of dietary fiber.

Viscous fibers help lower serum cholesterol by reducing the absorption of dietary

Table 4.9
Fluid-intake Recommendations During Exercise

2 hours prior to exercise, drink 500–600 mL (17–20 oz)
Every 10–20 minutes during exercise, drink 200–300 mL (7–10 oz)
Following exercise, drink 450–675 mL for every 0.5 kg body weight lost (or 16–24 oz for every pound)

Adapted with permission from Casa, D.J. et al. (2000). National Athletic Trainers'
Association:
Position statement: Fluid replacement for athletes. *Journal of Athletic Training,* 35, 212–224

cholesterol. They also help normalize blood glucose levels by slowing the rate at which food leaves the stomach to delay the absorption of glucose following a meal and by improving insulin sensitivity. As a result, viscous fibers play a potentially important role in the prevention and treatment of type 2 diabetes. In addition to their beneficial effects on glycemic control, viscous fibers promote a sense of satiety, or fullness, following a meal, which may help to prevent overeating and subsequent weight gain.

Incompletely fermented fibers, in contrast to viscous fibers, do not tend to bind with water, fluids, or cholesterol. These fibers, found in wheat bran, whole-grain breads and cereals, and vegetables, are called cellulose, hemicellulose, and lignins. They are believed to serve the function of "scraping" the sides of the bowel, thus helping to remove old gut-tissue cells. In addition, a major role of incompletely fermented fibers is to help maintain bowel regularity by increasing the bulk of the feces and decreasing the transit time of fecal matter through the intestines. Bowel regularity is associated with a decreased risk for colon cancer and hemorrhoids (when the hemorrhoids are related to straining and constipation).

The average American does not eat enough dietary fiber. The DRIs recommend that men and women (under age 50) consume 38 grams and 25 grams, respectively, of total fiber. Table 4.10 provides a list of suggestions to use with participants to help them include good sources of dietary fiber. Although fiber supplements are available, it is best to consume fiber with foods and with plenty of fluids. If a participant requests advice for problems with constipation that do not respond to increased dietary fiber and fluid intake, refer the participant to his or her physician.

Table 4.10
Tips for Increasing Dietary Fiber

- Increase intake of whole-grain breads and cereals
- Choose foods with as little processing as possible (whole-wheat breads and flours, brown rice)
- Include several servings of fresh fruits and vegetables daily
- Include legumes (beans and peas) in the diet on a regular basis
- Consume moderate amounts of meat

Estimating Fiber Intake

Fresh, whole, and dried fruits: ~ 2 g/serving (fruit juice contains very little fiber)
Whole-grain breads: ~ 2 g/slice
Whole-grain cereals: 3–12 g/serving
Vegetables: ~1–4 g/serving

Phytochemicals

Most people have probably been told that fruits and vegetables are good for them. Instructors should know (and tell their participants) that whole-grain breads and cereals, fruits, and vegetables contain more than just vitamins, minerals, and fiber. Research has uncovered exciting news about those garden-fresh foods mothers have been pushing for centuries. Vitamins and minerals are extremely important to overall health, but these foods also contain other non-nutritive substances that seem to play amazing roles in protecting one's health. These special compounds are called phytochemicals, which are the biologically active compounds in plants that give them their color, flavor, and natural disease resistance. Phytochemicals offer many health benefits. Some are potent cancer-fighters, blocking one or more of the steps in the process that leads to cancer. Others help fight the process of heart disease by working as **antioxidants.** The chemistry of phytochemicals makes the biochemistry of vitamins and minerals look easy; there are just a few vitamins and minerals, but there are literally thousands and thousands of phytochemicals.

125

Introduction to Nutrition

Supplements of these compounds are available in health-food stores, but they are not recommended. While most phytochemicals protect health, some *encourage* the cancer process. Keeping dietary intake in a natural balance is the best way to reap the benefits of phytochemicals without upsetting the natural balance between them. While it is hard to overconsume phytochemicals from foods, it is easy to get too much from a pill. The research is not yet sufficient to be sure about safety and efficacy. Instead, encourage participants to fill their shopping baskets with phytochemical-packed fruits, vegetables, and whole grains every time they shop. See Table 4.11 for some examples of phytochemical-rich foods.

Table 4.11
Phytochemicals from Food

Food	Phytochemical	Action
Broccoli	Sulforaphane	Helps remove carcinogens from cells
Citrus fruits and berries	B10, flavonoids	Blocks the cancer-promotion process; may boost immune-system function
Soybeans	Genistein, daidzein	Works against tumors by preventing the formation of capillaries needed to nourish them
Cruciferous vegetables (broccoli, cabbage, brussels sprouts, and cauliflower)	Indoles	Increase immunity and make it easier for the body to excrete toxins
Tomatoes	Lycopene (Carotenoid antioxidant)	May fight prostate and lung cancer by reducing cancer-cell proliferation; may prevent or slow atherosclerotic plaque development
Cherries, citrus fruits, strawberries, blueberries	Monoterpenes (polyphenols), catechins, ellagic acid (powerful antioxidant in strawberries)	May inhibit growth of early cancers
Greens (turnip, collard, mustard, kale, spinach)	Lutein and zeaxanthin (Carotenoid antioxidants)	Protect cells from free radical damage
Orange fruits and vegetables (carrots, sweet potatoes, pumpkin, squash, cantaloupe)	Beta-carotene (antioxidant)	Protects cells from free radical damage in vitro
Garlic, onions, leeks, chives	Allium, ajoene, and allicin (thioallyls)	Slows or prevents growth of tumor cells; prevents the formation of blood clots

Putting Together a Healthy Diet

With a basic understanding of macro- and micronutrients, how does an instructor guide participants in making healthy food choices? The **MyPyramid Food Guidance System** and the Dietary Guidelines for Americans 2005 are two tools that can help the instructor translate all of this complex nutrition information into simple-to-follow, healthy eating guidelines (Figure 4.1, Tables 4.1, 4.6, and 4.12).

From the MyPyramid.gov Web site, a person can print out recommended eating plans for many different caloric levels. The new pyramid graphic is intended to represent the variety, moderation, and proportions of foods that make up a healthy diet, as represented by the width of the colored bands. The majority of calorie and food intake should come from whole-grain breads and cereals, fruits, vegetables, and low-fat dairy products. The importance of daily physical activity is explicitly emphasized in the MyPyramid graphic, as is the importance of making small steps on the path to permanent behavior change.

As part of the 2005 Dietary Guidelines, the United States Department of Agriculture and the United States Department of Health and Human Services have developed healthy eating guidelines for calorie-intake levels starting at 1,600 kcal/day. This information is summarized in Table 4.12.

When individuals do not consume adequate servings from a food group, or miss one entirely, they are at risk of getting inadequate nutrients as well. Over time, this can have devastating consequences on a person's health. Table 4.13 illustrates the nutritional components at risk when daily patterns do not meet the recommended guidelines. The next section discusses the health implications of eating an unbalanced diet.

There are no perfect teaching tools, and the MyPyramid Food Guidance System is no exception. It may not provide enough information for people who already know a lot about nutrition, and everyone must still be aware of fats. For example, ice cream and milk appear in the same food group, as do french fries and broccoli. Obviously, ice cream and milk are not nutritionally equivalent. And no matter how much people might wish it were so, french fries are just not as good for the body as broccoli. Thus, fat-gram counting is a good tool for helping people make wise choices (see Table 4.6 for information on reasonable fat-gram intakes). There are many fat-gram guides available to help participants track their fat intake. Be careful, however. Just as a person can get too much of a good thing, he or she can get too little of a "bad" thing as well. In general, most adults should have a fat intake of 20 to 35% of total calories. Sixty grams is a reasonable intake for many adults. Being too restrictive on fat intake can lead to dissatisfaction with the diet, feelings of hunger, and "throwing in the towel" on making dietary changes. Moderation is the key, even when it comes to limiting fat.

Diet and Disease

Of course, eating well on a day-to-day basis will help people feel their best, have energy, and think clearly. However, eating well on a month-to-month and year-to-year basis can also save or prolong a person's life. There is a strong relationship between diet and disease. Four of the 10 leading causes of death are diet-related, which means that they are preventable to a large extent. Fitness professionals have the opportunity to affect peoples' health in a pro-

Table 4.12
Sample Diets for a Day at Three Calorie Levels

	Daily Amounts from Food Group		
	1,600 kcal	2,200 kcal	2,800 kcal
Bread/grains*	5 oz-eq	7 oz-eq	10 oz-eq
Vegetables	2 c (4 srv)	3 c (6 srv)	3.5 c (7 srv)
Fruits	1.5 c (3 srv)	2 c (4 srv)	2.5 c (5 srv)
Milk and dairy	3 c	3 c	3 c
Lean meat and beans	5 oz-eq	6 oz-eq	7 oz-eq
Oils	22 g	29 g	36 g
Discretionary calories†	132	290	426

Source: *Dietary Guidelines for Americans 2005*. U.S. Department of Agriculture/U.S. Department of Health and Human Services.
Note: srv = serving; c = cup; oz-eq = ounce-equivalent
* 50% of grains should be whole grains
† Discretionary calories are the additional calories a person can have only if he or she has chosen foods with no added sugar or fats to meet nutrient needs

found way by the information they give and the examples they set.

The link between diet and disease is a complex medical relationship. The principles instructors can employ via the MyPyramid Food Guidance System, the Dietary Guidelines, and awareness of fat intake (such as using fat-gram counting) can help lower the risks for many chronic diseases. Of all the nutrients, fat is most related to chronic disease.

Cardiovascular Disease

Cardiovascular disease, more commonly known as heart disease or CVD, is the most common killer of adults in the United States. The types and quantity of foods included in the diet have a strong influence on the risk of developing CVD. The nutrient of most concern

Table 4.13
Daily Intake Patterns With Increased Nutritional Risk

Food Group	Daily Intake	Deficiency
Dairy	<3 servings	Calcium
Protein	<5 oz-eq	Protein and iron
Vegetables	<4 servings	Vitamins, minerals, fat
Fruit	<4 servings	Energy, minerals, fiber, vitamins
Bread & whole grains	<5 oz-eq	Energy, minerals, fiber, vitamins

Note: oz-eq = ounce-equivalent

Introduction to Nutrition

is, of course, fat. A high total dietary-fat intake is associated with increased rates of CVD in all ages. One of the early and major biological indicators of CVD is elevated blood cholesterol, called "serum cholesterol." When total serum cholesterol is above 200 mg/dL, the risks of developing CVD are increased. Measuring serum cholesterol is usually referred to as measuring **"serum lipids."** Lipids are fats in the blood—and there is more than just cholesterol to think about. **Low-density lipoprotein, or LDL, cholesterol** is the type known as "bad" cholesterol. It is very much involved in the artery-blocking process. Risk of heart disease is elevated when LDL cholesterol is >100 mg/dL. **High-density lipoprotein, or HDL, cholesterol** is often called "good" cholesterol because it helps move body lipids from places of storage to places of use. Athletes often have very high HDL levels because they have trained their bodies to be efficient fat-burning machines and to produce more HDL cholesterol. It is desirable for HDL levels to be >40 mg/dL. Triglycerides are another type of blood fat, and they are often elevated right after eating. It is desirable for triglyceride levels to be <150 mg/dL after an overnight fast.

Where do all of these types of cholesterol come from? Cholesterol is made in the livers of animals. For the most part, the cholesterol in the blood is the cholesterol that the body manufactured, not the cholesterol in what a person may have eaten. Although there is some relationship between eating a high-cholesterol diet and having high serum cholesterol, the much stronger relationship is with saturated fat. Saturated fat is solid at room temperature, except for some tropical oils, and is found in animal and plant foods. Saturated fat biochemically signals the liver to increase its cholesterol production. In individuals with a strong genetic predisposition to

heart disease, this effect may be particularly potent. Therefore, for all individuals, it is recommended that saturated fat be kept to less than 10% of total caloric intake.

Some saturated fats are made from plant sources, such as stick margarine or solid shortening. These fats, used in food preparation or at the table, are made by blowing hydrogen gas through the liquid vegetable oil. During this process, a type of fat known as trans fatty acid is created. Some research indicates that trans fatty acids may provoke heart disease even more than saturated fats of animal origin.

Since tracking saturated fat grams in addition to total fat grams can be too confusing for many individuals, instructors can safely recommend the tips listed in Table 4.14 for lowering both total and saturated-fat intake.

Table 4.14
Tips for Lowering Both Total and Saturated-fat Intake

- Read food labels to track total fat-gram intake, keeping intake within reasonable limits.

- Choose low-fat (1% or less) dairy products.

- If you choose margarine, choose one with "liquid vegetable oil" as the first ingredient; try jam or jelly on breads instead of butter or margarine.

- In cooking, use moderate amounts of canola or olive oils. You can usually cut about half the fat out of recipes without changing their quality.

- Use cooking methods that do not use fat (bake, broil, steam, roast, poach) or use very little fat (stir fry).

- Eat meats in moderation, choosing the leanest selections; trim all visible fat and remove any skin.

- Keep protein portions to about 6 oz/day (the size of two decks of cards).

- Choose red meats once or twice a week at most; choose seafoods or poultry for the majority of your meals with meat.

- Limit egg yolks to fewer than three per week.

- Consume several meatless meals per week for lunches and dinners.

- Avoid organ meats and processed-meat products, such as bacon, sausage, hot dogs, etc., or choose the nonfat, very-low-fat, or meatless alternatives.

The unsaturated fats consist of polyunsaturated and monounsaturated fats. Polyunsaturated fats can help lower LDL cholesterol, but the monounsaturated fats have little to no independent effect. Why then are monounsaturated fats touted as being so healthful? Because while the polyunsaturated fats can help lower cholesterol, they lower all cholesterol: HDL and LDL. Higher HDL levels are linked with lower CVD risk. Therefore, protecting the HDL level is important. Some research shows that monounsaturated fats help raise HDL cholesterol, thus improving lipid profiles and lowering CVD risk. Overall, total fat should be kept between 20 and 35% of total caloric intake, with <10% coming from saturated fats.

There is one more type of fat worth mentioning: **omega-3 fatty acids.** These are the fats found in cold-water fish, including salmon, mackerel, menhaden, sardines, herring, and tuna. Research has shown that diets rich in these marine oils can lower blood cholesterol. Further, these oils can help prevent blood clots (the instigators of heart attacks and strokes) and may also lower high blood pressure. Some research has shown that consumption of cold-water fish just once a week cut rates of heart disease by 50%. Supplements have not been shown to have these protective benefits and can have some side effects. Therefore, while it is not advisable to take these oils as a supplement, it is advisable to consume deep-sea cold-water fish regularly.

Antioxidants protect membranes, lipid-rich organelles, and **lipoproteins,** like HDL, from being attacked by destructive agents known as free radicals. Vitamins A, C, and E, selenium, and omega-3 fatty acids all function as antioxidants in the body. They are interdependent and perform complementary functions, which in part explains why supplements seem to be less effective in preventing heart disease than eating foods rich in these nutrients.

Elevated **homocysteine** is now being recognized as a risk factor for heart disease, much in the same way as cholesterol. Although high homocysteine levels are in part due to genetics, diets poor in folate and vitamins B6 and B12 can also play a contributing role. Use the information in Tables 4.7 and 4.8 to help guide participants to healthy food selections.

Obesity

Diets high in fat can also lead to obesity, which is a complex and poorly understood disease that has several contributing factors. Certainly diet is one contributing factor, but so are physical inactivity and genetic predisposition, among others. One pound (0.45 kg) of excess body fat stores about 3,500 kcal of energy. To lose this fat, the stored energy must be burned. This is called creating an **energy deficit.** To lose 2 pounds (0.9 kg) per week, a person must burn 1,000 more calories per day more than he or she takes in. To lose 1 pound (0.45 kg) per week, a 500-kcal deficit must be created each day (500 kcal/day x 7 days = 3,500 kcal).

The rate of weight loss should average no more than 2 pounds per week (0.9 kg/week) after the first week (a greater amount of fluid is lost initially, which accounts for larger weight losses typically seen in the first week of a weight-loss attempt). Losing weight at a faster rate can be harmful to some individuals and it has not been shown to be associated with successful long-term weight loss.

Small changes in lifestyle that are sustainable are more likely to result in the permanent

Introduction to Nutrition

changes participants are seeking. Therefore, discourage participants from engaging in starvation or low-calorie diets when they attempt to lose weight. Instead, encourage a 500-kcal deficit from the energy intake needed to maintain body weight—half created by decreasing food intake and half created by increasing physical activity. For most people, cutting out 250 to 300 kcal of food is easy; almost everyone has some higher-fat, less-nutritious food choices they could substitute with fruits, vegetables, and whole grains. Similarly, for most people who need to lose weight, there are opportunities for increasing energy output, even without planned exercise. Planned or structured exercise sessions can make obese individuals uncomfortable or nervous due to physical discomfort on exertion, shortness of breath, joint pain, or other somatic complaints. Physical activity can be increased by simple walking, parking the car farther away, taking the stairs instead of the elevator, and limiting television watching. All obese individuals should be cleared by their physician before starting a vigorous exercise program.

In general, most obese or overweight individuals do not need severe caloric restriction. Many will be able to improve their health dramatically by following the principles of a healthy lifestyle, which apply to everyone. Overweight or obese individuals are no different from healthy individuals, in that they should consume only 20 to 35% of their total calories as fat, choose a wide variety of fruits, vegetables, and whole grains, consume protein foods in moderation [~6 oz/day (170 g/day)], and include low-fat dairy products. Weight loss is not easy, however, as the body seems to store energy more easily than it mobilizes it from storage. But with patience, persistence, and an eye toward overall health improvements

(not just weight on a scale), the overweight or obese individual has great power to improve his or her health.

Hypertension

One disease common in obese people and older adults is **hypertension,** or high blood pressure. Hypertension can damage the eyes, kidneys, liver, and the nervous system, and increases the risk for heart attacks and strokes. It is particularly common in people of African-American descent and is more prevalent in African-American women than men. Although genetic predisposition plays a big role in whether someone has hypertension, so do many lifestyle factors: obesity, high-sodium diets, alcohol consumption, and smoking. It is estimated that with weight loss, 80% of people with hypertension will have lower blood pressure. The Dietary Approaches to Stop Hypertension (DASH) trial showed that diet can lower blood pressure even without weight loss. Diets low in total and saturated fat and rich in fruits, vegetables, and low-fat dairy products had as strong an effect on blood pressure as some drugs (Appel et al., 1997; www.nhlbi.nih.gov; www.DashforHealth.com). Diets like these are rich in calcium, potassium, and magnesium, and when cold-water fish is chosen as a protein source, they are rich in omega-3 fatty acids as well.

A high intake of sodium in the diet can aggravate blood pressure in about 40% of hypertensive individuals. Sodium is most commonly found in table salt and in many processed foods, canned soups, cured meats, and cheeses. Although not all individuals are sodium sensitive, advise participants to avoid adding salt at the table or during cooking and to limit the number of highly processed foods they choose. Some hypertensive individuals are sensitive to alcohol as well. They can greatly reduce their blood pressure by limiting or eliminating alcohol. Caffeine has been found in some studies to raise blood pressure mildly throughout the day.

By far the most effective way to lower blood pressure in overweight or obese individuals is through weight loss. For many individuals, achieving and maintaining a healthy body weight can mean being able to discontinue medications. Hypertension should never be ignored; it should be managed by the participant working with his or her physician, using strategies like healthy nutrition, exercise, smoking cessation, and medications as needed.

Diabetes

As body weight increases, **diabetes** may also develop, particularly in individuals with abdominal or upper-body obesity. Remember that all carbohydrates eaten are transformed into blood sugar, called glucose. In diabetes, the body cannot control the blood glucose level, which can have serious short- and long-term consequences, including impaired vision, numbness in the extremities, nonhealing ulcers and wounds, heart disease, and death.

Diabetes is a very serious condition if left untreated and half of all individuals with diabetes do not know they even have the disease because they have never been tested. Most of these individuals suffer from the obesity-related condition called type 2 diabetes. Type 1 diabetes usually strikes younger individuals and is not related to being overweight. Type 1 diabetes is caused by the nonfunctioning of the insulin-producing beta cells in the pancreas. Type 2 diabetes is the most common form of diabetes, resulting from an inability of the body's cells to properly use insulin produced by the pancreas. Helping participants to achieve and maintain a healthy body weight can help prevent them from developing type 2 diabetes.

A commitment to exercise and a healthy eating plan is vital to managing diabetes once an individual has been diagnosed. The 2005 dietary guidelines are appropriate for most individuals with diabetes. However, these people should be monitored by their physician and a registered dietitian (R.D.) or certified diabetes educator (C.D.E.).

Cancer

Diet is one of the many factors that influence the development of **cancer.** Cigarette smoking is one of the strongest promoters of lung and oral cancers. Diet is more closely related to cancers of the esophagus, stomach, colon, rectum, breast, lung, liver, pancreas, endometrium, ovaries, bladder, and prostate. Although not all of these associations are clearly understood and some of the data are still debated, experts do agree that the way a person eats affects the risk of developing cancer. In countries where the typical diet is similar to accepted dietary recommendations, the incidence of cancer is about half of that in the U.S. (Woteki & Thomas, 1992). The components of food that are particularly important are fats, folic acid, vitamins A, C, and E, selenium, zinc, fiber, and the phytochemicals discussed previously. Fruits, vegetables, and whole grains are low in fats and rich in these food components.

Some foods can raise the risk of developing cancer. For example, salt-cured, smoked, and nitrate- or nitrite-containing foods should be avoided or consumed only in limited amounts. Foods preserved with **nitrates** and **nitrites,** such as lunch meats, hams, and hot dogs, can increase the risk for stomach cancers because they can be converted to **nitrosamines,** which are carcinogenic. Charbroiling or grilling foods generates a broad spectrum of compounds that increase cancer risk, such as **polycyclic aromatic hydrocarbons** and **heterocyclic**

Introduction to Nutrition

amines. Enzymes in the liver (called Phase I enzymes) activate these compounds, which form **DNA adducts** (i.e., attach themselves to DNA) and may cause mutations. Although charbroiling adds attractive flavors, it is recommended that these foods be consumed in moderation. Some of the phytochemicals in fruits and vegetables enhance the liver's Phase II enzymes, which help the body deactivate polycyclic aromatic hydrocarbons and heterocyclic amines. Alcohol intake has also been associated with increased risk for cancers of the mouth, esophagus, stomach, liver, and breast.

Some food components are often blamed for increasing cancer risk, but the data do not support those assertions. Artificial sweeteners are safe when consumed in moderate amounts. Food additives other than nitrates and nitrites are generally regarded as safe because no studies have shown any added risk of cancer. Irradiation of foods kills harmful organisms and increases the shelf life of foods. It does not increase cancer risk. While pesticides and herbicides are toxic in high doses, there is no current evidence linking them to an increase in cancer rates. However, it is good advice to thoroughly wash all produce before consuming it to remove dirt and any pesticide residue. While organic foods may be a personal preference, they are not thought to reduce the risk for cancer to any greater extent than consuming non-organic fruits and vegetables.

Physical inactivity may play a role in cancer development as well. Statistically, sedentary women are three times more likely to develop breast cancers than active women (McArdle, 1987). The risk of developing colon cancers in men may also decrease as physical activity increases. More scientific work needs to be done before a direct link between physical activity and cancer prevention can be made;

it may be that people who exercise regularly are more likely to have better overall health habits, thus lowering risk. Regardless, regular exercise is fundamental to achieving optimal health.

Osteoporosis

Osteoporosis is yet another important chronic disease related to nutrition and exercise. It affects 55% of people 50 years of age and older in the U.S. alone, most of them women. In osteoporosis, the bones become soft and later brittle, making them very prone to breaking at the spine, wrist, and hip area, sometimes even spontaneously (without a causative event or accident). Once osteoporosis has set in, it is almost too late to make significant improvements in bone mass, although research is advancing in this area.

Peak bone mass is achieved by about age 25. It is important to optimize the amounts of hard mineral deposited into bone by providing sufficient calcium and vitamin D intake during the growing years. After age 30, calcium intake and exercise are still important to maintain bone-mass density. Adult women need 1,000 to 1,300 mg of calcium per day, depending on age and condition (e.g., postmenopausal, pregnant, and lactating women will need more). One cup of milk, yogurt, or calcium-fortified orange juice provides about 300 mg of calcium. An ounce of cheese can contain from 70 mg (parmesan) to 270 mg (swiss) of calcium. Some green leafy vegetables, such as collards (179 mg per ½ cup) and turnip greens (138 mg per ½ cup), are also good sources of calcium. Without sufficient dietary calcium, the bones cannot grow strong and maintain their integrity.

There are some other nutritional factors that play a role in bone development. Vitamin D, which is found in fortified milk and can be synthesized by the body during sun exposure, is integral to the process of forming hard bones. About 30 minutes of sun on the face and hands can meet the daily needs for vitamin D. Weightbearing exercise (walking, aerobic dance, weight lifting, tennis, stair climbing) also promotes good bone density, but nonweight-bearing exercises (swimming, cycling) do not. A high-protein or a high-sodium diet can increase calcium loss in the urine, which lowers the amount of calcium available to the bones. Excessive alcohol intake impairs calcium absorption as well.

Teas, cocoa, spinach, asparagus, beet greens, and swiss chard are all high in chemicals called **oxylates.** Legumes and cereals high in bran are rich in **phytates.** Oxylates and phytates bind with calcium in the intestines, thus interfering with absorption. These foods should not be eliminated from the diet because they contain many other beneficial compo-

nents, but it is a good strategy not to rely on the calcium contained in them, as it might not be absorbed. It is not thought that the oxylates and phytates interfere with other sources of calcium eaten at the same time. Smoking also contributes to bone loss. See Table 4.15 for a list of tips to increase calcium intake.

Anemia

Iron-deficiency anemia is the most common nutritional deficiency in the United States, affecting about 2 to 5% of adolescent girls and women in the U.S. (Looker et al., 1997). Iron is a part of hemoglobin synthesis; hemoglobin carries the oxygen to the cells, allowing them to function. A decrease in red cells in the blood is called **anemia.** Anemia is diagnosed when hemoglobin concentrations fall below 12 g/dL for women and below 13.5 g/dL for men. Individuals with anemia often feel tired and listless, their endurance capacity is diminished, and their immune system is weakened, making them less resistant to colds or infections.

Most cases of anemia are due to poor iron intake, although poor intake of either folate or vitamin B12 can also result in this condition. Another cause is blood loss, either naturally (e.g., menstrual losses) or through injury or infection (e.g., gastrointestinal bleeding). The

Table 4.15
Tips for Increasing Calcium Intake

- Add nonfat milk powder to milk, soups, shakes or smoothies, meat loaf, baked goods, and mashed potatoes.

- Use milk or evaporated skim milk in cream soups, sauces, cocoa, and casseroles instead of cream.

- Top angel food cake, fruit, or gelatin with nonfat yogurt.

- Choose calcium-rich desserts such as frozen yogurt, puddings, and custards.

- Freeze milk in ice cube trays to use in shakes or smoothies.

- Substitute nonfat plain yogurt for sour cream or mayonnaise in dips, salad dressings, or as a baked potato topping.

- Sprinkle low-fat cheese on vegetables, salads, soups, or popcorn, or choose low-fat cheeses instead of meats.

- Use calcium-fortified products (orange juice, breakfast bars, etc.).

- Use tofu in meals [a 4 oz (113 g) serving has 150 mg of calcium].

Table 4.16
Tips for Increasing Iron Intake and Absorption

- Because acids enhance iron absorption, people should eat foods rich in vitamin C (particularly citrus foods) with each meal. Orange juice with breakfast can increase iron absorption by nearly 300%.

- Avoid coffee and tea with meals; they contain tannins, which inhibit iron absorption.

- Use cast iron cookware, as elemental iron will transfer to the foods, particularly when those foods are acidic. For example, the iron content of ½ cup of spaghetti sauce increases from 3 mg to 88 mg when simmered in a cast iron pot for three hours.

- Red meats and the dark meats of poultry are excellent sources of iron.

- Choose iron-rich fruits and vegetables, such as raisins, dried apricots, prunes, strawberries, dark green leafy vegetables, and legumes.

- Combine vegetable sources of iron with animal sources of iron (e.g., meat and vegetable or bean burritos, meat and bean soups and stews).

RDA for iron is 8 mg/day for adult males and postmenopausal women and 18 mg/day for premenopausal women. The average woman consumes only 12 mg/day, which does not meet this guideline. Table 4.16 presents tips for increasing iron intake and absorption. Because of the difficulty of obtaining sufficient dietary iron, individuals might be tempted to take an iron supplement. If a person chooses to do so, it is best to take small amounts, such as that contained in a general-purpose daily multivitamin/mineral supplement.

Iron supplementation will not improve endurance or performance in an individual with normal iron stores. Participants should be warned that feelings of fatigue can have many causes and may be completely unrelated to iron status. Iron overload is also a possibility and a serious medical concern. Excessive iron supplementation can also result in deficiencies of copper and zinc. Individuals concerned

about anemia should be tested by their physician and referred to a registered dietitian for assessment and dietary counseling.

There are different nutritional concerns at each stage of the lifecycle. See Table 4.17 for a listing of what an instructor should be aware of for participants at these different stages.

Special Topics of Concern

Alcohol

Moderate alcohol consumption (defined as one drink per day for women and two drinks per day for men) in most cases is considered safe and may actually have some health benefits, such as reducing the risk for cardiovascular disease. Because alcohol increases fluid loss, many serious athletes find it better to avoid alcohol during training and competition periods. Although alcohol contains carbohydrate, it is not something people should use to increase carbohydrate intake, as the

Table 4.17
Nutritional Concerns of Different Age Groups

Age Group	Nutrition-related Risk	Related Nutritional Component
Children	Anemia	Inadequate iron, folate, vitamin B12 intake
	Obesity	Excess caloric consumption, fat intake
	Eating disorders	Inadequate total intake
Young adults	Anemia	Inadequate iron, folate, vitamin B12 intake
	Obesity	Excess caloric consumption, fat intake
	Neural tube defects in offspring during pregnancy	Folate and vitamin B12 deficiency during the first 28 days of pregnancy
Middle-aged adults	Obesity	Excess caloric consumption, fat intake
	Hypertension	Excess body fat; inadequate calcium, magnesium, or potassium; excess sodium intake in salt-sensitive individuals (roughly 40% of all hypertensives)
	Diabetes	Excess body fat; possible other components (e.g., diet, inactivity)
	Cancer	Excess body fat and dietary fat; poor intake of vitamins and minerals (for antioxidant nutrients), fiber, and phytochemicals
Older adults	Cardiovascular disease	Excess body fat and dietary fat, poor intake of vitamins and minerals (for antioxidant nutrients), fiber, and phytochemicals
	Hypertension	Excess body fat; inadequate calcium, magnesium, or potassium; excess sodium intake in salt-sensitive individuals (roughly 40% of all hypertensives)
	Diabetes	Excess body fat; possible other components (e.g., diet, inactivity)
	Cancer	Excess body fat and dietary fat; poor intake of vitamins and minerals (for antioxidant nutrients), fiber, and phytochemicals
	Osteoporosis	Inadequate calcium and vitamin D intake

effects of alcohol actually impair performance. See Table 4.1 for recommendations from the Dietary Guidelines regarding alcohol.

Lactose Intolerance

Lactose intolerance is relatively common in adults. It can lead to symptoms such as bloating, distention, cramps, and flatulence following the consumption of dairy products. It is caused by a deficiency of the enzyme lactase, which is responsible for digestion of the milk sugar lactose. Many people who are lactose intolerant can actually digest small amounts of lactose with no problem, and yogurt and hard cheeses are usually well-tolerated. Over-the-counter lactase enzymes are very effective, and many reduced-lactose products are on the market. If an individual avoids dairy foods completely, he or she should be referred to a registered dietitian for a complete dietary assessment.

Caffeine and Other Ergogenic Aids

There are many agents that act as stimulants on the body, caffeine being the most widely consumed. **Caffeine** is a naturally occurring substance found in about 63 different species of plants, most notably coffee beans, cocoa beans, cola nuts, and tea leaves. Unless a food is processed for its removal, caffeine is present in any products made from those foods, such as coffee, tea, chocolate, and some soft drinks. Caffeine stimulates the central nervous system, making some people feel more awake and giving others the "jitters." Although it is relatively harmless, caffeine's side effects can include headache, nausea, muscle tremors, anxiety, nervousness, irritability, and insomnia. Though caffeine was once thought to be an "energy-enhancing" or **ergogenic aid,** research has not supported that idea.

Caffeine is one of the substances restricted by the U.S. Olympic Committee. This chemi-cal acts in the body as a diuretic and will contribute to fluid loss unless habitually used. Because the body quickly develops a tolerance for caffeine, the diuretic effect is not always notable in regular caffeine users. Caffeine can also contribute to elevated blood pressure in some individuals.

Many athletes, following the advice of coaches, friends, parents, or other athletes, will turn to some type of ergogenic aid to boost their performance capabilities. Examples include creatine, amino acids, steroids, and DHEA. Many of these dietary supplements have not been studied for safety or effectiveness. Some are downright harmful and many are ineffective. They can also be expensive. Just because a supplement is "natural" or available over-the-counter does not mean it is risk-free. The Dietary Supplement Health and Education Act of 1994 eliminated Food and Drug Administration (FDA) control over vitamins, minerals, amino acids, and herbs. Individuals should check with their doctors before using any supplements. See Appendix E for ACE's position on recommending nutritional supplements.

Nutrition for Athletic Performance

Many active individuals use nutrition to enhance athletic performance. Adequate nutritional status is an important part of a training program, just as it is an important part of general health. However, there is no secret to healthy nutrition for the athlete. Supplements, special diets, and food fads have not been shown to significantly impact endurance or strength. The guidelines for healthy eating can benefit all physically active individuals, from the moderately active to the elite athlete. In fact, people who exercise regularly will need more food to meet their energy needs. They are more likely to actually

Table 4.18
Nutrition Goals for Athletes

Energy	Ensure adequate total energy intake to support physical activity; maintain appropriate body weight
Carbohydrate	6–10 g/kg/day
Protein	1.2–1.4 g/kg/day for endurance-based sports 1.6–1.7 g/kg/day for strength-based sports

consume more nutrients as they consume a greater amount and a wider variety of foods. Nutritional recommendations for athletes are summarized in Table 4.18. The general advice is to consume a diet rich in carbohydrates, particularly complex carbohydrates, and moderate in protein and fat. Following the 2005 dietary guidelines and pattern outlined in Tables 4.6 and 4.12 will more than adequately meet the needs for protein and should meet the needs for the vitamins and minerals and other nutrients as long as the individual makes reasonable food choices (the french fry/broccoli example).

Consuming a high-carbohydrate diet also promotes glycogen storage. As discussed previously, glycogen is the storage form of carbohydrate in the muscles and is used for energy during physical activity. Adequate glycogen stores promote better endurance. For most recreational athletes, carbohydrate loading per se is not necessary; they will have enough glycogen to fuel even moderate-intensity physical activity. However, many serious athletes will want to ensure appropri-

ate intake before, during, and after intense, long-duration exercise, as shown in Table 4.19. The pre-event meal should be consumed far enough in advance so that glycogen reserves are maximized, but much of the food is digested before the event.

Even for individuals who are working to add lean body mass and build their muscles, excess protein is not necessary. A healthy diet can provide more than the needed amino acids, which are the building blocks of body protein. Protein powders and supplements are not cost-effective and excess protein intake is converted to glucose for the brain, burned for energy, or stored as body fat.

Eating Disorders

The alarming increase in the incidence of **eating disorders** is of great concern to every health and fitness professional. An eating disorder is a disturbance in eating behavior that jeopardizes a person's physical or psychological health. Eating disorders affect both men and women, although they are more common in women. These problems stem in part from unrealistic standards for body weight and body proportions. Dancers, wrestlers, gymnasts, and other athletes who strive for low body fat are the most vulnerable, although these disorders have also been noted in swimmers and cyclists. **Anorexia nervosa, bulimia nervosa**, and **binge eating disorder** are the three types of eating disorders recognized by the medical community.

Anorexia nervosa is usually characterized by an extremely low body weight and a denial of both hunger and thinness. To individuals suffering from this disorder, eating normally feels "out of control" and a normal body shape and size often "feels fat." Anorexics are obsessed with resisting food and often engage in vigorous exercise as a

Table 4.19
Carbohydrate-intake Guidelines Related to Exercise

Approximately three to four hours prior to the event	Consume 200–350 g carbohydrate (4 g/kg body weight)
Approximately one hour prior to the event	Consume 1 g carbohydrate/kg
During the event	Consume approximately 30 g carbohydrate every 30 minutes
Within 30 minutes following exercise	Consume 100 g carbohydrate

way to control both their eating and their body weight. Anorexia nervosa can be fatal. Eating disorders have the highest mortality rate of all the psychiatric illnesses.

Bulimia nervosa is characterized by a cycle of binging and purging. Typically, huge amounts of food are consumed prior to purging, which could include vomiting, fasting, and diuretic or laxative use. Like the anorexic, the bulimic is trapped by an obsession with thinness and a preoccupation with food.

Binge eating disorder (sometimes called compulsive overeating) is the least understood of the eating disorders. In this disorder, individuals usually consume large amounts of food without purging, yet they feel the same degree of guilt and emotional trauma as individuals with anorexia or bulimia. Although these individuals are quite often overweight or obese, not all overweight/obese individuals have a compulsive eating disorder.

On the surface, it may not be easy to tell the difference between a participant's healthy concern for body composition and athletic performance and an obsessive, destructive concern for being thin. A fitness professional cannot treat a person with an eating disorder; he or she should be seen by a medical team specializing in this field. However, by providing sound nutritional guidance, supporting realistic weight goals, and acknowledging that bodies come in many shapes and sizes, an instructor might be able to help prevent someone from developing an eating disorder.

Pregnancy

Following approval from their obstetricians, most women can remain active during pregnancy, especially if they were physically active pre-pregnancy. Some women may be advised to do moderate exercise during pregnancy, for the health of the baby or if they are gaining

weight too quickly. The energy needs associated with pregnancy require approximately 300 additional kcal per day. It is important that the energy requirements of exercise are also considered. In addition, pregnant women have lower fasting glucose levels than non-pregnant women and utilize carbohydrates during exercise at a greater rate (ACOG, 2002; 1994). As a result, pregnant women are at a higher risk of becoming hypoglycemic at rest and during exercise. Pregnant women should be sure to consume about 15 g of carbohydrate one hour prior to exercise to avoid low blood sugar levels during activity. They should also remain well-hydrated and meet their total energy needs. Women should seek their doctors' advice for guidance regarding proper nutrition and appropriate weight gain during pregnancy.

Summary

People who are interested in fitness are often interested in nutritional health as well. This interest makes them susceptible to many of the diet, supplement, and food fads constantly promoted in today's media and marketplace. Providing accurate information about the basics of nutrition can save participants time and money, as well as improve their health.

Decades of research have found that there is no "quick fix" to safely and legally improve health or athletic performance. If a person could "fix" his or her health, weight, or athletic performance overnight, he or she could just as easily put it in jeopardy. Fortunately, the human body is far more resilient than that. In a healthy diet, there is room for all foods in moderation, just as there is room for some sedentary activities, like watching a movie, in an active lifestyle.

Unfortunately, many people do not practice moderation when it comes to nutrition or exercise. Instead, they live an unbalanced lifestyle consuming nutrient-poor, high-calorie foods and engaging in little physical activity. While dietary fat intake exceeds recommended guidelines, fruit, vegetable, and whole-grain consumption are far too low in the population in general, resulting in low dietary fiber intakes. All of these nutritional issues can create significant health problems over just a few decades of life. Balance is the key to avoiding chronic health conditions such as obesity, heart disease, and diabetes on the excess side, and eating disorders such as anorexia nervosa on the other.

Help participants set realistic and achievable goals by making lifestyle changes they can live with for a lifetime. Group fitness instructors will be able to use their knowledge of nutrition to help participants achieve balance in their lives, help prevent or manage chronic disease, and improve the quality of their lives.

References

American College of Obstetricians and Gynecologists (1994). *ACOG Technical Bulletin #189.* Washington, D.C.: American College of Obstetricians and Gynecologists.

American College of Obstetricians and Gynecologists (2002). *ACOG Committee Opinion #267: Exercise During Pregnancy and the Postpartum Period.* Washington, D.C.: American College of Obstetricians and Gynecologists.

Appel, L.J. et al. for the DASH Collaborative Research Group (1997). A clinical trial of the effects of dietary patterns on blood pressure. *New England Journal of Medicine, 336,* 1117–1124.

Casa, D.J. et al. (2000). National Athletic Trainers' Association: Position statement: Fluid replacement for athletes. *Journal of Athletic Training, 35,* 212–224.

Institute of Medicine: Food, and Nutrition Board (2006). *Dietary Reference Intakes: The Essential Guide to Nutrient Requirements.* Washington, D.C.: National Academy Press.

Looker, A.C. et al. (1997). Prevalence of iron deficiency in the United States. *Journal of the American Medical Association, 277,* 12, 973–976.

McArdle, W. (1987). *Building Endurance.* New York: Time-Life Books.

U.S. Department of Agriculture/U.S. Department of Health and Human Services (2005). *Dietary Guidelines for Americans 2005.* www.healthierus.gov/dietaryguidelines

Woteki, C. & Thomas, P. (1992). *Eat for Life.* Washington, D.C.: National Academy Press.

Suggested Reading

American College of Sports Medicine (1996). Position stand on exercise and fluid replacement. *Medicine & Science in Sports & Exercise, 28,* i–vii.

American College of Sports Medicine, American Dietetic Association, Dietitians of Canada (2000). Joint position statement: Nutrition and athletic performance. *Medicine & Science in Sports & Exercise, 32,* 2130–2145.

American Diabetes Association and the American Dietetic Association (2003). *The Exchange Lists for Meal Planning.* www.diabetes.org/nutrition-and-recipes/nutrition/exchangelist.jsp

Clark, N. (2003). *Nancy Clark's Sports Nutrition Guidebook* (3rd ed.). Champaign, Ill.: Human Kinetics.

Dalton, S. (1997). *Overweight and Weight Management: The Health Professional's Guide to Understanding and Practice.* Gaithersburg, Md.: Aspen Publishers.

Krauss, R.M. et al. (2000). AHA Dietary Guidelines: Revision 2000: A statement for healthcare professionals from the Nutrition Committee of the American Heart Association. *Circulation, 102,* 18, 2284–2299.

Rosenbloom, C.A. (Ed.) (2000). *Sports Nutrition: A Guide for the Professional Working with Active People.* Chicago: The American Dietetic Association.

Sifton, D.W. (Ed.) (1995). *PDR Family Guide to Nutrition and Health.* Montvale, N.J.: Medical Economics.

Wardlaw, G.M. (2004). *Perspectives in Nutrition* (6th ed.). Boston: McGraw-Hill.

References and
Suggested Reading

Credible Sources for Nutrition Information

Federal Trade Commission—www.ftc.gov

Food and Drug Administration—www.fda.gov

Food and Nutrition Information Center—www.nal.usda.gov/fnic/

MyPyramid Food Guidance System—www.mypyramid.gov

National Cancer Institute—www.cancer.gov

National Heart, Lung and Blood Institute—www.nhlbi.nih.gov

National Institutes of Health—www.nih.gov

Shape Up America!—www.shapeup.org

U.S. Department of Agriculture—www.usda.gov

U.S. Department of Health and Human Services—www.dhhs.gov

Scientific and Professional Organizations Offering Credible Nutrition Information

American Academy of Pediatrics—www.aap.org

American Cancer Society—www.cancer.org

American College of Sports Medicine—www.acsm.org

American Diabetes Association—www.diabetes.org

American Dietetic Association—www.eatright.org

American Heart Association—www.americanheart.org

American Medical Association—www.ama-assn.org

American Society for Clinical Nutrition—www.faseb.org/ascn

Reputable Consumer Organizations

Better Business Bureau—www.bbb.org

Consumer Union—www.consumerreports.org

National Council Against Health Fraud—www.ncahf.org

Industry Groups that Provide Reputable Nutrition Information to the Public

Food Marketing Institute—www.fmi.org

National Dairy Council—www.nationaldairycouncil.org

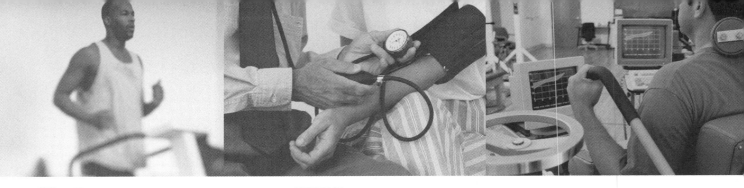

Chapter Five

David C. Nieman, Dr.P.H., F.A.C.S.M., has been a professor of health and exercise science for more than 25 years. He currently teaches at Appalachian State University in Boone, N.C. He is the author of several books, including *Fitness and Sports Medicine: A Health-Related Approach, Nutritional Assessment,* and *Fitness and Your Health,* and has written more than 200 articles that have appeared in such publications as the *Journal of the American College of Nutrition, Medicine & Science in Sports & Exercise, Women's Sports and Fitness,* and *ACE FitnessMatters.*

Health Screening

By David C. Nieman

The modern-day fitness movement began in 1968 when Kenneth Cooper, at that time a physician for the Air Force, published *Aerobics* (Cooper, 1968). In this book, Cooper challenged Americans to take personal charge of their lifestyles and counter the epidemics of heart disease, obesity, and rising healthcare costs through regular exercise. Millions took up the "aerobic challenge" and began running, cycling, walking, and swimming their way to better health.

Health Screening

Much has been learned about exercise and health during these nearly 40 years. In general, exercise has been found to be both safe and beneficial for most people (American College of Sports Medicine, 2006). However, there are some individuals who can suffer ill health from exercise. There is probably not a single fitness enthusiast in America who has not read the reports of famous athletes dying on basketball courts, runners found dead with their running shoes on, executives discovered slumped over their treadmills, or middle-aged men suffering heart attacks while shoveling snow.

Whether exercise is beneficial or hazardous to the heart depends on the person. For most people, regular exercise reduces the risk of heart disease by about 30 to 50% compared to those who are physically inactive (U.S. Department of Health and Human Services, 1996). However, for those who are at high risk for heart disease to begin with, vigorous exercise bouts can be potentially harmful. About 75,000 Americans suffer heart attacks during or after exercise each year (American College of Sports Medicine, 2006). Studies show that these victims tended to be men who were sedentary, over age 35, already had heart disease or were at high risk for it, and then exercised too hard for their fitness levels. And for patients with heart disease, the incidence of a heart attack or death during vigorous exercise is 100 times greater than for otherwise healthy individuals (American College of Sports Medicine, 2006). According to the Centers for Disease Control, more than one-third of all Americans have some form of **cardiovascular disease** (including high blood pressure) by age 55, and prevalence rises with age (NHANES IV, 1999–2000).

Also of concern is **congenital** cardiovascular disease, now considered a significant cause of athletic death in high school and college. In one study of 158 athletes who died young (average age 17) and in their prime, 134 had heart or blood vessel defects that were present at birth (Maron et al., 1996). In other words, when a young athlete dies during or shortly after exercise, it is most often due to a birth defect of the cardiovascular system (American Heart Association, 1996; Cantwell, 1998).

Health screening is a vital process for identifying and stratifying cardiovascular risk factors and referring individuals to appropriate healthcare providers, when necessary (American College of Sports Medicine, 2006). According to the American College of Sports Medicine (ACSM), the incidence of cardiovascular problems during physical activity is reduced by nearly 50% when individuals are first screened, and those identified with risk factors or disease are referred to appropriate healthcare providers and supervised medical activity programs (American College of Sports Medicine, 2006). Despite the proven benefits of screening, efforts to screen new members upon enrollment into health and fitness facilities are limited and inconsistent (American College of Sports Medicine/American Heart Association, 1998).

Several agencies and organizations recommend that every person participate in at least moderate-intensity physical activity for 30 minutes or more on most, if not all, days of the week (U.S. Department of Health and Human Services, 1996; American College of Sports Medicine, 2006). Efforts to promote physical activity will result in increasing numbers of individuals, with and without risk of heart disease, joining health and fitness facilities and community exercise programs.

Surveys reveal that 51% of health and fitness facility members are over the age of 45 (International Health, Racquet, & Sportsclub Association, American Sports Data, 2003; International Health, Racquet, & Sportsclub Association, American Business Information, Inc., 2004; IDEA & Modern Research & Communications, 2004).

This chapter focuses on procedures that group fitness instructors can implement to help protect participants when initiating exercise or athletic programs and emphasizes several key issues:

- Always obtain a medical history or pre-exercise health-risk appraisal on each participant and identify cardiovascular risk factors.
- Stratify individuals according to their disease risk.
- Refer high-risk individuals to appropriate healthcare providers for additional evaluation. Some moderate-risk individuals may also require a referral to appropriate healthcare providers for additional evaluation.

The Pre-exercise Health Appraisal Questionnaire

A preparticipation screening should be performed on all new participants, regardless of age, upon entering a facility that offers exercise equipment or services (American College of Sports Medicine/American Heart Association 1998; Tharrett & Peterson, 2006). The screening procedure should be valid, simple, cost- and time-efficient, and, most importantly, appropriate for the target population. Screening procedures range from self-administered questionnaires to elaborate tests.

Prior to commencing any self-guided physical activity (i.e., activity initiated and guided by the individual with little or no input or supervision from a qualified fitness professional), the individual should complete a minimal Health Appraisal Questionnaire (American College of Sports Medicine, 2006). The **Physical Activity Readiness Questionnaire (PAR-Q),** designed in the 1970s by Canadian researchers, has been used very successfully when testing large numbers of individuals in a short period of time or in health and fitness facility settings where a short, simple medical and health questionnaire is needed. After years of successful use and a revision in 2002, the PAR-Q (Figure 5.1) is recognized by experts as a minimal, yet safe pre-exercise screening measure for low-to-moderate intensity (but not vigorous) exercise training (Canadian Society for Exercise Physiology, 2002). Participants are directed to contact their personal physician if they answer "yes" to one or more questions.

In 1998, the American College of Sports Medicine and the American Heart Association published another screening questionnaire, which is slightly more complex than the PAR-Q (American College of Sports Medicine/American Heart Association, 1998). The American College of Sports Medicine/American Heart Association Health/Fitness Facility Preparticipation Screening Questionnaire (Figure 5.2) investigates an individual's history, symptoms, cardiovascular risk factors, and other health issues to direct him or her to either initiate an exercise program or contact a physician. Persons at higher risk are directed to seek facilities providing appropriate levels of staff supervision. This questionnaire takes only a few minutes to complete and more effectively identifies high-risk participants.

The screening questionnaires should ideally be interpreted and documented by qualified

Health Screening

Figure 5.1
The Physical Activity Readiness Questionnaire

The Physical Activity Readiness Questionnaire—PAR-Q

(revised 2002)

PAR-Q & YOU (A Questionnaire for People Aged 15 to 69)

Regular physical activity is fun and healthy, and increasingly more people are starting to become more active every day. Being more active is very safe for most people. However, some people should check with their doctor before they start becoming much more physically active.

If you are planning to become much more physically active than you are now, start by answering the seven questions below. If you are between the ages of 15 and 69, the PAR-Q will tell you if you should check with your doctor before you start. If you are over 69 years of age, and you are not used to being very active, check with your doctor.

Common sense is your best guide when you answer these questions. Please read the questions carefully and answer each one honestly: check YES or NO.

YES   NO

☐   ☐   1. Has your doctor ever said that you have a heart condition *and* that you should only do physical activity recommended by a doctor?

☐   ☐   2. Do you feel pain in your chest when you do physical activity?

☐   ☐   3. In the past month, have you had chest pain when you were not doing physical activity?

☐   ☐   4. Do you lose your balance because of dizziness or do you ever lose consciousness?

☐   ☐   5. Do you have a bone or joint problem (for example, back, knee, or hip) that could be made worse by a change in your physical activity?

☐   ☐   6. Is your doctor currently prescribing drugs (for example, water pills) for your blood pressure or heart condition?

☐   ☐   7. Do you know of *any other reason* why you should not do physical activity?

If you answered YES to one or more questions:

✔ Talk with your doctor by phone or in person BEFORE you start becoming much more physically active or BEFORE you have a fitness appraisal. Tell your doctor about the PAR-Q and which questions you answered YES.

✔ You may be able to do any activity you want—as long as you start slowly and build up gradually. Or, you may need to restrict your activities to those that are safe for you. Talk with your doctor about the kinds of activities you wish to participate in and follow his or her advice.

✔ Find out which community programs are safe and helpful for you.

If you answered NO honestly to all PAR-Q questions, you can be reasonably sure that you can:

✔ Start becoming much more physically active—begin slowly and build up gradually. This is the safest and easiest way to go.

✔ Take part in a fitness appraisal—this is an excellent way to determine your basic fitness level so that you can plan the best way for you to live actively. It is also highly recommended that you have your blood pressure evaluated. If your reading is over 144/94, talk with your doctor before you start becoming much more physically active.

Delay becoming much more active:

✔ If you are not feeling well because of a temporary illness such as a cold or a fever—wait until you feel better; or

✔ If you are or may be pregnant—talk to your doctor before you start becoming more active.

Please note: If your health changes so that you then answer YES to any of the above questions, tell your fitness or health professional. Ask whether you should change your physical-activity plan.

Informed Use of the PAR-Q: The Canadian Society for Exercise Physiology, Health Canada, and their agents assume no liability for persons who undertake physical activity, and if in doubt after completing this questionnaire, consult your doctor prior to physical activity.

No changes permitted. You are encouraged to copy the PAR-Q but only if you use the entire form.

Note: If the PAR-Q is being given to a person before he or she participates in a physical activity program or a fitness appraisal, this section may be used for legal or administrative purposes.

I have read, understood, and completed this questionnaire. Any questions I had were answered to my full satisfaction.

Name

Signature   Date

Signature of Parent   Witness
or Guardian (for participants under the age of majority)

Note: This physical activity clearance is valid for a maximum of 12 months from the date it is completed and becomes invalid if your condition changes so that you would answer YES to any of the seven questions.

© Reprinted with permission from the
Canadian Society for Exercise Physiology
Societe canadienne de physiologie de l'exercice   Supported by: Health   Santé
www.csep.ca/forms.asp   Canada   Canada

Figure 5.2

American College of Sports Medicine/American Heart Association Preparticipation Screening Questionnaire
American College of Sports Medicine (2006). *ACSM's Guidelines for Exercise Testing and Prescription* (7th ed.).
Philadelphia: Lippincott Williams & Wilkins.

Assess your health needs by marking all true statements

History
You have had:
- ☐ a heart attack
- ☐ heart surgery
- ☐ cardiac catheterization
- ☐ coronary angioplasty (PTCA)
- ☐ pacemaker/implantable cardiac
- ☐ defibrillator/rhythm disturbance
- ☐ heart valve disease
- ☐ heart failure
- ☐ heart transplantation
- ☐ congenital heart disease

Other health issues:
- ☐ You have musculoskeletal problems.
- ☐ You have concerns about the safety of exercise.
- ☐ You take prescription medication(s).
- ☐ You are pregnant.

Symptoms
- ☐ You experience chest discomfort with exertion.
- ☐ You experience unreasonable breathlessness.
- ☐ You experience dizziness, fainting, or blackouts.
- ☐ You take heart medications.

Recommendations

If you marked any of the statements in this section, consult your healthcare provider before engaging in exercise. You may need to use a facility with a medically qualified staff.

Cardiovascular risk factors
- ☐ You are a man older than 45 years.
- ☐ You are a woman older than 55 years or you have had a hysterectomy or you are postmenopausal.
- ☐ You smoke.
- ☐ Your blood pressure is greater than 140/90 mmHg.
- ☐ You don't know your blood pressure.
- ☐ You take blood pressure medication.
- ☐ Your blood cholesterol level is >200 mg/dL
- ☐ You don't know your cholesterol level.
- ☐ You have a blood relative who had a heart attack before age 55 (father/brother) or 65 (mother/sister).
- ☐ You are diabetic or take medicine to control your blood sugar.
- ☐ You are physically inactive (i.e., you get less than 30 minutes of physical activity on at least 3 days per week).
- ☐ You are more than 20 pounds (9 kg) overweight.

If you marked two or more of the statements in this section, you should consult your healthcare provider before engaging in exercise. You might benefit by using a facility with a professionally qualified exercise staff to guide your exercise program.

- ☐ None of the above is true.

You should be able to exercise safely without consulting your healthcare provider in almost any facility that meets your exercise program needs.

staff to limit the number of unnecessary medical referrals and avoid barriers to participation.

There are many other types of detailed preparticipation screening tools. A comprehensive questionnaire should include the following (American College of Sports Medicine, 2006):

- Past and current medical diagnoses
- Previous physical-examination findings
- History of symptoms
- Recent illness, hospitalization, or surgical procedures
- Orthopedic problems
- Medication use and drug allergies
- Lifestyle habits
- Exercise history
- Work history
- Family history of disease

Disease Risk Stratification

These questionnaires are designed to provide more information regarding risk stratification and the need for medical clearance prior to beginning a program of physical activity. While this information is crucial in classifying a potential exercise participant according to disease risk, it will also facilitate the exercise programming process, as the background information obtained from the questionnaire improves the instructor's ability to meet individual needs.

Stratification of risk is important for several reasons:

- To identify those in need of referral to a healthcare provider for more extensive medical evaluation
- To ensure the safety of exercise testing and participation
- To determine the appropriate type of exercise test or program

Using age, health status, symptoms, and risk-factor information, exercise participants can be classified into three primary risk stratifications as defined by ACSM: Low Risk, Moderate Risk, and High Risk (Table 5.1).

While it is recommended that persons classified as Moderate Risk, and especially High Risk, undergo a medical exam (or have had one within the past 12 months) and consider a medically supervised exercise test before engaging in vigorous exercise, no restrictions are required for individuals in the Low Risk category.

Group fitness instructors should take special care in accommodating the specific needs of low-risk individuals by selecting, modifying, and adapting activities when planning and supervising a safe and effective exercise class.

The 2006 American College of Sports Medicine guidelines also present a more detailed method for identifying the presence of major coronary risk factors and major signs and symptoms suggestive of cardiovascular, pulmonary, or metabolic disease.

Table 5.1
ACSM Risk-stratification Categories

1. Low Risk
- Younger individuals (men <45 years, women <55 years) who are asymptomatic and meet the threshold of no more than one risk factor

2. Moderate Risk
- Older individuals (men ≥45 years, women ≥55 years) or those who meet the threshold for two or more risk factors and are asymptomatic

3. High Risk
- Individuals with one or more signs and symptoms
or
- Individuals with known cardiovascular disease (peripheral vascular disease, cerebrovascular disease), pulmonary disease (chronic obstructive pulmonary diseases, severe asthma, cystic fibrosis) or metabolic disease (renal, liver, or thyroid disorder).

Signs or symptoms are not provided, as they must be interpreted by a qualified licensed professional within the clinical context in which they appear because they are not specific for cardiovascular, pulmonary, or metabolic disease.

American College of Sports Medicine (2006). *ACSM's Guidelines for Exercise Testing and Prescription* (7th ed.). Philadelphia: Lippincott Williams & Wilkins.

Health Screening

This procedure can include the use of the American College of Sports Medicine/ American Heart Association questionnaire or a more elaborate facility-specific medical and health-history questionnaire (American College of Sports Medicine, 2006). This process involves three basic steps:

1. Identify the American College of Sports Medicine coronary artery disease risk factor threshold (Table 5.2).

2. Stratify the risk category (see Table 5.1).

3. Determine the need for medical clearance and supervised testing prior to participation (Tables 5.3 and 5.4).

Candidates screened as unsafe for participation must be referred to their physicians

---

Table 5.2
Coronary Artery Disease Risk-factor Thresholds

Instructions:

Determine the total number of risk factors using the following risk-factor criteria, scoring a point for each risk factor identified. If high-density lipoprotein (HDL) levels exceed 60 mg/dL, subtract one point from the sum of positive risk factors, as high HDL levels lower the risk for coronary artery disease.

Positive Risk Factors

Family History +1
 • Myocardial infarction, coronary revascularization, or sudden death before 55 years of age in father
   or other first-degree male relative
 • Myocardial infarction, coronary revascularization, or sudden death before 65 years of age in mother
   or other first-degree female relative

Cigarette Smoking +1
 • Current cigarette smokers or those who quit within the previous six months

Hypertension +1
 • Systolic blood pressure ≥140 mmHg or diastolic blood pressure ≥90 mmHg, confirmed by measurements
   on at least two separate occasions, or on anti-hypertensive medications

Dyslipidemia +1
 • Low-density lipoprotein (LDL) cholesterol ≥130 mg/dL or HDL cholesterol <40 mg/dL, or on lipid-lowering medication
 • If serum cholesterol is all that is available, use serum cholesterol ≥200 mg/dL

Impaired Glucose Fasting +1
 • Fasting blood sugar ≥100 mg/dL confirmed by measurements on at least two separate occasions

Obesity +1
 • Body mass index of ≥30 kg/m²
   or
 • Waist girth >102 cm (40 inches) for men and ≥89 cm (35 inches) for women
   or
 • Waist/hip ratio ≥0.95 for men and ≥0.86 for women

As professional opinions vary regarding the most appropriate markers and thresholds for obesity, use additional valid markers to evaluate obesity as a risk factor (this may include a valid measure of percent body fat).

Sedentary Lifestyle +1
 • Persons not participating in a regular exercise program or not meeting the minimal recommendations from the Surgeon
   General's Report/USDA Guidelines

Negative Risk Factor

High serum HDL Cholesterol - 1
 • Score >60 mg/dL

TOTAL SCORE _____

American College of Sports Medicine (2006). *ACSM's Guidelines for Exercise Testing and Prescription* (7th ed.). Philadelphia: Lippincott Williams & Wilkins.

Table 5.3
Medical Exam (Within Past Year) and Exercise Test Recommendation

	Low Risk*	Moderate Risk[†]	High Risk[‡]
Moderate Exercise Intensity[¨]	Not necessary	Not necessary	Recommended
Vigorous Exercise Intensity[††]	Not necessary	Recommended	Recommended

* Younger individuals (men <45, women <55), asymptomatic and have no more than one risk factor
[†] Older individuals who have two or more risk factors and are asymptomatic
[‡] Individuals with one or more signs/symptoms or known cardiac (CVD, PVD, or CVA), pulmonary (COPD, asthma, cystic fibrosis, or interstitial lung disease) or metabolic (DM, thyroid disorders, liver or kidney) disease
[¨] Moderate exercise implies 40–59% $\dot{V}O_2$max or heart-rate reserve, or 11–12 on the rating of perceived exertion on the Borg 6–20 RPE for at least 45 minutes
[††] Vigorous implies ≥60% $\dot{V}O_2$max or heart-rate reserve, or an RPE ≥13 sustained for 20 minutes
Note: CVD = Cardiovascular disease; PVD = Peripheral vascular disease; CVA = Cerebral vascular accident; COPD = Chronic obstructive pulmonary disease; DM = Diabetes mellitus.

American College of Sports Medicine (2006). *ACSM's Guidelines for Exercise Testing and Prescription* (7th ed.). Philadelphia: Lippincott Williams & Wilkins.

for clearance and exercise guidelines. Refer each candidate to his or her physician for completion of a medical/physical examination and to obtain a physician's written medical release or clearance form.

The Medical/Physical Examination

The depth of the medical or physical examination for any individual considering an exercise program depends on the disease **risk stratification.** When a medical evaluation or recommendation is advised or required, written and active communication by the exercise staff with the individual's personal physician is strongly recommended. The form in Figure 5.3 can be used for this referral.

Table 5.4
Physician Supervision During Exercise Test

	Low Risk	Moderate Risk	High Risk
Submaximal	Not necessary	Not necessary	Recommended
Maximal	Not necessary	Recommended	Recommended

Cardiovascular Screening of Competitive Athletes

An average of 12 to 20 athletes, most of them high school students, die suddenly each year from congenital heart defects that are not detected during normal physical examinations (American Heart Association, 1996; Maron et al., 1996). About a third of the cases of sudden cardiac death are caused by a congenital heart defect called **hypertrophic cardiomyopathy** (thickened heart muscle), with the next most frequent cause being congenital coronary anomalies (American Heart Association, 1996).

In the United States there are nearly six million scholastic athletes. Although most states require a regular physical exam once a year or once every two years for these athletes, the cost for the more sensitive tests (e.g., two-dimensional **echocardiography**) that would detect heart defects ranges from $400 to $2,000 per screening. However, even with echocardiography, some athletes are incorrectly classified (e.g., false-positive or false-negative) (American Heart Association, 1996).

The sudden death of a young athlete is tragic, but the financial, ethical, medical, and legal issues involved in preparticipation screening have created huge barriers (Cantwell, 1998; Corrado et al., 1998). In 1996, the American Heart Association published a consensus statement on this issue from a panel of experts (American Heart Association, 1996). The group fitness

Figure 5.3
Sample Health History Form

Sample Health History Form

Name_____ Date_____

Age _____ Sex ☐ M   ☐ F

Physician's Name _____

Physician's Phone (_____) _____

Person to contact in case of emergency:

Name _____ Phone_____

Are you taking any medications or drugs? If so, please list medication, dose, and reason.

_____

_____

Does your physician know you are participating in this exercise program?

_____

_____

Describe any physical activity you do somewhat regularly.

_____

_____

Do you now have, or have you had in the past:	Yes	No
1. Heart problems, chest pain, or stroke	☐	☐
2. Increased blood pressure	☐	☐
3. Any chronic illness or condition	☐	☐
4. Difficulty with physical exercise	☐	☐
5. Advice from physician not to exercise	☐	☐
6. Recent surgery (last 12 months)	☐	☐
7. Pregnancy (now or within last 3 months)	☐	☐
8. History of breathing or lung problems	☐	☐
9. Muscle, joint, or back disorder, or any previous injury still affecting you	☐	☐
10. Diabetes or thyroid condition	☐	☐
11. Cigarette smoking habit	☐	☐
12. Obesity (more than 20% over ideal body weight)	☐	☐
13. Increased blood cholesterol	☐	☐
14. History of heart problems in immediate family	☐	☐
15. Hernia, or any condition that may be aggravated by lifting weights	☐	☐

Please explain any "yes" answers on the back.

Comments:

_____

instructor should support all efforts to encourage preparticipation screening of athletes. Here are the key recommendations from the American Heart Association (American Heart Association, 1996):

- Some form of preparticipation cardio-vascular screening for high school and collegiate athletes is justifiable and compelling, based on ethical, legal, and medical grounds.
- A complete and careful personal and family history and physical examination designed to identify cardiovascular prob-lems known to cause sudden death or dis-ease progression in young athletes is the best available and most practical approach to screening competitive athletes, regard-less of age. Such cardiovascular screening is an obtainable objective and should be mandatory for all athletes.
- Both a history and a physical examination should be performed before participation in organized high school (grades nine through 12) and collegiate sports. Screening should then be repeated every two years. In inter-vening years, an interim history should be obtained.
- The athletic screening should be per-formed by a healthcare worker with the requisite training, medical skills, and back-ground to reliably obtain a detailed cardio-vascular history, perform a physical exami-nation, and recognize heart disease.

Summary

For those who are at high risk for heart disease, vigorous exercise can trigger fatal heart attacks. These victims tend to be men who were sedentary, over 35 years old, already had heart disease or were at high risk for it, and then exercised too hard for their fitness levels.

Health screening is a vital process in first identifying individuals at high risk for exercise-induced heart problems, and then referring them to appropriate medical care. All facilities offering exercise equipment or services should conduct a health and cardiovascular screening of all new members and/or prospective users, regardless of age.

Several types of health appraisal question-naires are available, including the Physical Activity Readiness Questionnaire (PAR-Q) and the 1998 American College of Sports Medicine/American Heart Association Health/Fitness Facility Preparticipation Screening Questionnaire. When a medical evaluation or recommendation is advised or required, written and active communication by the exercise staff with the individual's personal physician is strongly recommended.

American College of Sports Medicine rec-ommends that participants be classified into three primary risk stratifications: Low Risk, Moderate Risk, and High Risk. Classifications are based on age, health status, symptoms, and risk-factor information. It is recommended that persons classified as Moderate Risk, and especially High Risk, undergo a medical exam (or have had one within the past 12 months) and consider a medically supervised exercise test before engaging in vigorous exercise. No restrictions are required for individuals in the Low Risk category.

Special care should be taken to accom-modate the specific needs of individuals when selecting, modifying, and adapting activities to ensure that all participants experience a safe and effective exercise class. The 2006 American College of Sports Medicine guidelines also present a more detailed method to identify the presence of major coronary risk factors and major signs and symptoms suggestive of cardiovascular, pulmonary, or metabolic disease. This procedure can include the use of the American College of Sports Medicine/ American Heart Association questionnaire or a more elaborate facility-specific medical and health history questionnaire (American College of Sports Medicine, 2006). This process involves three basic steps:

1. Identify the American College of Sports Medicine coronary artery disease risk-factor threshold.
2. Stratify the risk category.
3. Determine the need for medical clearance and supervised testing prior to participation.

Some form of preparticipation cardiovascular screening for high school and collegiate athletes is justifiable and compelling, based on ethical, legal, and medical grounds.

Appendix C details the general effects of several categories of medications on heart-rate response. This table should not serve as a substitute for consultation with a participant's physician.

References

American College of Sports Medicine (2006). *ACSM's Guidelines for Exercise Testing and Prescription* (7th ed.). Philadelphia: Lippincott Williams & Wilkins.

American College of Sports Medicine and American Heart Association (1998). Recommendations for cardiovascular screening, staffing, and emergency policies at health/fitness facilities. *Medicine & Science in Sports & Exercise,* 30, 1009–1018.

American Heart Association (1996). Cardiovascular preparticipation screening of competitive athletes. *Circulation,* 94, 850–856.

Canadian Society for Exercise Physiology. (2002). *The Canadian Physical Activity, Fitness & Lifestyle Appraisal.* Ottawa, Ontario.

Cantwell, J.D. (1998). Preparticipation physical evaluation: Getting to the heart of the matter. *Medicine & Science in Sports & Exercise*, 30 (suppl) S341–S344.

Cooper, K.H. (1968). *Aerobics.* New York: Bantam Books, Inc.

Corrado, D. et al. (1998). Screening for hypertrophic cardiomyopathy in young athletes. *New England Journal of Medicine,* 339, 364–369.

IDEA and Modern Research & Communications, Inc. (2004).

IHRSA and American Sports Data Health Club Trend Report (2003).

IHRSA and American Business Information, Inc. (2004).

Maron, B.J. et al. (1996). Sudden death in young competitive athletes: Clinical, demographic, and pathological profiles. *Journal of the American Medical Association,* 276, 199–204.

Tharrett, S.J., McInnis, K.J., & Peterson, J.A. (2006). *ACSM's Health/Fitness Facility Standards and Guidelines* (3rd ed.). Champaign, Ill.: Human Kinetics.

The 1999–2000 National Health and Nutrition Examination Survey IV, Part I (NHANES IV). Centers for Disease Control and Prevention, National Center for Chronic Disease Prevention and Health Promotion.

U.S. Department of Health and Human Services (1996). *Physical Activity and Health: A Report of the Surgeon General.* Atlanta, Ga.: U.S. Department of Health and Human Services, Centers for Disease Control and Prevention, National Center for Chronic Disease Prevention and Health Promotion.

Suggested Reading

Fletcher, G.F. et al. (2001). Exercise standards for testing and training: A statement for healthcare professionals from the American Heart Association. *Circulation,* 104, 1694–1740.

McInnis, K.J. & Balady, G.J. (1999). Higher cardiovascular risk clients in health clubs. *ACSM's Health & Fitness Journal,* 3, 19–24.

Nieman, D.C. (1999). *Exercise Testing and Prescription: A Health-Related Approach.* Mountain View: Mayfield Publishing.

Sharkey, B.J. (1979). *Physiology of Fitness.* Champaign, Ill.: Human Kinetics.

Shephard, R.J., Thomas, S., & Weller, I. (1991). The Canadian Home Fitness Test: 1991 update. *Sports Medicine,* 11, 358–366.

References and
Suggested Reading

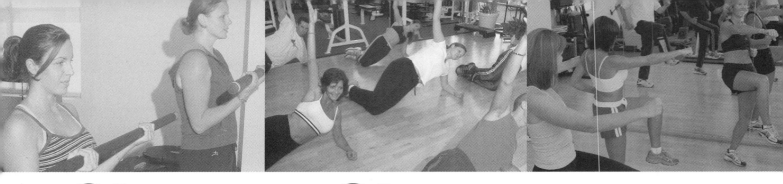

Chapter Six

Carol Kennedy, M.S., received her bachelor's degree in leisure studies from the University of Illinois and her master's degree in exercise and sport science from Colorado State University. For 20 years she worked in health clubs and recreational facilities as a fitness instructor and manager. She is now a full-time lecturer within the Department of Kinesiology's Fitness Specialist Undergraduate Curriculum at Indiana University. Kennedy teaches classes on group exercise leadership, one-on-one fitness training, and fitness management. She has produced videos on aquatic exercise and functional exercise progression, and has recently coauthored a research-based textbook, *Methods of Group Exercise Instruction.*

Group Exercise Program Design

By Carol Kennedy

The overall purpose of group exercise program design is to help people live happier and healthier lives through exercise. The underlying goal is to enhance the health-related components of fitness, which include a participant's cardiorespiratory endurance, muscular strength and endurance, flexibility, and body composition. It has been proven that exercising in a group can enhance overall adherence to exercise (Carron, Hausenblas, & Mack, 1996). Obesity is an ever-increasing problem in the United States, with physical activity seen as essential in the fight to combat obesity (Jakicic & Otto, 2005). Therefore, it is increasingly important that group exercise program design revolve around these health-related components of fitness.

Group Exercise Program Design

Group exercise has grown to include traditional high- and low-impact (hi/lo) classes, step, indoor cycling, kickboxing, sports conditioning, aquatic exercise, use of strength and conditioning equipment for group exercise, mind/body classes such as yoga and Pilates, stretching-only classes, and more. As these different types of group exercise workouts continue to be created and studied, the American College of Sports Medicine (ACSM) guidelines on exercise programming for healthy adults continue to be updated as well (American College of Sports Medicine, 2006). See Table 6.1 for a summation of the 2006 ACSM exercise programming guidelines for healthy adults. It is interesting that these guidelines validate a typical group exercise class format dating back to the inception of group exercise in the 1970s. The guidelines include cardiorespiratory, muscular strength and endurance, and flexibility recommendations, which have been a part of the group exercise experience for a very long time. A reminder: Cardiorespiratory duration still includes 20 to 60 continuous minutes or discontinuous 10-minute bouts that add up to 20 to 60 minutes total. Many group exercise class formats are set to be one hour in duration, with the cardiorespiratory segment being 20 to 40 minutes of continuous exercise to meet the old 1990 ACSM guidelines. Rethinking class schedules and offering a variety of times and activities is important for all successful fitness programs.

Some experts believe that group fitness instructors will continue to bring the group exercise experience out of facilities in the form of walking classes, training for adventure movement, and more (Hooker, 2003). According to Tharrett and Peterson (2006), future programs for group exercise include group classes "in a box" (e. g., BODYPUMP,™ BODYFLOW™), fusion fitness (blended styles such as spin/yoga or step/strength), extreme fitness (boot camp, SWAT fitness), and core and functional fitness classes. Many facilities offering group exercise are finding success with classes that are 30 minutes or shorter to help accommodate the busy schedules of participants. The

Table 6.1
2006 ACSM Exercise Programming Guidelines for Healthy Adults

Component of Training Program	Frequency (sessions per week)	Intensity	Duration	Activity
Cardiorespiratory	3–5	40%/50%–85% HRR or V̇O₂R 55%/65%–90% HRmax 12–16 RPE	20–60 minutes	Large muscle groups Dynamic activity
Resistance	2–3	Volitional fatigue (MMF) (e.g., 19–20 RPE) OR Stop 2–3 reps before volitional fatigue (e.g., 16 RPE)	One set of 3–20 reps (e.g., 3–5, 8–10, 12–15)	8–10 exercises that include all major muscle groups
Flexibility	Minimal: 2–3 Ideal: 5–7	Stretch to tightness at the end of the range of motion, but not to pain	15–30 seconds 2–4 reps per stretch	Static stretch all major muscle groups

Note: HRR = Heart-rate reserve; V̇O₂R = Maximal oxygen uptake reserve; HRmax = Maximal heart rate; MMF = Momentary muscular fatigue; RPE = Ratings of perceived exertion

American College of Sports Medicine (2006). *ACSM's Guidelines for Exercise Testing & Prescription* (7th ed.). Philadelphia: Lippincott Williams & Wilkins.

IDEA 2005 Fitness Trends survey (IDEA, 2005) lists core conditioning, indoor cycling, small group classes, dance, and combination (or fusion) classes as growing, while high- and low-impact and step classes are on the decline.

Finally, it is also important to consider the *Surgeon General's Report on Physical Activity and Health* (United States Department of Health and Human Services, 1996). This report focuses on the importance of physical activity in daily life, such as walking the dog or taking the stairs. It states, "Every U.S. adult should accumulate 30 minutes or more of moderate-intensity physical activity on most, preferably all, days of the week." It cannot be assumed that people are generally active. Guidelines for structured exercise as well as the activities of daily life need to be stressed. The challenge is to apply the information in this manual, current research, ACSM's exercise programming guidelines, and the Surgeon General's report into safe, effective, and highly motivating workouts to make a difference in the health and wellness of participants.

Group Exercise Professionalism and Attitude

Combining current research with participants' needs and designing a safe and effective class begins with the attitude and atmosphere established by the instructor. A comfortable environment can be influenced by a wide range of factors, from the quality of an instructor's communication skills to his or her attire. Each factor helps establish a professional and caring attitude. A group fitness instructor needs to be a motivator and an educator (Kennedy & Yoke, 2005).

Student-centered Instructor

The motivational and inspirational aspect of instructing includes having new moves, new music, and state-of-the-art equipment. The educational part of instructing includes having the knowledge of why certain moves are selected, making sure current research and knowledge are incorporated into the group exercise session, and making educated choices and decisions about the information given to participants. According to Westcott (1991), the most important characteristic of fitness instructors, as rated and ranked by participants, is knowledge of physical fitness.

It is important to compare and contrast a teacher-centered instructor with a student-centered instructor. The teacher-centered instructor can often foster dependence, intimidation, unattainable goals, and quick fixes (Table 6.2). The student-centered instructor, on the other hand, strives to establish an atmosphere of independence, encouragement, attainable goals, and realism (Table 6.3). Learning to take

Table 6.2
Teacher-centered Instructor

1. *Dependence:* You need me to be able to exercise. Here's a DVD of my class for when you go on vacation.
2. *Intimidation:* If you can't do 20 push-ups you don't belong in this class!
3. *Unattainable goals:* You'll see changes instantaneously from this class!
4. *Quick fixes:* 50 more outer-thigh leg lifts and you'll get rid of that extra "stored energy" on your thighs.

Table 6.3
Student-centered Instructor

1. *Independence:* Remember to work at your own pace. I will show modifications, but it will be your responsibility to monitor your intensity level accordingly. Here's how to do that ...
2. *Encouragement:* Awesome work! Remember, if there is pain, there will be little gain. Stay with it and you'll feel better.
3. *Attainable goals:* Learning to enjoy movement is a process that will take time. Try adding extra activity outside of class, like taking the stairs or mowing your yard. Those activities count as movement experiences also.
4. *Reality:* Outer-thigh leg lifts will strengthen your outer-thigh muscles, but there is no such thing as "spot reduction" of a specific area.

Group Exercise Program Design

responsibility for the health and well-being of participants starts with understanding the importance of establishing a positive attitude and atmosphere.

Creating a Healthy Emotional Environment

Another major factor in creating a comfortable environment for participants is establishing a healthy emotional environment. Education and motivation alone are not what keep participants coming back to group exercise. It is necessary to tap into the feelings and emotions of participants to impact adherence. One study concerning overweight women's perceptions of an exercise class revealed that the most powerful influences affecting their exercise behavior were concerns about embarrassment and judgment by others (Bain, Wilson, & Chaikind, 1989). Fox, Rejeski, and Gauvin (2000) found that enjoyment during physical activity is optimized when a positive and supportive leadership style is coupled with an enriched and supportive group environment. Instructors spend many hours preparing music, organizing the class flow, and selecting equipment, when, in fact, working on establishing a comfortable atmosphere can be just as important to participants. Try greeting participants as they enter the class, learn their names, or move the teaching platform to different parts of the room. If mirrors are utilized during the workout, it is important to face the participants when possible throughout the class to make direct eye contact. Looking at people through a mirror does not promote true interaction.

Instructors also need to realize that what they do and say has an impact on the class atmosphere. According to Goleman (2005), having "emotional intelligence" in any group

setting dictates the success of the group experience. Goleman believes that "the emotional economy is the sum total of the exchanges of feeling among us. In subtle (or not so subtle) ways, we all make each other feel a bit better (or a lot worse) as part of any contact we have; every encounter can be weighted along a scale from emotionally toxic to nourishing." A specific example of this within a group exercise setting would be announcing before class how great it feels to be in a group exercise class to improve overall health and well-being. Contrast this with telling an overeating indulgence story and stating specific intentions to "work it off" during the class. The first statement leaves participants with a health-related sense of purpose for the workout. The second statement can send a message that punishment through exercise is recommended after overindulging. Sending positive health messages throughout the group exercise experience is important for establishing the "emotional atmosphere" of the workout and utilizing the role-model aspect of teaching in a positive way.

An environment where instructors present a "body beautiful" can also be rather intimidating. Crawford and Eklund (1994) compared similar video exercise routines, with the instructor wearing a thong in one and the same instructor wearing shorts and a T-shirt in another. "High physique-anxious" participants rated the thong video more unfavorably than the shorts and T-shirt video. Instructors can help participants become more comfortable with their own bodies and keep them exercising by wearing a variety of exercise clothing. A study of 148 female fitness instructors at an instructor conference found that 64% of instructors perceived an ideal body as one that was thinner than their current body (Nardini, Raglin, & Kennedy, 1999). The average percent body fat of the instructors was 20.5%; the national average for this age group is 23.1%. Instructors' body-image perceptions are just that—perceptions. Perceptions can be changed, and this begins with the fitness instructor's self-awareness (Evans & Kennedy, 1993). If instructors are to make an impact on the health and well-being of participants, it will be important to address this issue on a personal level. Finally, be aware of the impact of the physical environment. Ginis, Jung, and Gauvin (2003) found that regardless of body-image concerns, women in mirrored environments felt worse after exercising than women in nonmirrored environments.

Physical-fitness Assessments

In most class situations, it is likely that group fitness instructors will be teaching new participants or individuals who attend sporadically. These circumstances make it difficult to measure participants' fitness through physical assessments, because the instructor has no control over the exercise program and follow-up testing. Additionally, many instructors are unknowledgeable about physical-fitness testing because conducting assessments is not a common practice. Furthermore, the format of a typical group fitness class does not allow instructors the freedom to use valuable class time for the performance of physical-fitness tests.

Despite the challenges facing instructors regarding the practice of conducting physical assessments in their classes, all fitness professionals should be aware of common exercise testing procedures and their role in a comprehensive exercise program. Developing skills in physical-fitness testing will be an overall advantage because it will help an instructor understand how to mea-

sure the important components of health-related fitness (i.e., cardiorespiratory endurance, flexibility, and muscular strength and endurance) and track participants' progress during a program. These skills will also become more useful as the trend of short-term group exercise programming takes hold. Many commercial fitness facilities and recreational community programs offer classes limited to time frames lasting six to eight weeks. In these situations, it is very likely that the same group of participants who started the program will also finish the program. These short-term programs lend themselves to physical-fitness testing, as long as it is made clear to participants that pre- and post-program fitness assessments will take place.

There are several good reasons to conduct physical-fitness assessments in the group fitness setting. First, performing pre-program baseline measurements, followed by reassessments using the same testing protocols, is one of the best ways to develop motivation in new exercise participants. Reports of high satisfaction are more likely when participants are able to look back to see how far they have come and see the extent of their fitness development. Second, fitness tests act as feedback. That is, what can be measured can also be managed. Performance feedback from periodic fitness assessments provides valuable data that let a participant know if he or she is on track to achieve the exercise-program goals. Third, fitness tests act as points of reference for program design. If the results of a battery of physical assessments reveal an area of fitness that is particularly lacking, the participant can work to improve the deficient area to enhance overall performance. Finally, being able to provide fitness-

Group Exercise Program Design

assessment services to participants sets an instructor apart from other group fitness instructors who do not have this skill set and shows that the instructor is a professional concerned about the safety and effectiveness of the participants' exercise programs.

When administering a battery of physical-fitness tests within one class period, it is important to sequence the order of the tests so that the effects of the previous tests have minimal impact on the performance of the subsequent tests. For example, the appropriate ordering of tests for a group fitness class would be cardiorespiratory endurance, muscular fitness, and finally flexibility.

Fitness Assessments and Health-related Components of Fitness

The following fitness-assessment tests are commonly utilized in a one-on-one setting. It is important to note that proper training is required to perform one-on-one assessments. This training is beyond the scope of this book and beyond the scope of practice of most group fitness instructors. However, being able to answer questions about these tests is important.

Body Composition

Hydrostatic weighing, also known as underwater weighing, is considered the "gold standard" of body-composition assessment. Body density is calculated from the relationship of normal body weight to underwater weight, with percent fat being calculated from body density. Though hydrostatic weighing is more precise and the choice of many researchers, it is often impractical in terms of expense, time, and equipment.

Bioelectrical impedance is another popular method for determining body composition. It is based on the principle that the conductivity of an electrical impulse is greater through lean tissue than through fatty tissue. Reliability using this method is problematic because environmental issues, such as hydration state, temperature, and humidity, can have an impact on the results and are hard to standardize. Assessing body composition via bioelectrical impedance requires minimal technical training with the analyzers, which range widely in price and quality.

Near-infrared (NIR) light interactance is another method of assessing body composition. The FUTREX 5000 is the most popular commercial NIR analyzer available. It emits near-infrared light at two frequencies into the biceps area of the dominant arm. At these frequencies, body fat absorbs the light while lean body mass reflects the light. Although convenient and easy to use, exercise physiologists have reported some problems with prediction errors (Neiman, 2003).

Anthropometric assessments for measuring body composition include circumference measurements using a tape measure, waist-to-hip circumference ratio, and skinfold caliper measurements. Skinfold caliper measurements require special training and are not practical for a group setting. They are therefore recommended for use in a one-on-one setting. It is important to keep in mind that there is a margin of error (plus or minus 3 to 4%) with each skinfold test, and all tests must be compared to identical tests performed by the same tester under identical testing situations for optimum results.

General body-fat percentage categories are listed in Table 6.4. Field tests for measuring body composition within a group exercise setting are discussed later in this chapter. These tests include waist-to-hip circumference and body mass index.

Table 6.4
General Body-fat Percentage Categories

Classification	Women (% fat)	Men (% fat)
Essential fat	10–13%	2–5%
Athletes	14–20%	6–13%
Fitness	21–24%	14–17%
Average	25–31%	18–24%
Obese	32% and higher	25% and higher

Cardiorespiratory Endurance

There are many different tests available for measuring cardiorespiratory endurance. The measurement of maximum oxygen uptake ($\dot{V}O_2$max) assesses the body's ability to take in oxygen via the pulmonary system, transport it via the cardiovascular system, and utilize it via the muscular system. Field tests and submaxi-

mal tests, such as the Rockport walking test or 12-minute walk/run test, indirectly estimate maximum **oxygen uptake.** Tests may vary in complexity from the relatively simple, such as **step tests,** walking tests, or running tests, which estimate $\dot{V}O_2$max, to those that use gas analyzers to measure oxygen uptake. Submaximal bicycle ergometer tests are a popular clinical alternative. These tests use heart-rate response to a given work intensity to predict $\dot{V}O_2$max. The direct measurement of $\dot{V}O_2$max using gas exchange can provide the most accurate results and is considered the gold standard. Direct $\dot{V}O_2$max tests may be prohibitive in cost and are generally not practical for instructors. Maximal oxygen consumption norms for men and women are shown in Table 6.5.

Table 6.5
Norms for Relative Maximal Oxygen Uptake (mL/kg)[2]

| Percentile | Age | | | | |
	20–29	30–39	40–49	50–59	60–69
Men					
90	54.0	52.5	51.1	46.8	43.2
80	51.1	48.9	46.8	43.3	39.5
70	48.2	46.8	44.2	41.0	36.7
60	45.7	44.4	42.4	38.3	35.0
50	43.9	42.4	40.4	36.7	33.1
40	42.2	41.0	38.4	35.2	31.4
30	40.3	38.5	36.7	33.2	29.4
20	39.5	36.7	34.6	31.1	27.4
10	35.2	33.8	31.8	28.4	24.1
Women					
90	47.5	44.7	42.4	38.1	34.6
80	44.0	41.0	38.9	35.2	32.3
70	41.1	38.8	36.7	32.9	30.2
60	39.5	36.7	35.1	31.4	29.1
50	37.4	35.2	33.3	30.2	27.5
40	35.5	33.8	31.6	28.7	26.6
30	33.8	32.3	29.7	27.3	24.9
20	31.6	29.9	28.0	25.5	23.7
10	29.4	27.4	25.6	23.7	21.7

Source: Adapted, with permission, from the *Personal Trainer Workshop Manual*, The Cooper Institute, Dallas, Tex. (revised 2006).
Study population for the data set was predominately white and college-educated. A modified Balke treadmill test was used with $\dot{V}O_2$max estimated from the last grade/speed achieved. The following may be used as descriptors for the percentile rankings: well above average (90), above average (70), average (50), below average (30), and well below average (10).

Group Exercise Program Design

Acquiring $\dot{V}O_2$max, whether it be from an indirect or direct method, is useful for quantifying percentage of workload by utilizing the metabolic equivalent (MET) system. Many cardiovascular machines (e.g., treadmills, elliptical machines, upright bikes) list METs on their display boards. With group exercise classes gravitating to this environment, it is important to have a basic understanding of the use of METs. The metabolic equivalent system is a simplified system for classifying physical activities in which one MET is equal to resting oxygen consumption, which is approximately 3.5 milliliters of oxygen per kilogram of body weight per minute (3.5 mL/kg/min). Maximal aerobic capacity is measured in mL/kg/min. Therefore, if $\dot{V}O_2$max was estimated to be 42 mL/kg/min, this number could be divided by 3.5 to obtain maximum METs, or 12 METs. Working at 50% of 12 METs would be 6 METs. A cardiovascular machine could then be set at 6 METs to accomplish this workload. This is one practical example of why cardiovascular testing can be useful for training in a group setting using cardio equipment. An instructor can also use a step test. A step test would be a good group test to administer to educate group exercise participants about their cardiorespiratory-fitness level in a more typical group exercise setting.

Muscular Strength and Endurance

Muscular strength and muscular endurance are two components of muscular-fitness testing. Muscular strength is the amount of force a muscle can produce in a single maximal effort. Muscular endurance is a muscle's ability to exert a force repeatedly over time. Tests to measure muscular strength include the one-repetition maximum (1 RM) test using weight equipment to overload, and isometric strength tests, which are usually done in a one-on-one setting. The grip-strength test using a hand dynamometer is also used to measure strength. The pull-up and the flexed arm hang are two muscular-endurance tests used by the President's Council on Physical Fitness. The YMCA also has a bench press test for muscular endurance. Muscular-endurance tests more commonly used by group fitness instructors are the push-up and half sit-up tests. It would be appropriate to administer these tests in a group setting to educate participants about the importance of muscular strength and endurance and to compare results over time to assess improvement.

Flexibility

Flexibility is defined as the range of motion around a joint or set of joints. Flexibility affects both health and fitness. Inflexibility increases the risk for joint and muscle injury, while excessive flexibility can lead to joint instability. There is no single flexibility test that predicts range of motion for all joints of the body. Therefore, each joint must be assessed individually. Flexibility testing is usually performed in a one-on-one setting using a goniometer to measure degrees of flexibility. These tests are often performed on an athletic training bench. The field tests covered in this chapter—sit-and-reach, or low-back and hamstrings flexibility, and shoulder flexibility—work well within a group exercise setting. Including field-test assessments in a group exercise setting is one way to establish an atmosphere of care and concern for the participants, as well as help them identify the health benefits of group exercise.

Field Tests for Group Fitness Instructors

Waist-to-hip Circumference

Waist-to-hip measurements are an easy way to teach participants about the risks associated with body-fat distribution. Provide a basic tape measure and instruct students on how to perform a waist-to-hip measurement appropriately. The waist measurement is the smallest waist circumference below the rib cage and above the umbilicus, measured while standing with the abdominal muscles relaxed (not pulled in). If there appears to be no "smallest area" around the waist, the measurement should be made at the level of the navel. Hip circumference is defined as the largest circumference of the buttocks–hip area taken while the person is standing. The waist-to-hip ratio is quick, easy, and focuses students on where they carry their body fat and whether this is a risk factor for diseases of the heart, diabetes, and some types of cancer (Figures 6.1 and 6.2; Table 6.6).

Body mass index (BMI) is another way to estimate body composition that is quick, easy, and does not require equipment or training. Of course, strictly speaking, BMI does not estimate body composition. Instead, it attempts to determine whether an individual is obese and how much their health risks are increased with increasing obesity. It is calculated as follows:

BMI = Weight in kilograms divided by height in meters squared

See Tables 6.7 and 6.8 for an example and reference chart. This test is a good one to include in a newsletter or handout for group exercise participants to do at home. Caution should be used whenever using total body weight instead of taking into

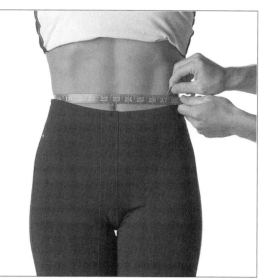

Figure 6.1
Abdominal circumference

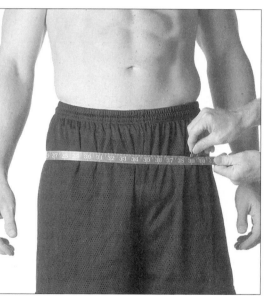

Figure 6.2
Hip circumference

Table 6.6
Waist-to-hip Ratios and Associated Levels of Health Risk

Classification	Men	Women
High risk	>1.0	>0.85
Moderately high risk	0.90–1.0	0.80–0.85
Lower risk	<0.90	<0.80

Adapted from Van Itallie, T.B. (1988). Topography of body fat: Relationship to risk of cardiovascular and other diseases. In: *Anthropometric Standardization Reference Manual*. Champaign, Ill.: Human Kinetics.

Group Exercise Program Design

Table 6.7
Body Mass Index Example

$$BMI = \frac{Weight\ (kg)}{Height^2\ (m)}$$

Convert weight from pounds (lb) to kilograms (kg) by dividing weight in lb by 2.2

Weight = 140 lb $\frac{140}{2.2} = 63.6$ kg

Convert height from inches to centimeters (cm), and then to meters (m), by multiplying height in inches by 2.54 and then dividing by 100:

Height = 58 inches
58 x 2.54 = 147.3 cm $\frac{147.3}{100} = 1.47$ m

$$BMI = \frac{63.6}{1.47^2} = 29.4$$

Table 6.8
Body Mass Index Reference Chart

Weight Category	BMI Range
Underweight	<18.5
Normal weight	18.5–24.9
Overweight	25.0–29.9
Grade I Obesity	30.0–34.9
Grade II Obesity	35.0–39.9
Grade III Obesity	>40

account fat and lean body weight. More muscular, athletic types may be calculated as overweight when in fact they simply have a lot of lean body weight. This is a major limitation of BMI testing.

Cardiorespiratory-fitness Testing

Maximal and submaximal exercise tests using the treadmill or bicycle ergometer are not well-suited for measuring the cardiorespiratory fitness of groups. In the group fitness setting, field tests for measuring cardiorespiratory endurance, such as the YMCA Submaximal Step Test, are more

appropriate because they are easy to administer, practical, inexpensive, and less time-consuming than the treadmill and bicycle ergometer tests. One important consideration for administering a cardiorespiratory field test with a group of individuals is that participants must be taught how to accurately measure their heart rates, which is covered later in this chapter.

YMCA Submaximal Step Test

Developed by Dr. Fred Kasch of San Diego State University, this three-minute step test requires participants to step on and off a 12-inch-high step bench to a standardized cadence. Although this test does not result in an estimation of maximal oxygen consumption, it gives an estimation of cardiorespiratory fitness in comparison to established norms.

Required items:
Step bench (12 inches in height)
Metronome set at 96 bpm
Stopwatch

Procedure:
Participants should perform a light warm-up prior to testing. Before beginning the test, demonstrate the correct stepping procedure. Set the metronome to 96 bpm and start stepping to a four-beat cycle (up, up, down, down). Both feet should come in complete contact with the top of the bench during the up portion of the cycle and touch the floor during the down portion of the cycle. Allow participants an opportunity to practice the movement cycle along with the metronome. It is acceptable for participants to change the lead foot during the test. Just before administering the test, notify participants that they will step continuously for three minutes and be seated immediately afterward for a one-minute pulse count.

Place the metronome in a location where it may be easily heard by all participants. Have the class start by simply marching on the floor in front of the bench to the rhythm provided by the metronome. Remind participants that they may use either foot to start the cycle and instruct them to begin stepping as the stopwatch is started. Check their stepping rhythm throughout the test and announce when one minute, two minutes, and two minutes and 30 seconds has elapsed. Immediately after completing three minutes of stepping, participants should be instructed to sit down on their benches and count their pulses for one minute. The one-minute post-exercise heart rate is used to score the test (Tables 6.9 & 6.10).

Muscular Strength and Endurance Testing

Group fitness instructors can measure participants' dynamic muscular fitness using calisthenic-type strength and endurance tests. These tests are based on specific exercises, such as the half sit-up and the push-up, and require the participant to perform a maximum number of repetitions for each exercise during the assessment.

Push-up Test

The push-up test is used to evaluate upper-body muscular strength and endurance (e.g., pectoralis major, anterior deltoids, triceps). The protocol calls for two different positions based on the sex of the

Table 6.9
Post-exercise Heart-rate Norms for the Three-minute Step Test (Men)

Rating	% Rating	Age (years)					
		18–25	26–35	36–45	46–55	56–65	66+
Excellent	100	50	51	49	56	60	59
	95	71	70	70	77	71	74
	90	76	76	76	82	77	81
Good	85	79	79	80	87	86	87
	80	82	83	84	89	91	91
	75	84	85	88	93	94	92
Above average	70	88	88	92	95	97	94
	65	90	91	95	99	99	97
	60	93	94	98	101	100	102
Average	55	95	96	100	103	103	104
	50	97	100	101	107	105	106
	45	100	102	105	111	109	110
Below average	40	102	104	108	113	111	114
	35	105	108	111	117	115	116
	30	107	110	113	119	117	118
Poor	25	111	114	116	121	119	121
	20	114	118	119	124	123	123
	15	119	121	124	126	128	126
Very poor	10	124	126	130	131	131	130
	5	132	134	138	139	136	136
	0	157	161	163	159	154	151

Source: *YMCA Fitness Testing and Assessment Manual* (4th ed.). © 2000. Reprinted and adapted with permission of the YMCA of the USA, 101 N. Wacker Drive, Chicago, Ill. 60606.

Group Exercise Program Design

Table 6.10
Post-exercise Heart-rate Norms for the Three-minute Step Test (Women)

Rating	% Rating	Age (years)					
		18–25	26–35	36–45	46–55	56–65	66+
Excellent	100	52	58	51	63	60	70
	95	75	74	77	85	83	85
	90	81	80	84	91	92	92
Good	85	85	85	89	95	97	96
	80	89	89	92	98	100	98
	75	93	92	96	101	103	101
Above average	70	96	95	100	104	106	104
	65	98	98	102	107	109	108
	60	102	101	104	110	111	111
Average	55	104	104	107	113	113	116
	50	108	107	109	115	116	120
	45	110	110	112	118	118	121
Below average	40	113	113	115	120	119	123
	35	116	116	118	121	123	125
	30	120	119	120	124	127	126
Poor	25	122	122	124	126	129	128
	20	126	126	128	128	131	129
	15	131	129	132	132	135	133
Very poor	10	135	134	137	137	141	135
	5	143	141	142	143	147	145
	0	169	171	169	171	174	155

Source: *YMCA Fitness Testing and Assessment Manual,* © 2000. Reprinted and adapted with permission of the YMCA of the USA, 101 N. Wacker Drive, Chicago, Ill. 60606

participant. Men are required to perform the test in the standard position with the hands and toes in contact with the floor. Women are required to use the modified position with the hands and knees in contact with the floor. Women who choose the standard push-up position (i.e., with the hands and toes in contact with the floor) must be notified that their scores will not be comparable to the standardized norms because the data represented in the norm table were produced from research using only the modified position for women.

Required items:

Exercise mat

Rolled towel (approximately 3 inches in height)

Procedure:

Participants should perform a light warm-up prior to testing. However, if this test follows a cardiorespiratory-fitness test, participants may proceed without a warm-up. A rolled towel should be placed on the center of the mat. Review the correct counting procedure—the push-up is complete when the chest touches the towel and returns to the start position with arms fully extended. Inform them of the proper breathing technique—to exhale with the exertion (when pushing away from the floor). Have participants assume the proper push-up position with the hands at, or slightly wider than, shoulder-width apart and their chests centered above the towel. Allow them to practice the push-up if they would like. Instruct them to begin the test by flexing the elbows and lowering the chest to the towel. This modified technique, which limits the depth of elbow flexion to 3 inches above the mat, has been provided to allow participation by more individuals. The traditional protocol (i.e., lowering the chest to the floor) puts undue stress on the glenohumeral joints, especially for individuals with a history of shoulder dysfunction. The score is the total number of push-ups completed without rest before the client reaches exhaustion (Table 6.11).

Half Sit-up or Partial Curl-up Test

The half sit-up test is used to evaluate abdominal muscle strength and endurance. It was developed to replace the traditional full sit-up test so that potential low-back problems could be eliminated and to better assess abdominal muscle function.

Required items:
Exercise mat
Stopwatch
Tape
Ruler
Metronome set at 50 bpm

Procedure:
Participants should perform a light warm-up prior to testing. However, if this test follows a cardiorespiratory-fitness test, participants may proceed without a warm-up. Place two strips of masking tape parallel to each other on a mat 10 cm apart. Review and demonstrate the proper half sit-up technique. Assume a supine position with the feet flat on the floor, shoulders relaxed, and knees flexed at approximately 90 degrees. The arms are at the sides, palms facing down with the middle fingers of each hand touching the first strip of masking tape. Alternative hand positions include: (a) having the hands held across the chest or (b) placing

Table 6.11
Push-up Test Fitness Categories

Gender	Age 20–29 M	20–29 F	30–39 M	30–39 F	40–49 M	40–49 F	50–59 M	50–59 F	60–69 M	60–69 F
Excellent	36 or more	30	30	27	25	24	21	21	18	17
Very Good	35	29	29	26	24	23	20	20	17	16
	29	21	22	20	17	15	13	11	11	12
Good	28	20	21	19	16	14	12	10	10	11
	22	15	17	13	13	11	10	7	8	5
Fair	21	14	16	12	12	10	9	6	7	4
	17	10	12	8	10	5	7	2	5	2
Needs improvement	16 or fewer	9	11	7	9	4	6	1	4	1

Source: The Canadian Physical Activity, Fitness, & Lifestyle Approach (3rd ed.). © 2003. *CSEP-Health & Fitness Program's Health-related Appraisal and Counseling Strategy* Reprinted with permission from the Canadian Society for Exercise Physiology.

the hands on the thighs and curling up until the hands reach the knee caps. Instruct participants that regardless of the hand position chosen, elevation of the trunk to 30 degrees is the important aspect of the movement.

Set the metronome to 50 bpm and instruct participants to perform slow, controlled curl-ups to lift the shoulder blades off the mat (the trunk makes a 30-degree angle with the mat) in time with the metronome (i.e., 25 curl-ups per minute). If using the tape method, instruct them to curl the upper spine until the fingertips touch the second strip of tape. Finally, instruct them to return to the original position with the shoulders touching the mat.

Place the metronome in a location where it may be easily heard by all participants. Allow participants an opportunity to practice the movement along with the metronome. Inform participants of the correct counting procedure—one curl-up is counted each time their shoulders return to the mat. Instruct participants to begin curling the trunk as the stopwatch is started. The score

169

Group Exercise Program Design

is the number of curl-ups performed in one minute (maximum of 25) without pausing (Table 6.12).

Table 6.12
Half Sit-up Test Fitness Categories

Norms for Men

Ages	20–29	30–39	40–49	50–59	60–69
Excellent	25 or more	25 or more	25 or more	25 or more	25 or more
Very Good	21–24	18–24	18–24	17–24	16–24
Good	16–20	15–17	13–17	11–16	11–15
Fair	11–15	11–14	6–12	8–10	6–10
Needs Improvement	10 or fewer	10 or fewer	5 or fewer	7 or fewer	5 or fewer

Norms for Women

Ages	20–29	30–39	40–49	50–59	60–69
Excellent	25 or more	25 or more	25 or more	25 or more	25 or more
Very Good	18–24	19–24	19–24	19–24	17–24
Good	14–17	10–18	11–18	10–18	8–16
Fair	5–13	6–9	4–10	6–9	3–7
Needs Improvement	4 or fewer	5 or fewer	3 or fewer	5 or fewer	2 or fewer

Source: The Canadian Physical Activity, Fitness, & Lifestyle Approach (3rd ed.). © 2003. *CSEP-Health & Fitness Program's Health-related Appraisal and Counseling Strategy* Reprinted with permission from the Canadian Society for Exercise Physiology.

Flexibility Testing

Evaluating participants' ranges of motion using flexibility tests is a great way to determine areas of the body that may need an emphasis on stretching. Stiff, inflexible muscles and joints pose a risk for injury and may adversely affect the performance of the simplest tasks. Inflexibility due to disuse, improper body alignment, or repetitive-task exposure is commonly seen in the areas of the hamstrings, lower back, and shoulders. To address these areas, two tests, the sit-and-reach test and the shoulder-flexibility test, will be covered.

Sit-and-Reach Test

The sit-and-reach test is used to assess low-back and hip-joint flexibility. Due to the possibility of injury to the low back and hamstrings, participants should refrain from fast, jerky movements during this assessment. Instead, they should perform the test trials slowly and with control. Participants with a history of low-back dysfunction and/or pain should avoid performing this test.

Required items:
Exercise mat
Tape
Yardstick
Procedure:
Participants should perform a light warm-up prior to testing. However, if this test follows a cardiorespiratory-fitness test, participants may proceed without a warm-up. Additional light stretching of the low back and hamstrings (e.g., modified hurdler stretch) is recommended before test administration. Place a yardstick on the floor and put a piece of tape at least 12 inches long on the 15-inch mark on the yardstick. Review and demonstrate the proper execution of the test. With the shoes off, sit on the floor with the yardstick parallel between extended legs. The zero mark of the yardstick should be toward the body. The feet should be placed approximately 12 inches apart with the heels aligned with the tape at the 15-inch mark. Extend the arms in front of the chest and place one hand on top of the other, with fingertips aligned. Inhale in the upright position and exhale while leaning forward, dropping the head toward or between the arms. The fingers should maintain contact with the yardstick and knees should remain in full extension (Figure 6.3).

Instruct participants to begin the test by slowly reaching forward with both hands as far as possible, holding this position for approximately two seconds. Remind them to keep their hands parallel and not to lead with one hand. The score is the farthest point on the yardstick reached after three trials (Table 6.13).

Shoulder-flexibility Test

This test measures the multirotational components of the shoulder joints. Participants with a history of shoulder dysfunction and/or pain should avoid performing this test.

Required items:

Measuring tape or ruler

Procedure:

Participants should perform a light warm-up prior to testing. However, if this test follows a cardiorespiratory-fitness test, participants may proceed without a warm-up. Instruct participants to sit or stand with the right arm extended straight up, letting the elbow bend so the hand comes to rest, palm down, between the shoulder blades. Next, have them reach behind the back with the left arm so the palm is facing up. Participants should attempt to bring the fingertips of both hands together behind the back. Repeat the test on the other shoulder. Scoring is based on the distance, if any, between the fingertips (Table 6.14).

Presenting the Results

An effective way to inform group fitness class participants of their physical-performance rankings is to have charts displaying the standardized norms for each test either hanging on the wall in a poster format or distributed in the form of a class handout. This method allows the individual to rank his or her performance without publicly discussing it with the instructor. However, for students who enjoy competition, publicly displaying their performance rankings and fitness goals can

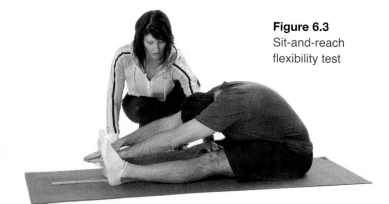

Figure 6.3
Sit-and-reach flexibility test

Table 6.13

Norms for Trunk-Flexibility Test Fitness Categories

	Men					
Ages	18–25	26–35	36–45	46–55	56–65	>65
% Rating						
90	22	21	21	19	17	17
80	20	19	19	17	15	15
70	19	17	17	15	13	13
60	18	17	16	14	13	12
50	17	15	15	13	11	10
40	15	14	13	11	9	9
30	14	13	13	10	9	8
20	13	11	11	9	7	7
10	11	9	7	6	5	4

	Women					
Ages	18–25	26–35	36–45	46–55	56–65	>65
% Rating						
90	24	23	22	21	20	20
80	22	21	21	20	19	18
70	21	20	19	18	17	17
60	20	20	18	17	16	17
50	19	19	17	16	15	15
40	18	17	16	14	14	14
30	17	16	15	14	13	13
20	16	15	14	12	11	11
10	14	13	12	10	9	9

Table 6.14
Evaluation of Shoulder Flexibility

Flexibility	Characteristics
Good	The fingers can touch.
Fair	The fingertips are not touching, but are less than 2 inches apart.
Poor	The fingertips are more than 2 inches apart.

Source: Adapted from Krepton, D. & Chu, D. (1984). *Everybody's Aerobics Book*. Oakland: Star Rover House. Reprinted with permission.

have a very motivating effect. Ideally, participants should have an option of whether to make their scores public or to keep the information private. In either situation, the instructor should educate the class about how to rank their performance scores based on normative data and what each ranking means. This facilitates effective goal-setting for both the instructor and the participant.

Follow-up Testing

Measurable fitness changes usually take a minimum of four weeks. Therefore, the first follow-up testing session is typically administered four to 12 weeks following the onset of exercise training.

Class Format

The next challenge is to take the student-centered approach to group exercise instruction into the development of the overall class format. No single class format is appropriate for every type of group exercise class. In a step class it is very appropriate to warm up using the steps; however, in a kickboxing class it would be more appropriate to practice kickboxing moves during the warm-up segment than to use a bench. Thermoregulation is important in an aquatic exercise class, so performing static stretches to enhance flexibility at the end of the workout may not be appropriate because participants can get cold. It may be suitable to perform some static stretching in the warm-up segment of a low-impact class for seniors, but not necessarily for young children. A 15-minute abdominal class may not even contain stretching, since the purpose of the class is confined to abdominal strengthening. These are just a few examples of why the same

class format may not be appropriate for all group exercise classes.

Here is a closer look at the general principles involved in each segment of group exercise—**pre-class preparation,** warm-up, cardiorespiratory, muscular strength and endurance, and flexibility/cool-down. These general principles apply to all types of group exercise, including hi/lo impact, step, aquatic exercise, indoor cycling, kickboxing, and sports conditioning.

Typically, most group exercise classes begin with pre-class preparation followed by a warm-up, which includes using specific movements to prepare for the cardiorespiratory activity. These movements are performed at a low-to-moderate speed and range of motion. They are also designed to specifically warm up the body for the activity to follow and to increase blood flow to the muscles. The cardiorespiratory segment that follows the warm-up is aimed at improving cardiorespiratory endurance and body composition and keeping the HR elevated for 10 to 30 minutes. Following the cardiorespiratory workout, a gradual cooldown reduces the HR toward resting levels and prevents excessive pooling of blood in the lower extremities. A muscular strength and endurance segment can also be included either before or after the **cardiorespiratory segment**, depending on the activity. The class ends with a flexibility/cool-down component that includes stretching and relaxation exercises designed to further lower HR, help prevent muscle soreness, and enhance overall flexibility.

In "fusion" classes, the segments might include 30 minutes of indoor cycling followed by 30 minutes of strength work. These classes may be combined or offered individually. Regardless of format, the focus should be on providing a safe and effective workout that addresses the health-related components of fitness.

Offering Options

Notice how the four components—warm-up, cardiorespiratory endurance, muscular strength and endurance, and flexibility—common to most group fitness classes are similar to the health-related components of fitness. It is important to note that the emphasis given to each aspect will vary depending on the objective of the class as well as the fitness level, age, health, and physical skill of its participants. It is difficult to schedule a specific type of group exercise class to meet everyone's needs. For example, putting beginners with advanced participants can be challenging for instructors. Therefore, calling a yoga class that features 30 minutes of activity "yoga-30" is helpful for beginners, while another class called "yoga-60," which features 60 minutes of activity, will attract more advanced participants. The number-one reason people do not exercise is lack of time, so it's a good idea to let participants know the duration of each session. Beginning classes should be shorter in duration and focus on less-intense movements; the skills needed to perform the cardiorespiratory segment also need to be basic. Using words like "complex movement patterns" to describe longer-duration sessions that contain more skills for the cardiorespiratory segment would help the advanced exerciser locate an appropriate class. Keep in mind that participants may walk to work in the morning and only need a flexibility or muscular strength and conditioning class. Offering different options and not staying with the typical hour-long format that encompasses all components is likely to meet more people's health goals.

Pre-class Preparation

There are a few common principles in the pre-class preparation for any group exercise class. They are listed below and will be reviewed in this section.

Ideally, the instructor:

- Knows participants' health histories and surveys new participants (see Chapter 5)
- Is available before class and orients new participants
- Discusses and models appropriate attire and footwear
- Has music cued up and equipment ready before class begins
- Acknowledges the class and introduces him- or herself
- Previews class format and individual responsibilities
- Brings fluids to classes and encourages participants to do the same

Know the Participants

Chapter 5 provided an in-depth review on acquiring health information and discussed waivers. It is important to note that the information gathered from these sources needs to be transferred into making a safe and effective class. For example, if two participants say they have occasional lower-back pain, incorporating abdominal and low-back strengthening as well as hamstring stretching into the class format on a regular basis would help their conditions. Make sure participants are aware that the time they took to fill out the health information form was worthwhile by asking questions and informing them about any modifications that have been made to the class as a result. Of course, some modifications will need to be explained directly to an individual participant if it is not appropriate to address the issue with the entire class.

Group Exercise Program Design

Orient New Participants

A professional, student-centered group fitness instructor takes the time to meet and orient new participants as well as be available if any participants have questions. Participants tend to respond more sincerely to questions, such as, "Who has been to an indoor cycling class three times or less?" rather than, "Who has never been to indoor cycling?" This orientation is such an important part of customer service, and it is also a time when instructors get the most feedback about the class in general. Instructors need to learn to be open to input and also take the time to get to know new participants. This is a part of continuing to establish a positive, comfortable class environment and is also essential to the adherence of the participant.

Choose Appropriate Attire

It is important that an instructor's attire be appropriate for the specific group exercise class. For example, when teaching a senior class, it would not be appropriate to wear a midriff outfit, as it might be intimidating. Observe what the participants wear to class and try to match their attire so they will feel more comfortable. Ask what attire they prefer. However, as a fitness professional, try to balance the comfort level of the class with functional wear. Correct spinal alignment and form should be visible with each movement that an instructor demonstrates. Make sure to notice and discuss appropriate footwear for the various group exercise classes. For example, some indoor cycles have cageless pedals that require specific cycling shoes for the workout. Encourage first-time step-class participants to wear cross-training shoes with adequate cushioning rather than running shoes that may catch on the tracked platform. Finally, in aquatic exercise, it is important to note that a regular swimsuit often does not provide adequate support to perform water exercise effectively. Be ready to supply new participants with information on where to locate appropriate shoes and attire for your classes.

Prepare Equipment

With all the different "toys" available for group exercise (e.g., stability balls, handheld weights, resistance bands, balance devices, weighted bars, yoga blocks), it's important to be prepared ahead of time and inform participants about what equipment will be used. Posting a note close to the entrance of the room to inform participants which equipment will be used also works well. Consider playing welcoming music before the beginning of class and always make sure to have music cued and the microphone ready to go. It is also important to use good quality tapes/CDs and plan for minimal changes to have a better class flow. Prior preparation can make the actual class run much more professionally.

Acknowledge Class Participants

Creating a positive attitude and atmosphere begins with the instructor making sure to welcome people before class begins and introducing him- or herself, especially when teaching in a facility where different people come to class every week and there is no set class list. For example, "Hi, my name is Mary. Welcome to the 45-minute strength class. Always check out the board to see what equipment we will be using in class."

This concept may sound minor, but it establishes an attitude of "we're in this together." Also, if participants are aware of the instructor's name, they will be more likely to come up and ask questions afterward. New people coming to a group exercise class are often afraid to ask questions or may feel out of place. Understanding this and asking for feedback will create a more open, safe environment for all participants, not just the ones who come to class every week.

Preview Class Format

An overview of the specific class format should accompany the instructor introduction. With so many different classes being offered, people often find themselves in the wrong class, which they may not realize until halfway through. Therefore, make sure to introduce the class format before each class begins. For example, "This is a 30-minute stretching class. There will not be an aerobic component to it." After previewing the class format, it is also important that the instructor makes participants understand their individual responsibilities. There is nothing worse than having a participant come up after class and say, "That workout wasn't hard enough." Intensity is the responsibility of the participant, not the instructor. It is your responsibility to make sure that modifications are given for various intensities to allow participants to make a choice. Encourage, demonstrate, and promote various exercise choices so participants are comfortable working at their own pace. This is one of the most important aspects of a group exercise class.

Warm-up

There are a few common principles behind the warm-up for any group exercise class. They are listed below and will be reviewed in this section.

- The beginning segment must include an appropriate amount of dynamic movement.
- The warm-up should focus largely on rehearsal moves.

- All the major muscle groups (if appropriate) must be stretched after a dynamic warm-up; stretches are held briefly (five to 10 seconds).
- Verbal directions should be clear and the volume, tempo, and atmosphere created by the music must be appropriate.

Appropriate Dynamic Movement

The purpose of the warm-up is to prepare the body for the more rigorous demands of the cardiorespiratory and/or muscular strength and conditioning segments by raising the internal temperature. For each degree of temperature elevation, the metabolic rate of cells increases by about 13% (Astrand & Rodahl, 2003). In addition, at higher body temperatures, blood flow to the working muscles increases, as does the release of oxygen to the muscles. Because these effects allow more efficient energy production to fuel muscle contraction, the goal of an effective warm-up should be to elevate internal temperatures 1 or 2° F, so that sweating occurs.

Increasing body temperature has other effects that are beneficial for exercisers as well. The potential physiological benefits of the warm-up include:

- Increased metabolic rate
- Higher rate of oxygen exchange between blood and muscles
- More oxygen released within muscles
- Faster nerve impulse transmission
- Gradual redistribution of blood flow to working muscles
- Decreased muscle-relaxation time following contraction
- Increased speed and force of muscle contraction
- Increased muscle elasticity

Group Exercise Program Design

- Increased flexibility of tendons and ligaments
- Gradual increase in energy production, which limits lactic-acid buildup
- Reduced risk of abnormal heart rhythms

Many of these physiological effects may reduce the risk of injury because they have the potential to increase neuromuscular coordination, delay fatigue, and make the tissues less susceptible to damage (Alter, 2004). Therefore, the overall focus of the warm-up period should be to increase core body temperature, which can be accomplished by including appropriate dynamic movement.

Rehearsal Moves

Blahnik and Anderson (1996) define rehearsal moves as "movements that are identical to, but less intense than, the movements your students will execute during the workout phase." Anderson (2000) believes rehearsal moves should make up the majority of the warm-up, thus preparing participants mentally and physically for the challenges of the workout ahead. Examples of rehearsal moves include utilizing the bench to warm up during a step class, teaching participants how to hill climb briefly in an indoor cycling class, performing one water interval segment to prepare for the cardiorespiratory water interval-training segment, or using light weights in the warm-up to prepare for a muscle-conditioning class. The whole concept of rehearsal moves relates to the principle of specificity of training. This principle states that the body adapts specifically to whatever demands are placed on it.

Durstine and Davis (American College Sports Medicine, 2006) believe that specificity applies not only to energy systems and muscle groups, but also to movement patterns. Since motor units used during training demonstrate

the majority of physiological adaptations, movement patterns must also be specifically trained. In a group exercise session, one of the main reasons participants become frustrated is that they are not able to perform the movements effectively. Introducing these movement patterns in the warm-up will assist with waking up associated motor units.

Utilizing rehearsal moves in the warm-up not only specifically warms up the body for the movement ahead, but also can serve as a time to set down some neuromuscular patterns by introducing new skills. For example, in a hi/lo class where a grapevine half-turn movement is performed, use the warm-up to break down the move, identify the directional landmarks in the room, and name the specific move. Thus, when a grapevine half-turn is referred to in the cardiorespiratory segment, the class participants will know what to do. The same idea applies to a difficult skill in a kickboxing class such as a side kick movement pattern. Practice this side kick slowly, using the music at half tempo in the warm-up when maintaining a higher level of intensity is not the main focus. When the side kick comes up in the routine, it will have been "rehearsed," and this will make it easier for participants to maintain their cardiorespiratory intensity level. Rehearsal moves, therefore, ought to make up a large part of the warm-up.

Stretches, if Appropriate

To stretch or not to stretch during the warm-up is a much-debated issue, and there is no consensus in the current scientific literature. Taylor et al. (1990) found that gains in flexibility were most significant when a stretch was held for 12 to 18 seconds and repeated four times per muscle group. Another study found that stretching the hamstrings for 30 seconds produced significantly greater flexibility than stretching for 10 seconds (Walter, Figoni, & Andres, 1995). If these two studies were the complete story, stretching in a group exercise warm-up would probably not be recommended, since it is impossible to stretch a muscle group four times and hold it for 30 seconds and still accomplish the goal of warming up. Yet, another study looking at strength and flexibility training in older adults found that stretching before and after strength training did not increase flexibility when resistance training was involved (Girouard & Hurley, 1995). Finally, a literature review conducted by the Centers for Disease Control and Prevention (CDC) in 2004 found insufficient evidence to conclude that pre-exercise stretching prevented injuries. However, the CDC stated that "the evidence is not of sufficient strength, quality, and generalizability to recommend altering or eliminating pre-exercise stretching" (Thacker et al., 2004).

Most prominent exercise-leadership books (Neiman, 2003; Howley & Franks, 2003; McArdle, Katch, & Katch, 2006) and stretching books (Alter, 2004) recommend an active warm-up with rehearsal moves followed by brief stretching with a focus on the warm-up; enhancing flexibility should be reserved for the cool-down portion of the workout. While there is no conclusive evidence showing any inherent benefit to stretching during the warm-up, there are no studies to show that it is dangerous. With this in mind, the warm-up should contain mostly warm-up movements. If static stretches are included, they ought to be held briefly (five to 10 seconds) to lengthen the muscle in preparation for activity.

In terms of organizing a group exercise class format for the warm-up segment, perform several rehearsal movements and, if static stretches are included, try to focus on active movement as well. For example, while performing a standing hamstring stretch, keep the upper body moving with triceps extensions to stay warm. In a cycling class, keep the legs pedaling and perform some upper-body stretches. When teaching a 30-minute session, it might be better to save the stretching for the end when it will be most beneficial in terms of enhancing flexibility. In this situation, it might not be appropriate to do static stretching. When teaching a 60-minute class, in which there is more time for the warm-up segment, actively contract the hamstrings and then stretch them briefly for optimum effectiveness. A group of seniors, however, might prefer warming up and then performing several minutes of static stretching. For seniors, balance is also an issue. After they have warmed up, they can hold a stretch for increased flexibility. By the end of the class, fatigue may keep them from being able to perform static stretches appropriately.

Instructors are in the best position to know their participants and determine what is best for them. The decision on how to go about warming up and stretching is an individual one. It is definitively known that flexibility is a health-related component of fitness and needs to be included in the workout. Whether it is at the end of the workout, in the middle, or during the warm-up should be a choice made by the instructor based on feedback from the participants until more definitive research on the topic has been conducted. It is known that optimum flexibility is achieved at the end of the workout, and dynamic movement should be performed before any static stretching in the warm-up.

Use of Music

Many group exercise classes utilize music as a way to motivate participants and create more overall enjoyment in the experience. Several research studies have validated the

Group Exercise Program Design

idea that music is beneficial from a motivational standpoint (Gfeller, 1988; Boutcher & Trenske, 1990). In terms of using music to create a beat to follow, research has found that external auditory cues, such as rhythmic music and percussion pulses, favorably affect coordinated walking and proprioceptive control (Staum, 1983). Kravitz (1994) found that subjects regularly report that they believe their performance is better with music accompaniment. Moving to the beat of the music is not always necessary in a group exercise setting. In fact, some yoga and outdoor group exercise sessions do not even use music. However, while using the beat is important in most kickboxing, step, and hi/lo classes, music is often used as background sound to help motivate or set a mood in classes such as cycling, boot camp, and aquatic exercise. Keep in mind that even in a "beat-driven" step class, participants may benefit by sing-along, less beat-driven music during the strength or stretching segments. Also, in an indoor cycling class, the warm-up music might be something to sing along with that does not contain a lot of hard drums or fast-paced tempos. The mood the music establishes helps create and control the individual segments of the class.

It is important to balance music and verbal cueing. Music that is so loud that the verbal cueing is not heard can be a problem for participants. Seniors especially need to be asked about the volume of the music, as they often have the most opinions and feedback about volume. IDEA (1997) published an opinion statement on the volume of music based on standards established by the United States Occupational Safety and Health Administration (OSHA). It stated that music intensity during group exercise classes should measure no more than 90 decibels (dB) and, since the instructor's

voice needs to be about 10 dB louder than the music to be heard, the instructor's voice should measure no more than 100 dB. A decibel meter can be purchased at a local electronics store for less than $50. It is worth the investment because music volume is a common source of complaints for participants. According to Long and colleagues' (1998) study on voice problems among group fitness instructors, 44% of instructors surveyed experienced partial or complete voice loss during and after instructing. They also had increased episodes of voice loss, hoarseness, and sore throat unrelated to illness since they began instructing. To protect the voice of instructors, it is also important to have a microphone system available.

Cardiorespiratory Segment

There are a few common principles behind the cardiorespiratory segment of most group exercise classes. They are listed below and will be reviewed in this section.

A group fitness instructor should:
- Promote independence/self-responsibility
- Gradually increase intensity
- Give impact and/or intensity options
- Build sequences logically and progressively
- Incorporate exercises that target a variety of muscle groups
- Use music to create a motivational atmosphere
- Monitor intensity through HR and/or ratings of perceived exertion (RPE) checks
- Incorporate a post-cardio cool-down/ stretch segment

Promote Self-responsibility

Whether teaching a Pilates, group treadmill, or a boot camp class, it is impossible to be everywhere or help everyone simultaneously. Each participant is working at a different fitness level and has different goals. Ideally, it would be nice if all classes could be organized according to intensity and duration levels. The reality is that many participants come to a class because the time is convenient, not necessarily because the class length or intensity level is suitable. If participants try to exercise at the instructor's level or another participant's level, they may work too hard and sustain an injury or they may not work hard enough to meet their goals.

To help promote independence and self-responsibility, encourage participants to work at their own pace, use HR monitoring or RPE checks, and inform them how they should be feeling throughout the class. For example, during the peak portion of the cardiorespiratory segment, let them know that they should feel out of breath. During the postcardio cool-down, tell them that they should feel their HRs slowing down. Be as descriptive as possible about perceived exertion throughout the workout. Also, it is important to demonstrate high-, medium-, and low-intensity options to teach the class at various levels. Help participants achieve the level of effort they want to reach and continually remind them that this is their responsibility—the instructor cannot be responsible for participants' exercise intensity levels. Pointing out participants who work at higher or lower levels can also help. It is recommended that you maintain a medium intensity most of the time, but that you also present other options and intensities as the need arises. Mastering this concept is the true "art" of group exercise instruction and the reason why group exercise leadership is more difficult than one-on-one training.

Gradually Increase Intensity

Even though the human body adapts to exercise very efficiently, gradually increasing intensity is necessary for the following physiological reasons:

• It allows blood flow to be redistributed from internal organs to the working muscles.

• It allows the heart muscle time to adapt to the change from a resting to a working level. The hardest and most dangerous time for changes in the heart's rhythm is in the transition from resting to high-intensity work or from high-intensity activity back to resting levels. At rest, the cardiovascular system circulates about 5 liters of blood per minute. Imagine the contents of two-and-a-half 2-liter soft drink containers circulating through the body every minute. At maximal strenuous exercise, the increase in workload requires as much as 30 to 40 liters per minute to accommodate working muscles.

• It allows for an increase in respiratory rate. Remember that the diaphragm, the major muscle involved in breathing, is like any other muscle and needs time to shift gears. Without time to warm up properly, a rapid increase in breathing results in side aches and hyperventilation (rapid, shallow breathing). Some hyperventilation is a part of beginning exercise, but sudden increases in breathing mean that the transition into the cardiorespiratory segment was not gradual enough.

For example, to gradually increase intensity during a hi/lo class, reduce the size of the movements in the first few minutes, and travel less. In a step class, keep moves less intense by avoiding propulsion-type moves. In an aquatic exercise class, use moves that have a smaller range of motion or shorter lever length. Finally, in an indoor cycling class, keep the flywheel tension set at a lower resistance for the first few minutes.

Group Exercise Program Design

Impact and/or Intensity Options

In most group exercise classes, movement selection can increase impact and/or intensity. It is your job to make sure that this increase is balanced and appropriate for the participants. For example, in a boot camp or sports-conditioning class, you may elect to jump with both feet back and forth over lines on the floor. This is a high-impact movement. The next movement selection might then be a more moderate-impact movement like a brisk walk around the room. Impact is not as much an issue in an indoor cycling class, where intensity options become more important. For example, a hill climb out of the saddle at a high resistance that lasts longer than three minutes is considered a higher-intensity option. This might be followed by a lower-resistance seated movement. All group exercise sessions have movements that can vary impact and intensity. It is important to take this into consideration when choosing movement **combinations** and segments.

Building Sequences

Building sequences involves taking complex moves and breaking them down into smaller parts. In a hi/lo class, for example, building sequences logically would include teaching a group a grapevine move for the first time by breaking down the movement. Perform two step touches to the right followed by two step touches to the left. Then perform the same step touches, only this time step behind to make a grapevine move. In a complex choreography step class, this might mean teaching a complex series by breaking it down into segments of eight counts and then adding on until a series of four groups of eight counts is completed. Progressing properly in an aquatic exercise class would mean marking a specific move by performing it, then increasing the speed of movement, traveling with the move, and then resisting the movement. If sequences are logically and progressively put together, there is a certain "flow" to the class that makes participants want to come back. Participants know when the flow is not there—they usually end up standing and watching, feeling confused while doing the movement, or executing it improperly.

Target a Variety of Muscle Groups

Instructors often have base moves (a series of movements that appear over and over again in their routine) within the cardiorespiratory segment. These base moves often involve the use of the quadriceps and hip flexor muscle groups. Examples include the basic march in place, walk around the room, and the basic step. Many participants use these muscle groups exclusively in daily living activities; therefore, continuing to use the quadriceps and hip flexors repeatedly during exercise is unnecessary. Striving to balance daily flexion with other movements is important.

Although it is impossible to individualize within a group exercise setting, understanding how the body functions in daily movement can help instructors determine which muscles are stronger and which muscles need to be focused on during group exercise. For example, walking forward works the hip flexors. Focusing on movement selection that utilizes the hamstrings (the opposing muscle group to the hip flexors) would help with muscle balance. The abductors are important stabilizer muscles for posture. Incorporating some abductor moves within the cardiorespiratory segment is recommended. In aquatic exercise, muscle balance is automatically achieved since there is no gravity. If the hip is flexed in water, the iliopsoas and rectus femoris perform the work. When the hip is extended in the water, the hamstrings perform the work. On land, this movement would be an eccentric contraction of the quadriceps. With the exception of aquatic exercise, it is important to analyze what movements work which muscle groups and vary the selection to promote overall muscle balance.

Music

Most group exercise classes that contain a cardiorespiratory segment use music to motivate and inspire participants. Always ask participants about their preference for music. Just as many personal trainers make the mistake of giving "their" personal workout to potential clients, group fitness instructors often choose music that is motivating to them. Although it is important that music motivate the instructor, it is imperative that it motivate the participants. With the wide array of commercial tapes/CDs available, it is easy to find a variety of music. Take formal and informal surveys of participants' preferences to get feedback on music. Probably one of the most time-consuming parts of teaching group exercise is finding good music. However, it is worth the time, since music can make or break the experience for the participants. It is recommended that an instructor use pre-arranged fitness-specific workout tapes/CDs for group exercise classes.

Methods of Monitoring Cardiorespiratory Intensity

Monitoring exercise intensity within the cardiorespiratory segment is important. Participants need to be given instruction regarding the purpose of monitoring HR during exercise and information on how to obtain a **pulse rate.** Proper instruction on how to take the HR is the first step to monitoring intensity effectively. The following are a few recommended sites for taking the heart rate:

Carotid pulse *site.* This pulse is taken from the carotid artery just to the side of the larynx using light pressure from the fingertips of the first two fingers. Remember, never palpate both carotid arteries at the same time and always press lightly (Figure 6.4a).

Radial pulse *site.* This pulse is taken from the radial artery at the wrist, in line with the thumb, using the fingertips of the first two fingers (Figure 6.4b).

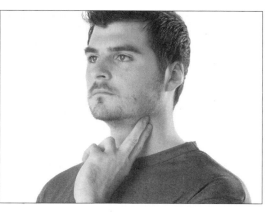

Figure 6.4a
Carotid heart rate monitoring

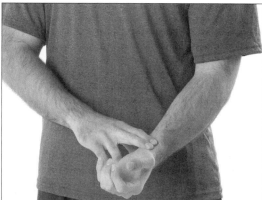

Figure 6.4b
Radial heart rate monitoring

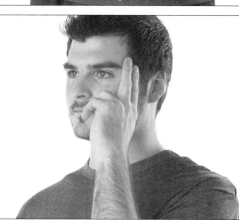

Figure 6.4c
Temporal heart rate monitoring

181

Group Exercise Program Design

Temporal pulse *site.* This pulse can sometimes be obtained from the left or right temple with light pressure from the fingertips of the first two fingers (Figure 6.4c).

Understanding the effective use of HR, RPE, the dyspnea scale, and the **talk test** is the next step in effectively monitoring exercise intensity. One method is not advocated over another, as all have applications depending on the type of activities participants will be performing during the group exercise class. However, research on group exercise has determined that HR taken in hi/lo classes represent a lower relative exercise intensity ($\dot{V}O_2$max) than that of running (Parker et al., 1989). Other research on different forms of group exercise (step, interval hi/lo, and progressive treadmill training) concluded that HR may not be an appropriate predictor of exercise intensity and that RPE is the preferred method (Roach, Croisant, & Emmett, 1994).

Many HR research studies were performed on runners and cyclists rather than group exercise participants. In a treadmill class or an indoor cycling class, use of HR monitors can be effective. However, in a kickboxing class, where arms and legs are moving in many different directions, RPE might be a better choice. Finally, there is research suggesting that utilizing HR in aquatic exercise in which the chest is submerged is not an appropriate technique (Frangolias & Rhodes, 1995). There is no one method that works for all different group exercise sessions or participants. It may be appropriate to utilize HR monitoring for beginners or advanced participants, but to use RPE more on a day-to-day basis. Many group fitness instructors have stopped using manual HR monitoring because it disrupts the flow of the class. Using HR monitors is always an option as well. There are no hard-and-fast rules for monitoring intensity other than that it

is an important responsibility of the group fitness instructor. Not monitoring intensity or failing to give constant intensity-monitoring gauges shows a lack of empathy for participants and may compromise their safety. A summary of how to use target HR, RPE, dyspnea scale, and the talk test is given below.

Percentage of Maximal HR

The percentage of maximal HR method is a very common and easy-to-calculate way to determine target HR. To use this method, **maximal heart rate** (HRmax) must first be determined from either a maximal stress test or the age-adjusted **maximal HR formula:**

Estimated maximal HR = 220 – age in years

The validity of the "220 – age" formula has been questioned, and its use as the sole method of determining HRmax should be avoided. Instead, use this formula in combination with the perceived exertion scale. Also, if a participant is taking medication that alters HR (e.g., beta blockers), measured maximal HR and/or RPE should be used. Target heart rate (THR) is calculated by taking a percentage of HRmax and adjusting it by about 15% to better reflect

Table 6.15
Using Percentage of Maximal HR to Determine Target Heart Rate (THR) Range

Example: 38-year-old participant who wants to exercise at 60–90% of HRmax:

Maximal HR = 220 – age

220 – 38 = 182 maximal HR x 0.60 to 0.90 = THR range

182	182
x 0.60	x 0.90
109	163.8 = 164

THR = 109–164
Corrected THR range =
1.15 (THR) = 1.15 (109–164) = 125–189

aerobic capacity or maximal oxygen uptake (Table 6.15). The formula is:

$$THR = (HRmax \times percent\ intensity\ desired) \times 1.15$$

Percent of HR Reserve

Another method to determine THR range is to use a percentage of HR reserve, which is found by using what is commonly known as the Karvonen formula. The recommended percent of HR reserve (50 to 85%) corresponds to a similar percent of maximal oxygen uptake (50 to 85%). This method differs from the HRmax method in that the **resting heart rate** is taken into account when determining THR. As in the HRmax method, the measured heart-rate response and/or RPE must be used in this method when the participant is taking prescribed medications that alter HR.

The key to this method is to take a percentage of the difference between maximal HR and resting HR (i.e., the heart-rate reserve), then add the resting HR to identify the THR. The reserve capacity of the heart reflects its ability to increase the rate of beating and cardiac output above resting levels to maximal intensity (Table 6.16). Current ACSM guidelines state

---

Table 6.16
Using HR Reserve (Karvonen's formula)
to Determine Target HR Range

220 – 38 years old=182		
Maximal heart rate (220-age)	182	182
minus resting heart rate (RHR)	−70 (RHR)	−70 (RHR)
	112	112
x 0.50 to 0.85	x .50	x .85
	56	95.2
+ RHR	+ 70 (RHR)	+70 (RHR)
= Target HR range	126	165.2=165

Target HR range = 126–165

---

that HR reserve is only a "guideline" used in setting exercise intensity (American College of Sports Medicine, 2006). That is why it is important to give participants an appropriate range of intensity to work within.

Ratings of Perceived Exertion (RPE)

Using RPE is another common method of determining exercise intensity. Based on subjective perceptions of intensity, clients rate the level of steady-state work, using the 6 to 20 RPE scale or 0 to 10 RPE scale developed by Borg (1998). Interestingly, RPE is both valid and reliable and is closely associated with increases in most cardiorespiratory parameters, including work, **maximal oxygen uptake,** and HR (Dunbar et al., 1992; Robertson et al., 1990). In a group exercise setting, RPE can be used independent of, or in combination with, HR to monitor relative exercise intensity of most participants. It must be understood that participants on medication that alters HR can use the RPE scale to monitor relative exercise intensity. The verbal description that reflects the intensity of work is important when using either numerical RPE scale (Table 6.17). For example, on the 6 to 20 scale, sitting at a desk is considered a 6 or 7, walking to the store is an 11, while beginning to breathe hard is a 13, and chasing a dog down the street is a 15. Relating real tasks in life with RPE helps participants understand how they should feel.

Dyspnea Scale

Dyspnea refers to difficulty in breathing or shortness of breath. The dyspnea scale is a subjective score that reflects the relative difficulty of breathing as perceived by the participant. Accordingly, this numerical scale can assist in monitoring exercise intensity:

+1 Mild, noticeable to participant, but not to observer

Group Exercise Program Design

Table 6.17
Category and Category-ratio Scales for Ratings of Perceived Exertion

RPE	Category Ratio Scale*	
6	0	Nothing at all
7 Very, very light	0.5	Very, very weak
8	1	Very weak
9 Very light	2	Weak
10	3	Moderate
11 Fairly light	4	Somewhat strong
12	5	Strong
13 Somewhat hard	6	
14	7	Very strong
15 Hard	8	
16	9	
17 Very hard	10	Very, very strong
18	*	Maximal
19 Very, very hard		
20		

Source: Adapted, with permission, from American College of Sports Medicine (2006). *ACSM's Guidelines for Exercise Testing and Prescription* (7th ed.). Philadelphia: Lippincott Williams & Wilkins.

+2 Mild, some difficulty that is noticeable to observer

+3 Moderate difficulty, participant can continue to exercise

+4 Severe difficulty, participant must stop exercising

The use of this scale is for participants who have pulmonary conditions (asthma, emphysema) and those who feel limited due to breathlessness. Participants should be instructed to use the scale as a guide to their exercise intensity and in conjunction with HR and RPE. Instructors should caution participants who use this scale to reduce their intensity levels when breathing becomes labored (+3). If the severity of the pulmonary condition seems to worsen over time, instructors should consult with the participant's physician and recommend a more appropriate exercise setting.

Talk Test

The talk test is another subjective method of gauging exercise intensity that can be used as an adjunct to HR and RPE. When participants exercise, it is highly recommended that breathing be rhythmic and comfortable. Particularly for newer clientele, talking while exercising can indicate whether an appropriate intensity is being achieved. If the participant is "winded" and gasps for breath between words when conversing, then the exercise intensity is too high and should be reduced. As higher-intensity activities are performed, it is expected that breathing rate will become faster and shallower. For higher fitness levels, the use of the talk test may not be appropriate.

Application of Intensity Monitoring to the Group Exercise Setting

Whether using target HR, RPE, the dyspnea scale, or the talk test to monitor exercise intensity, there are a few practical-application points to remember:

- If using music and measuring HR, turn off the music so the music beats do not influence the counting of heart beats.
- Peripheral pulses are encouraged over the use of the carotid pulse; if using the carotid pulse, press lightly.
- Check intensity toward the middle of the workout so the workout can be modified.
- Keep participants moving to prevent blood from pooling in the lower extremities when checking intensity (a slight stepping motion is enough).
- Utilize a 10-second pulse count if using target HR.
- Give modifications based on results and encourage participants to work at individual levels.

Incorporate a Post-cardio Cool-down and Stretch Segment

The last few minutes of any group exercise session that contains cardiorespiratory work should be less intense, to allow the cardiorespiratory system to recover. Because metabolic waste products get trapped inside the muscle cells, many people experience increased cramping and stiffness if they do not cool down gradually. Cooling down enables waste products to disperse and the body to return to resting levels without injury. It is also important to cool down to prevent blood from pooling in the lower extremities and to allow the cardiovascular system to make the transition to less-intense workloads. This is especially important if some type of muscle work will follow the cardiorespiratory segment. Encourage participants to relax, slow down, keep the arms below the level of the heart, and put less effort into the movements. Using less driving music, changing the tone of voice, and verbalizing the transition to the participants can create this atmosphere. Performing some static stretches at the end of this segment also works well. Participants often run off to their next commitment or go into the strength-and-conditioning area to perform muscle work, so they may risk missing the flexibility segment of the class if it is not included in this portion of the class format.

Muscular Strength and Endurance Segment

There are a few common principles in the muscular strength and endurance segment of most group exercise classes. They are listed below and will be reviewed in this section.

A group fitness instructor should:
- Promote muscle balance, functional fitness, and proper progression
- Maintain proper form and observe participants' form and suggest modifications for injuries and special needs
- Give verbal, visual, and physical cues on posture/alignment and body mechanics
- Use equipment (toys) safely and effectively
- Create a motivational and instructional atmosphere

Encourage Muscle Balance, Functional Fitness, and Proper Progression

Meeting the muscular strength and endurance needs of participants in a one-on-one personal-training setting is relatively easy. The program can be tailored directly to the participant, which gives personal trainers a distinct advantage. How, then, does a group fitness instructor determine which muscle groups to work and why during the muscular strength and endurance segment of the class format? Knowing how the body functions in daily movement can guide appropriate exercise selection for muscle groups that are not normally used in the daily routine.

Think of the group exercise class as an opportunity to balance out work from daily living. Stretching and strengthening muscles that are not regularly used can help improve participants' overall muscle balance. This approach brings the group fitness instructor's role closer to that of individualized trainer (Yoke & Kennedy, 2004).

For a summary of what muscles need strengthening and stretching for improved health, see Table 6.18. This table was created by analyzing the muscles most people use for routine living. For example, people normally pick things up using elbow flexion, which works the biceps concentrically (on the up phase). They then put things down working the biceps eccentrically (on the down phase)

185

Group Exercise Program Design

against gravity. Because of gravity, the triceps do not get worked a lot in daily living. In aquatic exercise, however, the same example would produce a concentric contraction of the biceps on elbow flexion and a concentric contraction of the triceps on elbow extension due to the relative absence of gravity in the water. Keep in mind that the list in Table 6.18 is for functional daily living for participants who are exercising for health and fitness. This does not mean the stronger muscles should not be worked in a group exercise setting; however, the instructor's focus needs to be on balancing the use of weaker muscle groups and stronger muscle groups.

Selecting exercises during the muscular strength and endurance segment can be a challenge. The wide variety of equipment and innovations available make it easy to get creative with exercise selection, but those choices must meet the needs of par-

ticipants. For example, triceps dips on a stability ball would not be a good choice for a beginning strength class. This is a very complex exercise that would not be appropriate for all participants. Many complex exercises need to be reserved for one-on-one training. If one person cannot perform the exercise properly, be sure to move closer and offer assistance or change the exercise. Select exercises that are more intermediate and then give options on the lower and higher end to make them easier or more difficult.

Instructor Responsibilities

Instructors are often selected because they naturally have excellent form. For example, potential hi/lo instructors are often picked from among the front-row participants who regularly attend class. Cyclists often instruct indoor cycling classes. It is important to note that "having" the skill and "teaching" the skill are two different things. Instructors who have good form may need instruction on teaching effective cueing for the skills they naturally have, whereas those instructors who need help developing good form may more readily be able to explain what good form looks like. As an instructor, it is essential to have good alignment in all exercises demonstrated, especially for the benefit of the visual learners in the class.

One of the most important differences between a teacher-centered instructor and a student-centered instructor is that a student-centered instructor can and will help participants with individual needs to make exercise safe and less painful or problematic. To facilitate this, an instructor must know the problems and limitations of participants and observe what the participants are doing. For example, if a participant has tight hamstrings and occasionally talks of back pain, he or she may deviate from the demonstrated exercise

Table 6.18
Key Muscles

Muscles that need strengthening
Anterior tibialis
Hamstrings
Rhomboids/middle trapezius
Pectoralis minor/lower trapezius
Shoulder external rotators (teres minor and infraspinatus)
Triceps
Latissimus dorsi
Gluteals
Posterior deltoid

Stabilizers that need strengthening
Erector spinae
Abductors
Adductors
Abdominals

Muscles that need stretching
Gastrocnemius
Quadriceps/iliopsoas
Upper trapezius
Pectoralis major
Hamstrings
Sternocleidomastoid
Anterior/medial deltoids

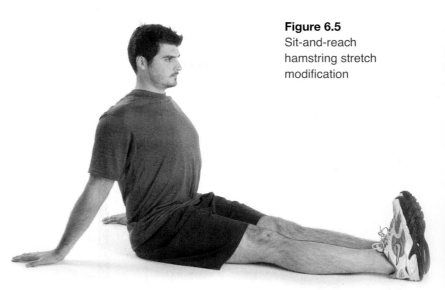

Figure 6.5
Sit-and-reach
hamstring stretch
modification

as shown in Figure 6.5. Verbalizing a modification that involves putting the hands back to support the back and then slowly inching the hands forward shows that the instructor is properly observing each participant's form and suggesting adaptations for special needs.

The point of this example is to encourage all group fitness instructors to get out on the floor and observe and assist, not just during the warm-up stretch segment but during the entire workout. Demonstrate a move, perform a few repetitions, and then get up and begin watching participants. Another option is to occasionally move around the room while demonstrating the movement. Staying in one place only gives one frame of reference to participants. Plus, being a coach is a large part of the group exercise experience. In general, when the instructor is nearby and observing, participants' listening skills and exercise technique improve. The skill of being a coach applies to all segments of the class format and needs to be evaluated throughout the class. It is important to allow participants to see that the instructor has empathy.

Verbal, Visual, and Physical Cues on Posture/Alignment

Eight out of 10 Americans will have back problems during their lifetime; therefore, it is essential to give verbal cues on posture/ spinal alignment in each segment of the class and in every movement during the muscular strength and endurance segment. Here are some points to remember when teaching posture in a standing position. (The numbers below correspond to those in Figure 6.6.)

1. The head should be suspended (not pushed back or dropped forward) with the ears in line with the shoulders, shoulders over hips, hips over knees, and knees over ankles.

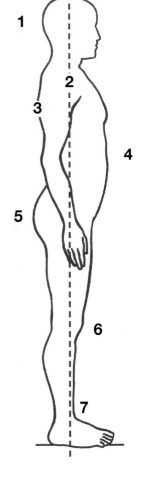

Figure 6.6
Visual cues on
posture/alignment

2. The arms should be suspended and hanging from the shoulders. Have participants circle the shoulder back and down. The arms should hang at the lowest point.

3. Participants must maintain the three natural curves of the spine. A decrease or increase in the low-back curve changes the amount of compression the spine can withstand.

4. Have the participants lightly compress the abdominal muscles to help support the spinal column, especially with lifting. Compression helps to distribute weight over the entire torso, not just the low back. Extreme compression, however, restricts breathing.

5. The hips can be tucked slightly, particularly for individuals with exaggerated lumbar lordosis, pregnant women, and participants with a large, protruding abdominal area.

6. The knees should be unlocked or soft. Hyperextended knees shift the pelvis, contributing to an increased low-back curve and back strain, along with decreased blood flow to and from the legs.

7. The feet should be shoulder-width apart with the weight evenly distributed. Participants who roll their feet to the inner or outer edges need to concentrate on keeping their weight over the entire bottom surface of each foot.

8. An imaginary plumb line dropped from the head should pass through the cervical and lumbar vertebrae, hips, knees, and ankles.

Giving appropriate verbal, visual, and physical cues is one of the most important aspects of the muscular strength and endurance segment. As a general rule, in most exercises, the stabilizers will be engaged. Give several posture cues (e.g., chin up, chest out, tighten the abdominal muscles) before giving instruction on the specific muscle group to be worked. For example, when performing a standing biceps strengthening exercise using resistance tubing, cue participants to soften the knees, get a good base of support with the feet apart comfortably, and contract the abdominals while keeping the spine in a neutral position. Then go on to cue the movement for the biceps.

A closer look at verbal, visual, and physical cues will reveal that there is more than one way to communicate and direct movement. Verbal cues include cueing movements with appropriate terminology and instruction. For example, when performing a standing outer-thigh leg lift to strengthen the gluteus medius, the following verbal cues could be included:

• Ask participants to contract the stabilizers.

• Give appropriate posture cues.

• Remind participants that the range of motion of the movement is around 45 degrees, so they should lift with the side of the heel. If the toe comes up, hip flexion occurs, and the already strong quads/hip flexor muscles become more activated. It is important to key into the muscle being worked for maximum effectiveness.

• Keep the movements slow and controlled and alternate sides to promote better participant comfort and balance.

Visual cues include the instructor's form. It is imperative that, when the verbal cues are given, the instructor also performs the movement effectively. In the above example, if the instructor is saying to keep the movement in a 45-degree range of motion, but is lifting higher than that, it is confusing to the participants. Whatever instructions are given need to be mimicked in the movement example by the instructor. Practice is one of the only ways to become good at being an effective visual demonstrator.

Physical cues are another way to give feedback to participants on their form. To give physical cues, it is important to walk around the room and actually observe participants. A good motivator/educator rarely is at the front of the class, but is instead moving around and observing participants from different angles. Most physical cues in group exercise classes are given by the instructor for the participants to perform, since the instructor cannot help everyone at once. For example, when leading an abdominal curl-up exercise with the elbows behind the head, it is important to cue "elbows out to the side." If the participant can see his or her elbows, the pectorals are also being worked. Walk around to check on this and visually demonstrate proper alignment.

These are just a few ways to give feedback to participants regarding proper form. It is important to note what style of communication comes easiest to the participant: verbal, visual, or physical. Working on the area that is most difficult for the participants will help the instructor improve. Giving and getting feedback is another important key to learning and growing. Fitness professionals who give a lot of feedback and ask participants for feedback on a regular basis are providing good customer service. It is important to practice student-centered instruction as opposed to teacher-centered instruction, especially in the area of verbal cues.

Utilize Equipment Safely and Effectively

Portable resistance-training equipment such as resistance tubing, stability balls, hand-held weights, and weighted bars are

to group exercise what toys are to children. They make the class more fun and provide the ability to overload the muscles in a more effective, individualized way. Some instructors actually refer to them as "toys" and the group exercise experience as "play." The most important part of having equipment is to make sure it is appropriate for various ability levels. Post information and tell participants to work at their own levels. Be sure to get information and education on any new equipment. Many vendors advertise their product as the "best, most effective" device. Only instructors and participants can determine this. Analyze the need for extra equipment and be sure to test it properly before introducing it to the class. Keeping the muscular strength and endurance segment separate from the aerobic portion is also important, unless it is an interval- or circuit-style class. Research has shown that the addition of light hand-held weights to the aerobic segment of a traditional hi/lo (Blessings et al., 1987; Yoke et al., 1988) and a step class (Kravitz et al., 1997) does not significantly increase energy expenditure. Therefore, it is recommended that instructors do not use, nor instruct others to use, hand-held weights during the aerobic segment to enhance cardiorespiratory fitness.

Create a Motivational and Instructional Atmosphere

Using music and/or the music beat during the muscular strength and endurance segment is optional. For example, a musical tempo of 130 beats per minute is too fast for leading abdominal crunches. Always slow the tempo down to half tempo to gain control first. Then, go to the full musical tempo. Choose music that does not have a lot of vocals so

Group Exercise Program Design

that cueing words can be heard and understood. A tempo of 110 to 120 beats per minute will enhance safe and effective movement. Reduce the volume of the music and set a tone that is more focused than that of the aerobic segment. Outlined below are some general cues for muscular-endurance exercises:

- Participants must perform each exercise slowly, smoothly, and with control.
- Have participants key into the muscle group being worked and try to relax other body parts.
- Tell participants to stop when they feel tired or change to the other side or alternate sides as desired.
- Correct form is more important than the number of repetitions, keeping to the music tempo, or the amount of resistance used.
- Participants must learn to concentrate on breathing and work to exhale on the effort and inhale on the relaxation portion.

Flexibility Segment

There are a few common principles in the flexibility segment of most group exercise classes. They are listed below and will be reviewed in this section.

- Stretching of major muscle groups is performed in a safe and effective manner.
- Relaxation and visualization concludes the flexibility segment.

Stretching

As mentioned earlier in this chapter, it is important to stretch the muscle groups that have been used in the group exercise activity as well as muscles that are commonly tight. For instance, after an indoor cycling class, stretching the quads, calves, and hamstrings makes sense because they are major muscles used for cycling. In a kick-boxing session it is important to stretch the muscles that surround the hip, as they are used in kicking movements. The stronger muscle groups people use all day for daily living activities (calves, hamstrings, pectorals, hip flexor, anterior deltoids) should also be stretched.

How long should the stretches be held? Shrier and Gossal (2000) suggested performing one static stretch per major muscle group and holding the stretch for 15 to 30 seconds. The ACSM guidelines (2006) suggest performing static stretches for 15 to 30 seconds, two to four repetitions per muscle group, a minimum of two to three days per week. It is not always possible to perform four repetitions. However, if leading a stretching-only class, this would be the ideal.

There are precautions for stretching. Ballistic (bouncing) stretching and passive overstretching can be potentially dangerous. Although certain athletic populations may benefit from ballistic stretching, ballistic stretches have been shown by some researchers to be significantly less effective than other stretching methods (Wallin et al., 1985). Passive overstretching and ballistic stretching initiate a stretch reflex. Special receptors within the muscle fiber detect sudden stretches (muscle spindles) and excessive stretching (Golgi tendon organ) of the muscle. There is a complicated and continual interplay between opposing muscle groups that leads to precision of control and coordinated movement. During this interplay, if a muscle is activated by a sudden stretch or if continued overlengthening of the muscle fiber occurs, the system stimulates the muscle to contract rather than lengthen and maintains the contraction to oppose the force of excessive lengthening.

Simply put, if a person overstretches or bounces a stretch, then the muscle shortens to protect itself. Keep pulling on a shortened muscle and it will either cramp up or rip and tear—but it will not lengthen. This process is often referred to as the myotatic stretch reflex. Keep in mind that this is an involuntary reflex that people do not have control over. It all happens at the spinal cord level and individuals cannot mentally override it, no matter how hard they try.

Therefore, stretching should be comfortable. Encourage proper form by using cues like "move to the position where you can feel the muscle pull slightly, then hold; your muscles should not feel like a rubber band ready to snap; find a comfortable stretch and hold; if you are shaking, then back off the intensity of the stretch." Also, as an instructor it is important to model average flexibility so that participants do not imitate form they cannot match. As with any other activity, it is important to progress participants appropriately. Yoga is a good example of an activity that has many high-risk stretches. They are taught progressively, however, so the body adapts to them over time. Putting some of these yoga moves into a traditional group exercise setting can be dangerous.

Reminding participants of proper posture throughout stretching helps to promote overall body stability and balance, and enhances the effectiveness of the stretching experience. At least two to three verbal cues are needed on every stretch to make sure body positioning is effective. For example, in a standing hamstring stretch, it is important to cue to tilt the pelvis anteriorly to lengthen the hamstring muscles (Figure 6.7). Sullivan, Dejulia, and Worrell (1992) performed a study on anterior and posterior pelvic tilt positioning using two types of stretching techniques and found that the anterior pelvic position was the most important variable for enhancing hamstring flexibility.

Relaxation and Visualization

During a group exercise class, participants have been working hard and increasing the blood flow of nutrients and oxygen to the exercising muscles. Stiffness and muscular tension are now gone. As each minute of the class passes, anxieties, worries, and stressors of the day are released. Participants have switched from logical and calculating functions to operating on spontaneity, with fluid thought. Many ideas come, but no one idea of concern stays in focus as the class progresses. The hardest part for participants is getting to an exercise class. When it is all over they usually feel good about coming. It is this feeling that keeps them coming back. They have taken time to care for themselves and thus taken another step toward healthier living. The relaxation and visualization segment is where the instructor can help participants complete their journeys. Take the last few minutes of every class to let participants experience a few moments of increased relaxation or an opportunity to reenergize before returning to their duties and commitments. These relaxation moments can be structured or free-flowing, philosophical or quiet.

Silence or quiet, slow, soothing music might be enough. Storytelling, guided imagery, or creative visualization might help deepen the sensation as the instructor describes quiet forests, gentle breezes, a warm fire, or a cozy room. Starbursts, bright, intense sunlight, or the power of a wave or waterfall might suggest the energy necessary to continue with the day's activities. Partner massage or group stories,

Group Exercise Program Design

deep breathing, or progressively tightening and releasing muscle groups may help participants find any remaining tensions, areas of pain, or resistance to change. While the participants are receptive, use the time to compliment them on their hard work and reinforce their positive lifestyles or help them perform a mental exercise to increase their levels of self-esteem and personal power. Consider reading inspirational quotes or poetry or announcements about upcoming events. An instructor can let the class in on his or her life outside of class to create a cohesive, family-like atmosphere. Instructors need to find a comfort area and use these last few minutes to end the exercise experience on a high note, allowing participants to take their positive feelings past the allotted time.

Summary

Safe, effective, and purposeful group exercise class design requires knowledge of fitness to help participants achieve their desired gains as well as good psychosocial skills. Outlined below is a summary of the class format segments reviewed in this chapter. Use this checklist as a reminder, as well as a potential evaluation tool. You will need to continually modify the different segments to meet the needs of the ever-changing fitness industry. It is important to know that group exercise carries with it a lot of power if participants feel welcome, learn, improve physically, get to know each other, and feel their time spent was worthwhile. One of the biggest challenges of being an effective group fitness instructor is

Figure 6.7
Standing
stretches

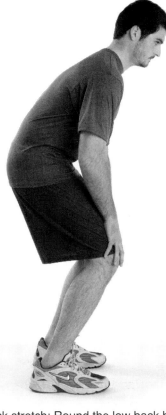

Low-back stretch: Round the low back by using the abdominal muscles to produce an extreme posterior tilt.

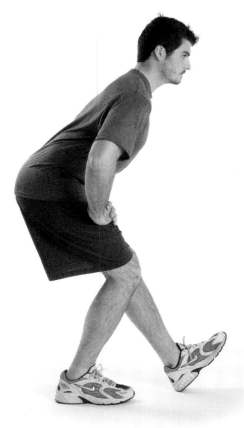

Hamstring stretch: Extend one leg and lean forward, using the hands for support.

being able to balance all of these challenges. It is important that instructors move beyond emphasizing the magnitude of fitness gains and future outcomes and understand that the real power of exercise lies in the experience itself.

Class Format Summary Checklist

Pre-class Preparation

The group fitness instructor:

- Knows participants' health histories and surveys new participants (see Chapter 5)
- Is available before class; orients new participants
- Discusses and models appropriate attire and footwear

- Has music cued up and equipment ready before class begins
- Acknowledges the class and introduces him- or herself
- Previews class format and individual responsibilities
- Brings water to classes and encourages participants to do the same

Warm-up Segment

- Includes an appropriate amount of dynamic movement
- Focuses on rehearsal moves as a large part of the movement selection
- Stretches major muscle groups (if appropriate) after the dynamic warm-up and holds stretches briefly (five to 10 seconds)

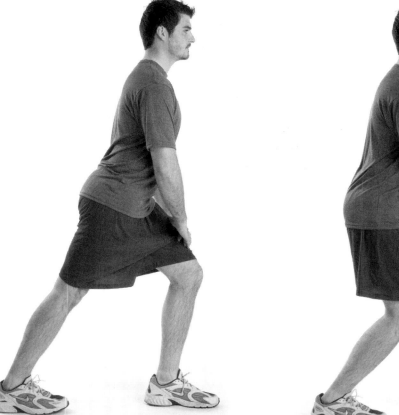

Gastrocnemius stretch: Keep the rear foot straight and the heel on the ground. Shift the body weight forward over the front foot.

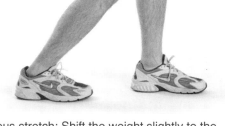

Soleus stretch: Shift the weight slightly to the back and bend the back knee.

- Offers clear verbal directions and ensures that the volume, tempo, and atmosphere created by the music are all appropriate

Cardiorespiratory Segment
- Promotes independence and self-responsibility
- Gradually increases intensity
- Gives impact and/or intensity options
- Builds sequences logically and progressively
- Utilizes a variety of muscle groups
- Uses music to create a motivational atmosphere
- Monitors intensity through HR and/or RPE checks
- Incorporates a post-cardio cool-down and stretch segment

Muscular Strength and Endurance Segment
- Encourages muscle balance and functional fitness
- Uses appropriate form, observes participants' form, and suggests adaptations for injuries and special needs
- Offers appropriate verbal, visual, and physical cues on posture and alignment and body mechanics
- Utilizes equipment (toys) safely and effectively
- Creates a motivational and instructional atmosphere

Flexibility Segment
- Performs stretching of major muscle groups in a safe and effective manner
- Concludes with relaxation and visualization

References

Alter, M. (2004). *Science of Flexibility* (3rd ed.). Champaign, Ill.: Human Kinetics.

American College of Sports Medicine (2006). *ACSM's Resource Manual for Guidelines for Exercise Testing and Prescription* (5th ed.) Philadelphia: Lippincott Williams & Wilkins.

American College of Sports Medicine (2006). *ACSM's Guidelines for Exercise Testing & Prescription* (7th ed.). Philadelphia: Lippincott Williams & Wilkins.

Anderson, P. (2000). The active range warm-up: Getting hotter with time. *IDEA Fitness Edge,* April 6–10.

Astrand, P. & Rodahl, K. (2003). *Textbook of Work Physiology* (4th ed.). New York: McGraw-Hill.

Bain, L., Wilson, T., & Chaikind, E. (1989). Participant perceptions of exercise programs for overweight women. *Research Quarterly,* 60, 2, 134–143.

Blahnik, J. & Anderson, P. (1996). Wake up your warm up. *IDEA Today,* June 1996, 46–52.

Blessing, D. et al. (1987). The physiologic effects of eight weeks of aerobic dance with and without hand-held weights. *American Journal of Sports Medicine,* 15, 5, 508–510.

Borg, G. (1998). *Borg's Perceived Exertion and Pain Scales.* Champaign, Ill.: Human Kinetics.

Boutcher, S. & Trenske, M. (1990).The effects of sensory deprivation and music on perceived exertion and affect during exercise. *Journal of Sport & Exercise Psychology,* 12, 167–76.

Carron, A, Hausenblas, H., & Mack, D. (1996). Social influence and exercise: A meta-analysis. *Journal of Sport & Exercise Psychology,* 18, 1–16.

Crawford, S. & Eklund, R. (1994). Social physique anxiety, reasons for exercise, and attitudes toward exercise settings. *Journal of Sport & Exercise Psychology,* 16, 70–82.

Dunbar, C. et al. (1992). The validity of regulating exercise intensity by ratings of perceived exertion. *Medicine & Science in Sports & Exercise,* 24, 1, 94–99.

Evans, E. & Kennedy, C. (1993). The body image problem in the fitness industry. *IDEA Today,* May, 50–56.

Fox, L., Rejeski, J., & Gauvin, L. (2000). Effects of leadership style and group dynamics on enjoyment of physical activity. *American Journal of Health Promotion,* 15, 5, 277–83.

Frangolias, D. & Rhodes, E. (1995). Maximal and ventilatory threshold responses to treadmill and water immersion running. *Medicine & Science in Sports & Exercise,* 27, 7, 1007–1013.

Gfeller, K. (1988). Musical components and styles preferred by young adults for aerobic fitness activities. *Journal of Music Therapy,* 25, 28–43.

Ginis, M., Jung, M., & Gauvin, L. (2003). To see or not to see: Effects of exercising in mirrored environments on sedentary women's feeling states and self-efficacy. *Health Psychology,* 22, 4, 354–361.

Girouard, C. & Hurley, B. (1995). Does strength training inhibit gains in range of motion from flexibility training in older adults? *Medicine & Science in Sports & Exercise,* 27, 10, 1444–1449.

Goleman, D. (2005). *Working with Emotional Intelligence* (10th ed.). New York: Bantam Books.

Hooker, S. (2003). The exercise/fitness professional's expanding role in promoting physical activity and public health. *ACSM's Health and Fitness Journal,* May/June, p. 7–11.

Howley, E. & Franks, B. (2003). *Health Fitness Instructor's Handbook* (4th ed.). Champaign, Ill: Human Kinetics.

IDEA (2005). 2005 *IDEA Fitness Programs & Equipment Survey.* San Diego, Calif.: IDEA.

IDEA (1997). Recommendations for music volume in fitness classes. *IDEA Today,* p. 50.

Jakicic, J. & Otto, A. (2005). Physical activity considerations for the treatment and prevention of obesity. *American Journal of Clinical Nutrition,* 82, 1, 2265–2295.

Kennedy, C. & Yoke, M. (2005). *Methods of Group Exercise Instruction.* Champaign, Ill.: Human Kinetics.

Kravitz, L. (1994). The effects of music on exercise. *IDEA Today,* October, 56–61.

Kravitz, L. et al. (1997). Does step exercise with handweights enhance training effects? *Journal of Strength & Conditioning Research,* 11, 3, 194–199.

Long, J. et al. (1998). Voice problems and risk factors among aerobic instructors. *Journal of Voice,* 12, 2, 197–207.

McArdle, W., Katch, F., & Katch, V. (2006). *Exercise Physiology* (6th ed.). Philadelphia: Lippincott Williams & Wilkins.

Nardini, M., Raglin, J., & Kennedy, C. (1999). Body image disordered eating: Obligatory exercise and body composition among women fitness instructors. *Medicine & Science in Sports & Exercise,* May Supplement.

Neiman, D. (2003). *Exercise Testing and Prescription* (5th ed.). Mountain View, Calif.: Mayfield Publishing.

Parker, S. et al. (1989). Failure of target heart rate to accurately monitor intensity during aerobic dance. *Medicine & Science in Sports & Exercise,* 21, 2, 230–234.

Roach, B., Croisant, P., & Emmett J. (1994). The appropriateness of heart rate and RPE measures of intensity during three variations of aerobic dance. *Medicine & Science in Sports & Exercise,* 26, 5, (Supplement).

Suggested Reading

Robertson, R. et al. (1990). Cross-modal exercise prescription at absolute and relative oxygen uptake using perceived exertion. *Medicine & Science in Sports & Exercise, 22, 5, 653–659.*

Shrier, I. & Gossal, K. (2000). Myths and truths of stretching. *Physician and Sportsmedicine, 28, 8, 57–63.*

Staum, M. (1983). Music and rhythmic stimuli in the rehabilitation of gait disorders. *Journal of Music Therapy, 20, 69–87.*

Sullivan, M., Dejulia, J., & Worrell, T. (1992). Effect of pelvic position and stretching method on hamstring muscle flexibility. *Medicine & Science in Sports & Exercise, 24, 12, 1383–1389.*

Taylor, D. et al. (1990). Viscoelastic properties of muscle-tendon units: The biomechanical effects of stretching. *American Journal of Sports Medicine, 18, 300–309.*

Thacker, S.B. et al. (2004). The impact of stretching on sports injury risk: A systematic review of the literature. *Medicine & Science in Sports & Exercise, 36, 3, 371–378.*

Tharrett, S. & Peterson, J. (2006). *Fitness Management.* Monterey, Calif.: Healthy Learning.

United States Department of Health and Human Services (1996). *Physical Activity and Health: A Report of the Surgeon General.* Atlanta, Ga. U.S. Department of Health and Human Services, Centers for Disease Control and Prevention, National Center for Chronic Disease Prevention and Health Promotion.

Wallin, D. et al. (1985). Improvement of muscle flexibility: A comparison between two techniques. *American Journal of Sports Medicine, 13, 4, 263–268.*

Walter, J., Figoni, F., & Andres, F. (1995). Effect of stretching intensity and duration on hamstring flexibility. *Medicine & Science in Sports & Exercise, 27, 5, Supplement S240.*

Westcott, W. (1991). Role-model instructors, *Fitness Management,* March, 48–50.

YMCA (2000). *YMCA Fitness Testing and Assessment Manual.* Champaign, Ill.: Human Kinetics.

Yoke, M. et al. (1988). The metabolic cost of two differing low impact aerobic dance exercise modes. *Medicine & Science in Sports & Exercise, 20, 2, (Supplement) (Abstract #527).*

Yoke, M. & Kennedy, C. (2004). *Functional Exercise Progressions.* Monterey, Calif.: Healthy Learning.

Suggested Reading

American College of Sports Medicine (2006). *ACSM's Resource Manual for Guidelines for Exercise Testing and Prescription* (5th ed.). Philadelphia: Lippincott Williams & Wilkins.

American Council on Exercise (2003). *Personal Trainer Manual* (3rd ed.). San Diego, Calif.: American Council on Exercise.

Bryant, C.X. & Franklin, B. A. (2007) *ACE's Guide to Exercise Testing and Program Design: A Fitness Professional's Handbook* (2nd ed.). Monterey, Calif.: Healthy Learning.

Jordan, P. (1997). *Fitness Theory and Practice.* Sherman Oaks, Calif.: Aerobics and Fitness Association of America.

Kennedy, C. & Yoke, M. (2005). *Methods of Group Exercise Instruction.* Champaign, Ill.: Human Kinetics.

Chapter Seven

Lorna L. Francis, Ph.D., previously a physical education professor at San Diego State University, is an internationally recognized speaker and the author of several fitness books. An ACE-certified instructor, Dr. Francis is an emeritus member of ACE's Board of Directors and was co-recipient of the 1989 IDEA Lifetime Achievement Award.

Richard J. Seibert, M.A., M.Ed., a fitness-industry consultant and ACE-certified Group Fitness Instructor, is an internationally recognized speaker and author specializing in group fitness instructor training. Seibert contributed toward the development and delivery of ACE's Practical Training Workshop Program and has served on several ACE Exam Development Committees.

IN THIS CHAPTER:

Teaching a Group Exercise Class

By Lorna L. Francis and Richard J. Seibert

Each year, millions of Americans participate in some form of group exercise class. They perform indoor cycling, water aerobics, cardio kickboxing, yoga, Pilates, and many other forms of group exercise. In every one of these situations, they rely on a group fitness instructor to help them learn and perform the necessary movements to be successful. The success of the class depends on the instructor's ability to apply sound instructional principles and practices. In fact, effective teaching may well be the most important aspect of the group fitness instructor's role. Inadequate leadership is often cited by participants as a reason for dropping out of formal exercise programs.

Teaching a Group Exercise Class

Unfortunately, many people believe that teaching is intuitive and spontaneous. However, an intuitive and spontaneous approach to teaching often results in ineffective leadership. Over the years, researchers have provided valuable information to help instructors effectively plan and implement their programs. Scientific investigation of teaching techniques has led to an understanding of the phenomenon of teaching and its impact on learning behavior. More importantly, when followed, teaching techniques provide the instructor with the necessary means to transfer their fitness knowledge, skill, and enthusiasm to their exercise participants. The purpose of this chapter is to provide a sound teaching foundation by exploring the elements of effective teaching and how they apply to a group fitness setting.

Systematic Class Design

Instructors need to follow a simple system to target the correct audience, design an effective class, and teach the correct exercises. The system works well in the correct order of application, and, conversely, can be disastrous when the instructor reverses the order of application. To teach the right class to the right set of participants, you must first understand the exercise participants. Next, the overall goals and objectives of the class should be determined to aid in exercise selection. After the class is over, you must determine the quality of the class. More specifically, you must evaluate how well the students met the goals and objectives of the class.

By reversing the order of application, an instructor may design the class around a set or style of movements. This method of class design can discourage class participation, except for those few participants who happen to be successful with the movements. By following the correct order, the instructor is determining the class through the selection of movements rather than determining the movements based on the class.

Understanding the Exercise Participant

Many instructors do not appreciate the complexity of the process required to learn a new exercise or movement pattern. In a matter of seconds, the student must perceive and react to the proper cues, remember similar situations and instruction on what to do, determine the proper strategy and make the correct response, and, finally, through feedback, determine whether he or she performed the exercise correctly. This section examines the learning process and describes learning strategies that will facilitate the teaching of motor skills.

Magill (2000) defines learning as an "internal change in the individual that is inferred from a relatively permanent improvement in performance of the individual as a result of practice." Instructors can therefore infer that learning has occurred when a person's performance shows less variability over time.

Learning takes place in three domains of human behavior: cognitive, affective, and motor. All three domains are important in the fitness field.

The **cognitive domain** describes intellectual activities and involves gaining knowledge. Studies have shown that education within an exercise program positively affects motivation and exercise compliance. Therefore, competent instructors should remain up-to-date on the latest research in exercise and related fields in an effort to inform their students and respond intelligently to their questions or concerns.

The **affective domain** describes emotional behaviors. Motivation to exercise depends on a person's feelings about exercise. Instructors are therefore instrumental in helping participants develop positive attitudes toward exercise.

Finally, the **motor domain** refers to those activities requiring movement. Learning motor skills is the foundation of exercise classes.

Within the fitness profession, the motor domain has been heavily emphasized and limited attention has been given to the affective and cognitive domains. However, research has shown that teaching within all three domains is critical to exercise compliance.

Stages of Learning

To teach effectively, an instructor must be aware of the various stages of learning. One of the most commonly cited learning models was developed by Fitts and Posner (1967), who theorized that there are three stages of learning for a motor skill: cognitive, associative, and autonomous. Within the **cognitive stage of learning,** learners make many errors and have highly variable performances. They know they are doing something wrong, but they do not know how to improve their performance. At this stage, participants seem terribly uncoordinated and consistently perform exercises incorrectly.

Those in the **associative stage of learning** have learned the basic fundamentals or mechanics of the skill. Their errors tend to be less gross in nature and they can concentrate on refining their skills. During this stage, exercise participants are able to detect some errors and the instructor needs to make only occasional corrections.

During the **autonomous stage of learning,** the skill becomes automatic or habitual. Learners can perform without thinking and can detect their own errors. Driving a car, for example, is a very complex motor skill that over time is performed in the autonomous stage. The driver often is concentrating elsewhere and is able to recognize when mistakes are made.

The type and amount of information that exercise participants can understand depend on their current stage within the learning process. Beginning aerobic exercisers may be concentrating fully on performing the skill correctly. They may forget to perform even the most basic tasks, like breathing regularly or watching out for obstacles. Because beginners are less skilled at determining what information they must attend to, the instructor must provide them with specific information about what is important. For example, since maintaining appropriate posture is necessary to properly execute many exercises and movement patterns, the instructor must constantly remind beginners to maintain correct exercise posture. Advanced aerobic exercisers are more likely to understand and respond to fine motor-skill adjustments. For example, relaxing a grip or contracting an antagonist muscle group has more meaning to an advanced exerciser. However, advanced participants may require more information when a routine or sequence has changed from a habitual pattern. To employ appropriate teaching strategies, the instructor must be aware of each participant's stage of learning.

The following instructor guidelines will facilitate the movement of the exercise participants from the beginner level to the advanced level.

• **Enhance motivation to learn.**
Wlodkowski (1998) describes how a

motivated learner will surpass a nonmotivated learner in performance and outcome. Without motivation, there is little effort and participation. Simply stated, instructors need to develop classes that strongly appeal to their participants. Instructors must avoid the pitfall of developing classes that have greater appeal to them than to their participants.

- **Progress gradually from simple to complex.** It is important to ensure that exercise participants master movements and movement patterns in their simplest forms before moving on to complex movements. For example, if a participant is displaying poor posture and form during standing lunges, he or she would be ill advised to move on to standing lunges utilizing additional resistance.
- **Offer feedback.** Participants tend to view corrective feedback as informative rather than critical, especially when they can use the feedback to improve performance. Feedback that equally focuses on successes and errors can help move participants into an advanced stage in which they can monitor their own performance. A more thorough discussion of feedback is provided at the end of this chapter.

Participant Needs

Many group fitness classes are composed of participants with varying levels of fitness and skill. In smaller communities, special populations, such as pregnant women, obese individuals, or people with disabilities, are mainstreamed into regular group fitness classes. This state of affairs presents a challenging teaching environment for instructors. To effectively plan a group exercise class, it is important that an instructor first be familiar with the health history and fitness level of each class participant. Having this information will help the instructor develop modifications to the exercise plan that can reduce a participant's risk of developing health complications during exercise. For example, participants with a history of high blood pressure should be reminded not to perform static strength exercises and to avoid holding the arms at or above shoulder level for an extended period of time. A pregnant woman should be advised not to perform exercises on her back after the fourth month of pregnancy. Mainstreaming special populations can be done as long as these individuals are apprised of specific exercise modifications and are periodically reminded of those modifications during the class session. For more information on modifying exercise for special populations, see Chapter 9.

Program Implementation

Establishing Class Goals

The effective use of goal-setting facilitates both learning and performance of motor skills. The competent group fitness instructor establishes **program goals** and aids participants in developing their personal goals. Program goals should reflect what the instructor expects students to gain from the program. Examples of program goals might include the following:

- The participant will maintain adequate aerobic fitness, or increase it, to acquire cardiorespiratory health benefits.
- The participant will maintain adequate and specific joint range of motion, or increase it, to prevent muscle imbalances and to provide appropriate range of motion for exercise movements.
- The participant will maintain adequate and specific muscular strength, or

increase it, to prevent muscle imbalances and to provide adequate strength to effectively perform exercise movements.

Lesson Planning

Planning and class preparation result in the efficient use of time, smooth progression of activities, and greater program variety. Instructors who do not plan their lessons often present the same music, exercises, and movement patterns day in and day out. Participants and instructors alike become bored with this daily routine.

It is particularly important that inexperienced instructors write out their daily class activities. While experienced instructors may no longer need to write a daily lesson plan, they should at least spend time before each class mentally preparing class activities. A daily lesson plan should consist of class objectives, planned activities and the time allotted for each activity, necessary equipment, and patterns of class organization. Figure 7.1 contains a sample lesson plan that can be modified to meet the needs of individual instructors and the objectives of specific classes.

Class Objectives

Just as group fitness instructors need to establish program goals, they also need to develop more specific objectives for each class meeting. **Class objectives** state what the instructor expects participants to accomplish during each exercise session. The following are examples of class objectives:

- The participant will maintain or increase **cardiorespiratory fitness** by exercising aerobically for 15 to 30 minutes at an intensity of 50 to 75% of maximal **heart-rate reserve.**

- The participant will increase or maintain adequate and specific flexibility by performing the following stretching exercises to their fullest range of motion and holding them for 15 seconds: hamstrings, quadriceps, and so on.
- The participant will increase or maintain adequate and specific strength and endurance by performing two sets of eight to 12 repetitions of the following exercises: curl-ups, prone shoulder and hip extensions, and so on.

Objectives help the instructor focus on the purpose of each selected exercise and activity. In fact, novice instructors should list the purpose of each strength and flexibility exercise used in their classes. Knowing the purpose and benefits of each exercise will help an instructor select appropriate class activities.

Class Activities and Time Allocations

Class activities are planned to meet the objectives of each component of a group fitness class. Components of a class include:

1. Warm-up and prestretch
2. Aerobic conditioning
3. Aerobic cool-down
4. Resistance training
5. Poststretch

Strength and flexibility exercises should be carefully planned. Specific stretching and resistance-training exercises are discussed in Chapter 3. The selection of music and movement patterns for the warm-up, aerobic-conditioning, and cool-down segments of the class is one of an instructor's most challenging tasks. This very important activity is addressed in greater detail later in this chapter.

The time allotted for each activity varies according to the total class time available and the specific nature of the activity. Some activities will naturally require more time

Teaching a Group Exercise Class

Figure 7.1

Sample Lesson Plan

Class: Aerobic Exercise		**Date:**		**Time:** 9:00–10:15 a.m.	

Class Objectives:

1. Participants will improve or maintain cardiorespiratory fitness by performing aerobics movements for 15 to 30 minutes at 50 to 75% of HR reserve.

2. Participants will improve or maintain flexibility by performing specific stretching exercises, holding for 10 seconds at maximum range of motion.

3. Participants will improve or maintain strength by performing specific strength exercises for three sets of 12 repetitions.

Activities	Time (minutes)	Patterns of Class Org.	Equipment	Music	Comments
Warm-up	5			Will vary according to season, age group, and participant interest. 120–140 bpm	Slow and controlled rehearsal
Pre-aerobic stretch (Pectoralis major, hamstrings, hip flexors, erector spinae, quads, gastrocnemius)	5	(same as above)		120–140 bpm	Utilize active stretching rather than deep static stretching
Aerobic exercise (Freestyle technique using a linear progression)	25	(same as above)		120–140 bpm	Take ExHR; check ExHR with a show of hands
Cool-down	4	(same as above)		120–140 bpm	Take recovery HR
Muscle strengthening (Curl-ups, toe raises, prone hip extension, triceps extension, scapulae adduction)	20		Mats, rubber cords	110–130 bpm	Slow and controlled; breathe on exertion
Postaerobic stretch (Same muscle groups as pre-aerobic stretch)	10	(same as above)	Towels	100 bpm	Stretch to the point of tightness, not pain
Final note	1				Give praise/ encouragement

Note: bpm = Beats per minute; HR = Heart rate; ExHR = Exercise heart rate

than others. Minimum and maximum time requirements for the warm-up, conditioning, and cool-down segments are discussed in Chapter 6. The time allotted for stretching and strengthening depends on the number of exercises to be performed.

Beginning and ending class on time is also important. Instructors who methodically plan their lessons will know the precise length of time for each activity. However, since unforeseen events, such as a CD player malfunction, do occur, the competent instructor needs to be flexible and able to improvise at the last minute, if necessary.

Patterns of Class Organization

Group fitness classes should be arranged to ensure the safety of participants and enable everyone to hear the instructions and see the demonstrations. Patterns of class organization refer to the formations used by instructors to provide their students with maximum opportunities for learning and performing. In a typical group fitness class formation, the instructor stands at the front of the room and participants face him or her. While this formation can be effective, it has one major disadvantage. Usually the enthusiastic, experienced participants stand in the front of the room while the less experienced exercisers stay in the back. The result is a potentially unsafe situation, because it is difficult for an instructor to observe those in the back of the room. To resolve this problem, the instructor can periodically move from the front to the sides and to the back of the class, asking participants to turn and face him or her in each new position. It is further recommended that the instructor keep the level of complexity low when turning the class toward the back. Participants in the back row are likely to feel uncomfortable with the rest of the class behind them.

It is common for group indoor cycling classes to be laid out in a circular or horseshoe pattern. The instructor is at one end of the room and participants form a single or double circle around them. Group fitness instructors using this formation should change their point of focus to observe each person in class.

Facility and Equipment Considerations

Not all instructors can choose the facility in which they teach. Ideally, the exercise facility should have the following:

- Good ventilation, with a temperature range of 60 to 70° F (16 to 21° C)
- A floor that will effectively absorb shock and control undesirable medial-lateral motions of the foot. A hardwood sprung floor is ideal.
- Sufficient space for each student to move comfortably (with arms extended laterally, each participant should be able to take two large steps in any direction without touching another student)
- Mirrors for participants to observe their own exercise positions and postures. However, it should be noted that some overweight or obese individuals may perceive seeing their image in the mirror as a demotivating aspect of exercise participation. These participants may feel more comfortable exercising in an area where their reflection is not the main focus of the task performance. In these situations, an instructor's ability to cue effectively and provide timely feedback will improve the participant's chances of performing safe and effective exercise.
- In large classes, a raised platform for the instructor
- Access to drinking water

Basic equipment needs include music CDs, CD player and speakers, microphone, mats, and some form of resistance-training equipment, such as weights, pads and gloves, tubes, or rubber cords. Equipment for additional activities, such as circuit training, might include balls, hoops, jump ropes, and steps. Additionally, particular equipment-based formats, such as indoor cycling and Pilates reformer classes, call for their own specialized equipment and space considerations.

Always arrive early to check that all equipment is in working order before class begins. Class time should never be spent sorting through music CDs or searching for equipment.

One of the most important pieces of group fitness equipment is the sound system. Although instructors rarely have the opportunity to select the sound system, they should be familiar with the basic features of the equipment they are using. Before beginning class, always check the proper setting of the volume, bass, treble, and pitch controls. According to Price (1990), audiologists recommend that group fitness instructors keep their music volume under 85 decibels (dB) (normal conversation ranges from 60 to 70 dB, an alarm clock ringing 2 feet away is about 80, a chainsaw is 100, while a jet plane takeoff is around 120). The Occupational Safety and Health Administration (OSHA), which regulates noise standards for workers, states that ear protection must be provided for workers if noise level on the job averages 90 dB over an eight-hour period. Extended exposure to sound levels at 85 to 90 dB and above can eventually damage a person's hearing. Instructors who use loud music are not only at risk of damaging their own hearing and that of their participants, but they are also much more likely to suffer from voice injury, as they find themselves having to shout over loud music.

In addition to keeping the music volume at an appropriate level to protect the hearing of class participants, audiologists recommend that instructors turn up the bass and lower the treble, since high frequencies can be more damaging than low frequencies (Price, 1990). A higher bass setting can also be beneficial for class participants who have difficulty hearing the underlying beat. If a CD player has pitch control (a feature that allows the user to speed up or slow down the music tempo), it should be checked for proper positioning before class begins (the center position usually indicates normal speed). Nothing is more frustrating for an instructor than to begin a class and find that the music is much slower or faster than anticipated. Instructors should attempt to minimize the use of the pitch control, because extreme changes in the speed of the music distort the sound. If an instructor is constantly pitching the music speed up, he or she might want to consider selecting music that is performed at a faster tempo.

Selecting Appropriate Exercises

An effective group fitness instructor must develop skills to determine which exercises and movement patterns are effective and safe to use in the exercise class. A thorough knowledge of exercise science is essential in this decision-making process. An **exercise evaluation** must be done for each movement pattern to determine its effectiveness and safety. To determine exercise effectiveness, ask, "Does this particular exercise do what it is supposed to do?" In other words, what is the purpose of the exercise and does it meet the intended objective? When considering stretching exercises, ask, "Does this particular exercise effectively stretch the muscle(s) it is supposed to stretch?"

For example, while it is possible to stretch the erector spinae and hamstrings using a straight-legged sitting toe-touch exercise, class participants with tight erector spinae or tight hamstrings may be unable to put sufficient stretch on the targeted muscles. Compound stretches, in which several major muscle groups are being stretched at the same time, do not isolate a specific muscle or muscle group. Therefore, two different stretches might be used: one that targets the hamstrings and one that targets the erector spinae.

When considering the effectiveness of strength exercises, ask, "Does this exercise strengthen the intended muscle(s)?" Some group fitness instructors are confused about the direction in which the resistance is being applied when evaluating certain strength exercises. Consequently, they tend to teach exercises that do not target the intended muscle group. For example, holding a rubber cord in the right hand above the head while pulling the cord down toward the hips with the left hand (lat pull-down), will help strengthen the latissimus dorsi. However, performing this same movement with a hand-held weight will strengthen the deltoid. Knowledge of muscles and their actions and an understanding of the direction in which the resistance is being exerted are valuable in helping an instructor select effective strength exercises.

If an exercise does not fulfill the instructor's objective, it should not be selected for inclusion in the group fitness class. If an exercise is determined to be effective, the instructor must then decide if it is safe. "Does the selected exercise cause pain in the joints or does it put unnecessary stress on other vulnerable parts of the body?" For example, while unsupported, sustained for-

ward flexion in a standing position is often used to stretch the hamstrings, this particular position can be hazardous to the lumbar spine. Therefore, a safer alternative for stretching the hamstrings should be considered. While in many instances the instructor will probably choose to reject an exercise that is determined to be unsafe or contraindicated, there are times when the benefits of an exercise outweigh the risks. For example, to effectively stretch the quadriceps it is necessary to apply an external force to move the heel of the foot toward the buttocks. This position can be mechanically stressful to vulnerable structures of the knee. However, if the exercise is performed with care, the benefits often outweigh the risk for participants with healthy knees.

The ability to evaluate the effectiveness and safety of exercises will improve as an instructor learns more about the functional anatomy of the human body and the many factors that can affect efficient human movement.

An instructor must also be familiar with the specific mechanics of each exercise. For example, when using elastic resistance, there is a natural tendency to hyperextend the wrist joints when flexing and extending the elbow joint (this gives the exerciser a mechanical advantage). Since wrist **hyperextension** puts considerable stress on the tendons that cross the wrist joint, class participants must be frequently reminded to maintain a neutral wrist position. Careful attention must be given to avoid shoulder impingement. This condition can occur when class participants repeatedly use lateral movements of the arms above shoulder level with the palms facing downward (with or without weights). Students must be encouraged to turn the palms upward as the arms are raised above shoulder level. When performing lunging or squatting exercises, it is advisable that the load-bearing knees are not flexed deeper than 90 degrees, as this movement tends to place high levels of compression stress on the back of the kneecaps.

These are just a few examples of common technique errors performed by exercise participants. To effectively teach and correct exercises, the instructor must have a good understanding of sound mechanics for every exercise selected.

Selecting Appropriate Teaching Techniques

To become proficient at teaching group exercise, an instructor must be familiar with methods for selecting appropriate exercises and movement patterns, analyzing exercise skills, and modifying exercise for various fitness levels and special populations. He or she must also be knowledgeable concerning techniques for increasing participant motivation and exercise adherence (see Chapter 8). The following section addresses these important teaching strategies.

Teaching Styles

The teaching style chosen is an important factor in determining success in effectively presenting class activities. The instructor should be familiar with a variety of teaching styles. Mosston (2001) has identified eight specific teaching styles. Each accomplishes a different set of objectives, and it is both possible and desirable to use several styles in a group fitness class. The five styles directly applicable to an exercise class are command, practice, reciprocal, self-check, and inclusion. Each style is described and

discussed in terms of its practical application to aerobic exercise.

An instructor using the **command style of teaching** makes all decisions about posture, **rhythm,** and duration, while participants follow his or her directions and movements. This style is most appropriate when instructors want to achieve the following objectives:

- Immediate participant response
- Participant emulation of the instructor as a role model
- Participant control
- Safety
- Avoidance of alternatives and choices
- Efficient use of time
- Perpetuation of aesthetic standards

The command style has been perhaps the most commonly used style in group fitness classes. While this style is particularly suited to warming up, cooling down, and learning new routines and exercises, it leaves no room for individualization. The participant has little say in decisions about personal physical development and few opportunities exist for social interaction. To achieve these objectives, an instructor must rely on other teaching styles.

The **practice style of teaching** provides opportunities for individualization and includes practice time and private instructor feedback for each participant. While all exercisers are working on the same task, individual participants can choose their own pace and rhythm. The practice style is particularly suited for classes in which the fitness levels of participants vary greatly. Using this style, instructors can encourage students to perform the maximum repetitions suitable to their skill or fitness level. The real key is that once instructors determine the task, such as curl-ups, they are free to move around and give individual feedback when necessary. A disadvantage to this style is that not all participants are sufficiently motivated to achieve their maximum potential.

The **reciprocal style of teaching** involves the use of an observer or a partner to provide feedback to each participant. This style enables everyone to receive individual feedback, an often impossible task for the instructor. The reciprocal style can best be used for fitness assessment. For example, tests evaluating posture, girth measurements, strength, and flexibility can be quickly administered by partners. Using a criteria card that describes the test, the criteria for passing, and the performance level achieved allows students to monitor their own progress. A sample criteria card is presented in Figure 7.2. Aside from providing the participant with important feedback, the reciprocal style encourages social interaction, which is one reason people choose to participate in organized exercise programs. One major disadvantage of this style is that the observer or partner may not provide appropriate feedback.

The **self-check style of teaching** relies on participants to provide their own feedback. Participants perform a given task and then record the results, comparing their performance against given criteria or past performances. This style lends itself nicely to the recording of **target heart rate, recovery heart rate,** and number of floor-exercise repetitions. Instructors must provide a record card for each participant. A sample record card is presented in Figure 7.3. Because a key component of motivation and exercise compliance is self-monitoring of progress, it is desirable to incorporate the self-check style into every exercise program.

The **inclusion style of teaching** enables multiple levels of performance to be taught within the same activity. Perhaps one of the most significant problems facing the group fitness industry is teaching multiple skill and fitness levels in the same class. Skill and fitness level can vary in each segment of the exercise class, including stretching, strengthening, and aerobic work. Class should be designed to incorporate all levels so that each person can achieve maximum success. During the stretching and strengthening segments of the program, the instructor can offer alternate positions for the different levels. For example, during abdominal work the participant with weak abdominal muscles can choose to do pelvic tilts, while the person with stronger abdominals can perform curl-ups. The instructor can also offer different levels of difficulty during the aerobic segment. For example, participants who are new to kickboxing can perform front kicks while more advanced participants can perform front kicks followed by blocks and punches. Instructors periodically need to demonstrate each level of movement, spending more time on the patterns for beginners.

Teaching Strategies

When teaching an exercise or movement pattern, determine which teaching approach will be most effective. Use the following strategies separately or in combinations. An instructor should also use redundancy to help participants learn the movements more deeply.

Slow-to-Fast

The **slow-to-fast teaching strategy** allows participants to learn complex movement at a slower pace. Also known as rhythmic variation, this technique emphasizes the proper configuration of a movement pattern. For example, if an instructor was teaching a box step (left foot forward, right foot across left

Teaching a Group Exercise Class

Figure 7.2
Sample
criteria card

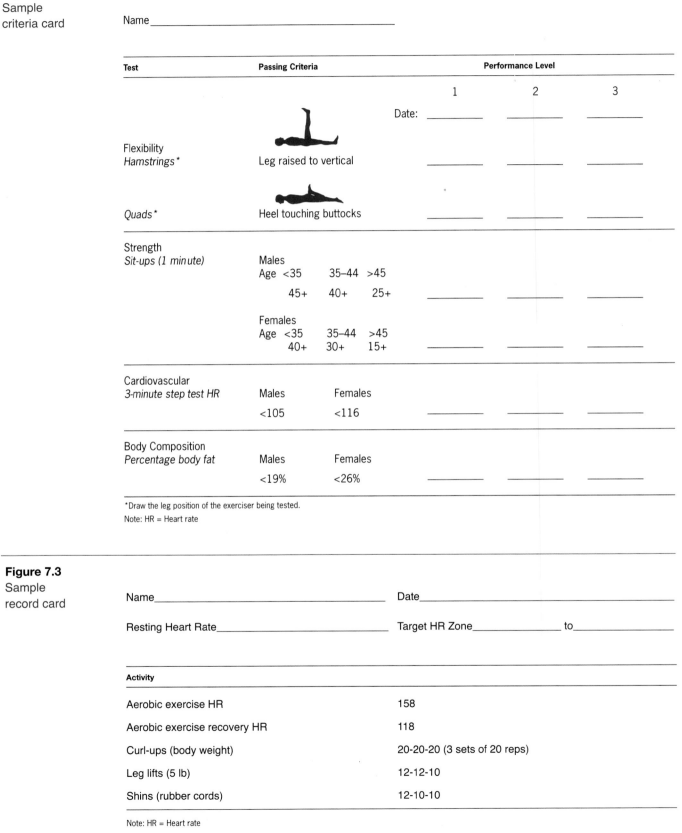

Name_____

Test	Passing Criteria	Performance Level		
		1	2	3
		Date: _____	_____	_____
Flexibility Hamstrings*	Leg raised to vertical	_____	_____	_____
Quads*	Heel touching buttocks	_____	_____	_____
Strength Sit-ups (1 minute)	Males Age <35 35–44 >45 45+ 40+ 25+	_____	_____	_____
	Females Age <35 35–44 >45 40+ 30+ 15+	_____	_____	_____
Cardiovascular 3-minute step test HR	Males Females <105 <116	_____	_____	_____
Body Composition Percentage body fat	Males Females <19% <26%	_____	_____	_____

*Draw the leg position of the exerciser being tested.
Note: HR = Heart rate

Figure 7.3
Sample
record card

Name_____ Date_____

Resting Heart Rate_____ Target HR Zone_____ to_____

Activity	
Aerobic exercise HR	158
Aerobic exercise recovery HR	118
Curl-ups (body weight)	20-20-20 (3 sets of 20 reps)
Leg lifts (5 lb)	12-12-10
Shins (rubber cords)	12-10-10

Note: HR = Heart rate

foot, left foot backward, right foot to the right), instead of performing individual steps on each beat of the music, two counts would be taken for each foot placement, thus taking eight counts to complete the movement pattern. The amount of time taken to perform the movement is increased so that the entire skill can be taught in sequence. Once participants have learned to perform the movement correctly, they can perform the movement on the beat. Because this strategy may reduce **exercise intensity,** refrain from using it for extended periods of time during the peak of the aerobic segment of class.

Repetition Reduction

The **repetition reduction teaching strategy** involves reducing the number of repetitions that make up a movement sequence. It is used for a movement pattern that has two or more distinguishable parts. For example, if an instructor wanted to use a combination of one jumping jack and two alternating punches, he or she might begin the sequence with four jumping jacks and eight alternating punches, reducing the movement pattern to two jumping jacks and four alternating punches, finishing with one jumping jack and two alternating punches. This technique allows participants to master each movement within a sequence. It should be noted that in this example, the number of music beats for the jumping jacks equals the number of beats needed to perform the punches. In this way, the movement fits smoothly into music written in eight-count phrases.

Spatial

The **spatial teaching strategy** is commonly used when introducing participants to a new body position. During the strength-training segment of the class, begin each new exercise by reviewing proper alignment. An instructor might say, "Begin with your feet about shoulder-width apart, knees slightly bent, and spine straight with supportive abdominals. Hold the dumbbells with the palms facing the body, elbows slightly bent, shoulders down, and head looking straight ahead." Note that the direction of alignment cues was given in a toe-to-head direction to prepare the class for a lateral dumbbell raise. The same cues can be offered in a head-to-toe sequence.

Part-to-Whole

The **part-to-whole teaching strategy** breaks a skill down into its component parts and each part is practiced. The instructor should teach each part in its simplest form. Once participants have mastered each component, they can be placed in proper sequence. When breaking movements down into parts, it is important to note any critical or advanced components. For example, a movement pattern may require pivoting on one or both feet. In this case, make sure that the class can perform the pivot safely before adding the pivot into the movement pattern. The simplest way of using the part-to-whole teaching strategy is the "add-on method." After introducing a movement pattern, "A," a new part is practiced and then added to make "A + B." After movement pattern "A + B" is mastered, a new movement, "C," is practiced and then added to the existing pattern to make "A + B + C." Additional parts are added to make a sequence of movement patterns.

Simple-to-Complex

The **simple-to-complex teaching strategy** treats a sequence of movement patterns as a whole, with small changes occurring at the pace of the class. Using this advanced

211

Teaching a Group Exercise Class

strategy, small amounts of complexity are added to a simple movement combination to slowly challenge participants. As an example, a movement pattern, "A + B," is introduced in its simplest form. Movement "A" is 16 counts of abdominal curls, and movement "B" is 16 counts of alternating oblique curls. Movements "A + B" are repeated until the entire class can perform them correctly. Movement "A" is then made more complex by adding a rhythmic variation to it of one count up and three counts down. This 16-count variation of "A" is followed by the original 16-count "B" movement. The added level of complexity is repeated until the entire class can perform it correctly. At this time, the instructor maintains the 16-count variation of "A" followed by an optional advanced movement variation for "B" in which the opposite knee lifts during the alternating oblique curl. This strategy is well suited for mixed-level classes, as it allows each participant to progress to a level that is comfortable for him or her.

Preparing and Teaching Class Activities

The majority of a group fitness instructor's preparation time is spent selecting music and developing movement patterns. The purpose of this section is to explain music selection, explore different choreographic techniques, and become familiar with successful cueing skills.

Selecting Music

Music not only provides the timing for exercise movements, it also makes a class enjoyable and helps to motivate participants. Because music plays an important role in most group exercise programs, an instructor should be familiar with its fundamental elements.

The music **beat** is made up of the regular pulsations that have an even rhythm and occur in a continuous pattern of strong and weak pulsations. Strong pulsations are called the **downbeat,** while weaker pulsations are called the **upbeat.** A series of beats forms the underlying rhythm of a song. The rhythm is the regular pattern of sound that is heard when listening to music. A **meter** organizes beats into musical patterns or measures, such as four beats per measure. A **measure** is a group of beats formed by the regular occurrence of a heavy **accent** on the first beat or downbeat of each group. Most group fitness routines use music with a meter of 4/4 time (the first "4" indicates four beats per measure while the second "4" shows that the quarter note gets the beat).

To successfully choreograph movement patterns, an instructor must be familiar with his or her music. Determining music **tempo** is the first requirement. The tempo, or speed, of the music determines the progression as well as the intensity of exercise. The beats per minute (bpm), or music tempo, for a song can be determined by counting each beat for one minute. Using experience and common sense, instructors have adopted general guidelines for selecting the appropriate music tempo for the various components of a group fitness session (see Figure 7.1). Slow tempos under 100 bpm without a strong underlying beat are generally used for poststretching, while tempos from 120 to 140 bpm are frequently used for warm-ups, prestretch, and cool-downs. Muscle-strengthening exercises are often performed to tempos of 110 to 130 bpm. The tempo for strengthening exercises should be slow enough for participants to control their movements. Aerobic activities are generally performed at a tempo of 120 to 160 bpm. Instructors must be

Preparing and Teaching
Class Activities

cautious when choosing music speeds over 150 bpm because participants need to move quickly at higher tempos.

Encouraging students to perform smaller movements will help them preserve the control necessary for safety when using high music speeds. Beginners should never be expected to move at fast speeds, because they are not yet proficient enough to perform quick movements under control. Another consideration with fast-paced music is that participants with long arms and legs need more time to cover the same spatial area as participants with shorter limbs. For example, people with short arms can bring their arms above their heads more quickly than can people with long arms. Consequently, participants with long arms often appear to be uncoordinated unless they bend their elbows to keep in time with the instructor and the music.

After determining the tempo, it is useful to break down the music into musical phrases. According to Bricker (1991), "as letters of the alphabet combine to form sentences, so beats of music combine to form measures, and measures combine to form phrases. A **phrase** is composed of at least two measures of music. To learn to recognize musical phrases, imagine where you would pause for breath if you were singing a song." Shyba (1990) likes to think of a musical "sentence" as a group of four phrases (usually 32 counts). Shyba recommends that instructors indicate on a piece of paper each musical phrase with a pen stroke crossing the set out with the last phrase in the sentence (卅). Therefore, if a person were listening to 32 measures (four beats per measure) making up 16 musical phrases (eight beats per phrase) or four musical sentences (32 beats per sentence), there would be four sets of three vertical pen strokes crossed by one diagonal pen stroke (each

pen stroke representing an eight-count phrase: 卅 卅 卅 卅). Musical phrasing is ideal when it groups into musical sentences of 32 counts. However, there are times when a phrase may be subdivided, and it becomes awkward if the instructor is in the middle of a 32-count combination when the musical phrasing becomes inconsistent. Shyba (1990) recommends that instructors use phrasing inconsistencies to introduce a new step or perform simple free-form footwork until the musical sentences reestablish themselves.

When choreographing movements to music, take care to begin the movement pattern on the downbeat of the measure (the first count of the measure). Combining eight-count movements, such as eight marches or four jumping jacks to make up a 32-count combination, helps participants anticipate movement changes on the downbeat, thus giving them a feeling of success (Figure 7.4).

While many movement patterns can be performed on each beat of the music, it is possible to change the rhythm of the movement so that it is being performed double-time to the basic beat (one and two and three and four and), half-time (two counts per movement), or in **syncopation,** where the accent is temporarily displaced from the naturally occurring accent in the music (one AND two AND, with

---

Figure 7.4

A sample 32-count movement pattern

Phrase Number (8 counts)	Music	Movement
#1	Mary had a little lamb,	8 march forward
#2	Little lamb, little lamb,	4 jumping jacks
#3	Mary had a little lamb,	8 march back
#4	Whose fleece was white as snow.	4 jumping jacks

Teaching a Group Exercise Class

the accent occurring on the AND rather than on one or two).

The rhythm of the music can often dictate the style of movement. Instructors will find it easiest to work with music that has a steady rhythm and a strong beat. The type of music selected will depend on the demographics of the exercise group and the instructor's creativity. Staying open-minded is important. An instructor must not rely exclusively on his or her personal music preferences. The music selected should reflect, in part, the interests of the age group. For example, young people may enjoy Top 40 pop, while an older group may prefer swing or big band music. Age should not be the only criterion for selecting music, however. In some parts of the country, gospel, folk, and country music are more appealing than rock 'n' roll. Instructors may also want to consider the time of the year. At Christmas, for example, participants may be delighted to exercise to "Rudolph the Red-Nosed Reindeer." For further variety, select music for special "theme days"— square dance, clogging, and folk music for a country music day or cha-cha, rumba, and samba music for a Latin music day. The greater the variety of music, the more enjoyment most participants will derive from a group fitness program.

With some types of group fitness instruction, the music is used to set a mood rather than to mark movement patterns. In these cases, selecting music written in eight-count phrases with regular rhythms and beats is unnecessary. Indoor cycling, stretching, and yoga classes are just some of the classes that traditionally use music to enhance the mood of the exercise rather than to synchronize movements.

To keep participants interested, change music frequently. If an instructor has trouble

staying current with music selections, there are national music organizations that manufacture music CDs and tapes for group fitness classes. In addition, feel free to ask regular participants for music suggestions.

Choreography

The types of movements selected should reflect the goals and objectives of the class. The first consideration is whether the selected movement or the sequencing of movements is safe. Other chapters in this manual address high-risk and contraindicated exercises, but for review purposes, keep in mind the following general guidelines when selecting choreography:

- Avoid movements that result in hyperextension of any joint.
- Avoid excessive repetitions on one weightbearing leg; alternate legs frequently.
- Avoid flinging the limbs at any time.
- Make sure lateral foot movements are well-controlled to avoid tripping or falling (especially on carpet).
- Avoid contraindicated positions such as sustained and unsupported forward flexion.
- Avoid stretching muscles ballistically while performing movement patterns.
- Avoid changing direction rapidly. Transitions between complex step patterns may require a movement sequence in place before changing direction.
- Avoid continuous movement that requires participants to remain on the balls of their feet for extended periods.
- Avoid holding the arms at or above shoulder level for an extended period of time. Vary frequently low-, mid- and high-range arm movements.

• Balance routines so that the same movements are performed equally on both sides of the body.

Choreographic Methods

Two basic choreographic methods, known as **freestyle choreography** and **structured choreography**, are used to combine movement patterns and music. The structured method uses choreographed movements that are formally arranged and repeated in a predetermined order, usually to the same piece of music each time the routine is used. Examples of structured programs are Les Mills' BODY-PUMP® and Judi Sheppard Missett's Jazzercise.®

The freestyle method uses movements that are built and sequenced by the instructor during the exercise class. The pacing is often dependent on the success participants demonstrate with the sequences as well as the complexity of the movement patterns or combinations. Freestyle movements can be sequenced either by using a **linear progression** or by placing movements into patterns or combinations. A linear progression consists of one movement that transitions into another without cycling sequences. By changing only one variable at a time, such as arm or leg movement, direction of movement, or rhythm, students can practice movement patterns without the pressure of remembering sequences. Linear progressions are particularly useful for introducing new moves and for adding variations. The following is an example of a linear progression in which only one element of variation is changed at any one time:

Base movement: Knee-lift in place for eight counts (four knee-lifts)

Add arms: Arm curls for eight counts

Add direction: Travel forward for eight counts; travel backward for eight counts

Change the arms: Overhead press for 16 counts (still traveling)

Change the legs: Hamstring curls (same arms) for 16 counts (still traveling)

Change the arms: Push down for 16 counts (still traveling)

When using a freestyle approach, it is important to use effective teaching strategies so class participants can successfully follow the choreography to maintain appropriate levels of exercise intensity. Copeland (1991) recommends that instructors start with a base move, such as marches or step-touches, and change only one element of variation at a time. Examples of elements of variation recommended by Copeland include planes, levers, direction, and rhythm. Variations in planes include the horizontal or transverse plane, which divides the body into lower and upper parts and includes rotation around the long axis of the body; the frontal plane, which divides the body into anterior and posterior parts and includes abduction and adduction; and the sagittal plane, which divides the body into right and left sides and includes flexion and extension. An instructor can change the arms from lateral raises (frontal plane) to arm curls (sagittal plane).

Lever variations refer to the length of a lever or limb (short, long). Changing from an arm curl (short arm lever) to frontal raises (long arm lever) is an example of a lever variation. Directional variations add the element of travel, allowing participants to move forward, backward, left, right, diagonally, or in a circle. Variations in rhythm involve changing the rhythm of a movement. For example, varying a jumping jack to a slow jumping jack changes the rhythm of a similar movement.

Combinations are defined as two or more movement patterns combined and repeated in sequence several times in a row. The following is an example of a combination:

- Four lunges in place with upright rows—eight counts
- Four knee lifts traveling forward with overhead presses—eight counts
- Four jumping jacks with arms lifting laterally—eight counts
- Eight runs traveling backward with chest presses—eight counts

According to Copeland (1991), "There are many advantages to using patterns in your choreography. The human mind instinctively arranges events into patterns, so they allow the mind to relax and easily anticipate what will happen next. This repetition allows… students to commit to the movement more fully and to maintain a steady-state workout." However, an instructor must select movement patterns carefully. Complex routines can slow down the class and confuse participants, particularly in a beginning or multilevel class.

Finally, when putting the class together, movement patterns can be taught using a combination of teaching strategies. For example, an instructor may teach an oblique curl using the fast-to-slow teaching strategy, then add an abdominal curl movement using a part-to-whole teaching strategy to create a sequence of 32 counts of oblique curls followed by 32 counts of abdominal curls. He or she can then reduce the repetitions to 16 counts of oblique curls and 16 counts of abdominal curls to create the final movement pattern.

To keep track of the movement patterns or choreographed routines, it is helpful to maintain a card file, notebook, or computer file to record specific movement patterns and teaching strategies. Before teaching a new routine or series of movement patterns to a class, practice (preferably in front of a mirror) until the movement patterns are memorized and transitions and cues have been worked out. Practicing routines or combinations in advance helps instructors determine whether the sequence of movement patterns flows smoothly.

A slow progression is important to help participants learn a skill effectively and avoid musculoskeletal injuries. Encourage beginners to start slowly and progress gradually. In addition, movements must be selected so that most participants are successful. Some participants will learn new steps more quickly than others. Be patient and supportive of slower learners, reminding them that they will improve with practice. And always try to be available before and after class for individual help.

It is important that all movement patterns are effectively and safely sequenced to ensure smooth and comfortable transitions. A simple transition is one between two movements that are closely related. Simple transitions involve changes using either the legs or the arms. For example, punching up transitions easily into punching front. As the number of variations between movement patterns increases, so does the difficulty of the transition. Also, changing both legs and arms at the same time increases the difficulty of the transition.

The way an instructor sequences movements should be based on **physiological, biomechanical,** and **psychological balance** (Copeland, 1991). Intensity and duration are two physiological considerations when sequencing movements. To help class participants maintain heart rates within their training zones, the relative intensity level of each movement must be balanced. For example, if a high-intensity movement is chosen (e.g., jumping jacks or high-impact lunges), the next movement should be less intense (e.g., marches). If an exercise class is of long duration, too many high-intensity movements may fatigue participants before the end of the session.

Biomechanical balance is achieved by balancing the musculoskeletal stress of various movements. For example, if a movement is performed on one leg at a time, care must be taken to change the support leg before it is overly stressed. Similarly, if a movement, such as jumping jacks, is highly stressful to a joint, the next movement should not stress that same joint. Finally, be careful not to use too many complex movements, as doing so makes it difficult to achieve psychological balance. According to Copeland (1991), "Movement that is too complex is not only frustrating for the student but has a direct effect on the physiological and biomechanical balance. Form, technique, and safety can be compromised."

Cueing

Cueing is a crucial part of teaching group exercise classes. It serves as a notification system that allows class participants to follow movement patterns with ease and confidence. The success with which students perform movement sequences in a smooth and continuous manner depends on the instructor's ability to effectively cue changes in movement patterns.

When leading group exercise, face the class as often as possible, using mirroring techniques, such as moving to the participants' left when directing them to the right. An instructor can only monitor class safety by watching all participants at all times. All cues should be precise and timely.

Transitions play an integral part in cueing. If the transition is closely related, then the amount of information should be small. A long cue is only necessary when the transition is

difficult and involves a movement that is unrelated. The content of the cue may include the body part, the action, the direction, and/or any elaboration necessary to understand the movement. See Table 7.1 for examples of movement cues.

Table 7.1
Examples of Movement Cues

Body part	Action	Direction	Elaboration
Arms	Reach	Up	2 times
Hands	Push	Side	In place
Shoulders	Press	Front	Right
Knee	Lifts	Back	Forward
Foot	Taps	Diagonal	Double time
Head	Roll	Down	Slowly

Once the movement cue has been described, place the cue into the music using the following formula: "4 (gap) 3 (gap) tell me what to do (gap)." The cue begins on the heavy downbeat of the beginning of the phrase. The final gap represents the time between when the movement cue ends and the new movement begins. The final gap can be filled with a clap or vocal sound, like "now" or "go." For example, to introduce an arm pattern, use a cue similar to the following: "4 (gap) 3 (gap) arms press up (gap)." To modify or make a small change to the arm pattern, use "4 (gap) 3 (gap) alternate the arms (gap)." To view the timing of the cue, refer to Table 7.2.

Table 7.2
Verbal Cues and Timing

Music Counts	1	2	3	4	5	6	7	8
Example #1	4		3		arms	press	up	
Example #1 - *modified*					arms	press	up	Clap
Example #2	4		3		alter-	nate the	arms	
Example #2 - *modified*					alter-	nate the	arms	HUP!

Using this formula, plug in the important descriptive words to guide the exercise participant into the next movement. Once the movement is established, only small cues are necessary if the changes are closely related.

Here are some additional guidelines for effective cueing:

- Count down, 4, 3, 2...rather than up, 1, 2, 3...
- Avoid words with more than one meaning, like "out."
- Refer to objects around the room to help with directional cues. The cue "face the window" may have more meaning than "turn right."
- Count out difficult rhythms (e.g., 1 - and - 2 - 3 - and - 4).
- Be consistent with names of movements and timing of cues.
- Avoid tagging on extra words with little meaning, such as, "now take it to a..." or "I wanna see a..."

As students become proficient at executing movement patterns, they will need fewer verbal cues from the instructor. Instead of cueing every movement, limit verbal cues to transitions between movements. Visual cues are also helpful to communicate movement expectations. The use of visual cues has several advantages, including lowering the risk of voice injury, allowing the instructor to communicate in facilities with poor acoustics or with a large number of class participants, and providing opportunities for the hearing-impaired to join a group fitness program.

There are currently two formalized sets of visual cues in use among group fitness instructors. According to Webb (1989), who promotes a series of hand/arm visual cues called the Aerobic Q-Signs (Figure 7.5), verbal cues can be used to call out the name of the step while visual cues are used to indicate the direction or number of repetitions. Webb recommends that instructors practice visual cue signs in front of a mirror, making sure that visual cues are given four counts before the movement change is to occur. She also suggests that instructors introduce a few signs at a time into their classes so that participants can gradually adapt to their use.

Oliva (1988) promotes visual cues based on the principles of Visual-Gestural Communication and American Sign Language to include persons who are deaf or hard of hearing (Figure 7.6). Oliva maintains that visual cues must be "visually logical" and clearly visible to viewers. For example, instructors should indicate lower-body moves by patting the lead leg. A strong distinction needs to be made between moves that travel and moves that simply change direction (within one step of original position). Specific visual cues that match specific low-impact foot moves are available (Oliva, 1988). Oliva recommends that visual cues for turns should be indicated directly above the floor space that the turn will cover. Finally, the timing and command sequence for visual cues should be the same as for verbal cues.

Verbal and visual previews are particularly useful when introducing a complex movement pattern. Each of these previews is given by the instructor while the class performs a given movement. When using a verbal preview, the instructor explains in detail the next step or arm pattern. When using a visual preview, the instructor demonstrates the next movement sequence, while the class continues to perform the current movement.

When using verbal cues, it is imperative that the instructor learns to use his or her voice properly to avoid vocal injuries. According to MacLellan, Grapes, and Elster (1980), voice injuries among group fitness instructors occur

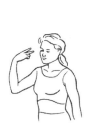
Watch me

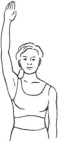
Hold/stay

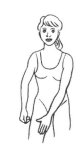
Left leg

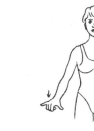
Stay in place

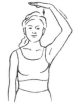
From the top

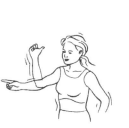
Forward/backward

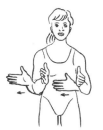
Shift to face this direction

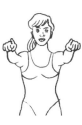
March in place

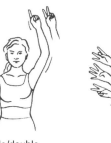
Single/double

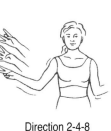
Direction 2-4-8

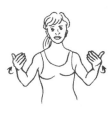
Move it forward

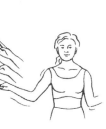
Move it back

Figure 7.5
Aerobic Q-signs (Source: Webb, 1989)

Figure 7.6
Visual cues for exercise classes (Source: Oliva, 1988)

from "the improper use of the voice, interference of muscular tension with vocalization, attempts at projection over loud music, and a poor work environment." They recommend the following techniques to prevent voice injury:

- Keep cues short and avoid unnecessary vocalization.
- Keep music at a decibel level that does not require the instructor to shout over the music.
- Frequently take small sips of water to keep the vocal mechanism lubricated.

- Avoid cueing in positions that inhibit abdominal breathing (such as during curl-ups) or constrict the vocal tract (such as when performing push-ups). It is preferable to give the cues before the exercise is executed.
- When using a microphone, speak in a normal voice.
- Do not lower the pitch of the voice to sound louder, as this leads to vocal fatigue (producing a hoarse, weak, and strained voice).
- Avoid frequent clearing of the throat.

Analyzing Performance and Providing Alignment Cues

An important role of the group fitness instructor is to effectively analyze the movement skills of class participants. An exercise that is performed incorrectly will not achieve the desired goal, but more importantly, improper exercise execution could result in injury. Body alignment is crucial to proper exercise execution. An instructor must therefore have a thorough knowledge of appropriate body alignment.

Most exercises require participants to maintain a neutral pelvis. Class participants should be frequently reminded of mechanically sound posture—neutral head, shoulders back, chest up, neutral pelvis, and relaxed knees (standing posture). See Chapter 3 for more information on proper body alignment.

When teaching exercise technique, communicate important alignment and execution cues. It is also recommended that the instructor walk around the room as much as possible to make appropriate corrections. This is particularly important during the muscular-strength and poststretch phases of the exercise class. Unless appropriate feedback is provided, few participants, especially beginners, will have any idea that they are not performing an exercise properly.

Be very cautious with hands-on corrections. Pushing a participant's limb into proper position during a stretch could result in a serious injury for the exerciser, especially if he or she is inflexible. As a rule of thumb, do not perform hands-on corrections for exercises that require the manipulation of a muscle being stretched. Instead, demonstrate proper execution of the exercise and offer verbal corrections. However, if a participant is hyperextending a joint, for example, it might be beneficial for the instructor to lightly touch the exerciser's knees or elbows as a reminder to soften them. If the instructor deems a hands-on correction appropriate, he or she must be sure to ask permission to place the hands on the participant prior to the correction. Common sense must always be applied when making decisions about whether to physically correct an inappropriate exercise position.

The most common modification that has to be addressed by group fitness instructors is that of modifying exercise intensity to provide safe and effective activity for all fitness levels. Factors that affect exercise intensity include music tempo and the size of arm and leg movements. In a multilevel program, the speed of music must be selected to accommodate the less-fit individuals in the class. It is hazardous for individuals with a poor level of fitness to exercise to fast music. However, a person with a higher level of fitness can manipulate the exercise by performing larger leg and arm movements to increase exercise intensity. An instructor can assist in this process by demonstrating movement modifications for each level of fitness found in the class.

One way to meet the intensity needs of each level of fitness is to be familiar with the energy expenditure for different types of movements. For example, the following is a four-level system based on the fact that both locomotion and large leg movements increase energy expenditure.

- **Level one:** small leg motions, in place
- **Level two:** small leg motions, traveling
- **Level three:** large leg motions, in place
- **Level four:** large leg motions, traveling

Using this system, advanced participants can be shown how to increase intensity by increasing the leg motions and the amount of traveling. Likewise, beginner participants can be shown how to decrease intensity by decreasing the leg motions and the amount of traveling.

Arm movements can also be adjusted, though to a lesser degree than leg movements, to increase or decrease intensity. While it is true that an overhead press is more intense than an arm curl, this is because the arm curl is performed with a shorter lever and fewer muscle groups and therefore requires less energy expenditure to perform than an overhead press, which moves from a shorter lever to a longer lever and involves more musculature. However, the side arm raise (a long-lever exercise that involves shoulder abduction to shoulder height with the elbows extended) requires about the same energy expenditure as an overhead press, even though the side arm raise is performed at a lower level than an overhead press.

Teaching to two or three levels requires some skill on the part of the instructor, who needs to demonstrate each of the levels every time a new movement is introduced. While it is tempting to spend most of the class time demonstrating the more intense version of a movement, it is probably the least-fit or beginner student who requires constant visual cues. It is not surprising that deconditioned individuals (who, more often than not, are also less skilled at movement performance) emulate the more intense choreography being demonstrated by the instructor, even when the instructor tells participants to move at their own pace. Unfortunately, beginning level participants are not skilled enough to perform movements without visual cues. After intensity options are given and each of the levels has been demonstrated, come back to performing to the level of the beginner participants. Do not forget that an instructor's primary

objective as an exercise leader is to teach rather than to perform.

It is the responsibility of both the instructor and the participant to monitor exercise intensity. The instructor controls intensity according to the music tempo selected and the types of movements demonstrated. The participant manipulates the exercise intensity by controlling the size of the movements performed. Encourage beginners to take their heart rates frequently, and be aware of the progress participants are making. One approach is to ask for a show of hands for those above, below, or within their **target heart-rate range.** Advise those participants who are above their target zone to keep their feet closer to the ground and reduce the size of their arm movements. Those students exercising below their target zone should be encouraged to take larger steps and increase the size of their arm movements if they are ready to do so.

Make sure that exercise heart rates can be reported in a nonthreatening and noncompetitive environment to ensure honesty. Accurate reporting is particularly important for participants who must maintain strict exercise heart rates due to specific medical conditions.

To avoid injury, it is extremely important that participants adjust the intensity of their movements to their cardiorespiratory fitness levels. Within a multilevel class, beginners should be encouraged to progress slowly in both the intensity and duration of exercise. After deconditioned exercisers have reached their aerobic goal for the day, request that these individuals lower the intensity by "walking" through the rest of the movements while more experienced participants continue to exercise at a higher intensity. Be very careful not to give conflicting messages to

Teaching a Group Exercise Class

participants. If everyone is expected to work at his or her own intensity level, an instructor must avoid general phrases such as, "Get your feet up higher," "Push through it," or "Just do one more." Participants will feel compelled to work at higher intensities regardless of whether they are ready to do so.

Providing Feedback

During class, the group fitness instructor has many opportunities to provide immediate **feedback** to participants. Wlodkowski (1998) defines feedback as information that learners receive about the quality of their performance on a given task. Generally speaking, feedback should be informational, based on performance standards, specific, and immediate. Quality feedback can be used to either reinforce performance or make the necessary corrections to improve performance.

Informational Rather Than Controlling

Feedback is for the participant's benefit, not the instructor's. Therefore, it should be filled with information about the participant's performance. An instructor should act like a mirror, reflecting the information about the performance back to the participant. Feedback that is perceived as pressure to perform or to please the instructor can ultimately decrease motivation to perform (Ryan, 1982). For example, the statements, "Your knee is at belt level, which is just the right place" and, "Your knee is at chest level, move it down to belt level" are better than, "I am so pleased you got it right" or, "I'd like it better if you lowered your knee to belt level."

Once a participant has made an improvement in performance, a positive statement like, "That's it" or, "Now you have it" can help

reinforce the new performance. Kaess and Zeaman (1960) demonstrated that positive feedback (i.e., knowledge that one is right) is more effective than negative feedback (i.e., knowledge that one is wrong). Instructors should seek to find positive performances from each participant throughout the class.

Based on Performance Standards

An instructor relies on kinesiological principles, past experience, and aesthetic standards to determine the correctness of a performance (Mosston, 2001). Kinesiological principles are used to determine which postures and movements are mechanically correct. For example, curl-ups are performed with the knees bent to reduce stress on the lower back and to isolate the abdominal musculature. Past experience is often used to correct a movement based on subtleties accumulated from observing many exercisers perform the same movement. Experienced instructors can often find just the right word or phrase to correct consistently inappropriate performances. Aesthetic standards are used to correct movements and postures determined to be culturally attractive. Group fitness movements are often corrected on the basis of aesthetic standards.

Specific

Feedback should be specific for the same reason movement cues should be. Exercise participants cannot correct mistakes unless they are clear about their errors and the correct performance standards. A nonspecific statement like, "You did that great," may not clearly communicate what was great about the exercise. Instead, use the specific details of the performance standard to explain what was observed. For example,

"You kept breathing throughout the exercises. Great job!"

Immediate

Delivering feedback as soon as possible allows the exercise participant to make a connection between the performance and the feedback. It also can be applied right away. If the feedback is delivered later, the exercise participant may not be as motivated to apply the information.

In addition to feedback regarding what was observed compared to the performance standard, an instructor may add rationales and corrective teaching statements. A rationale explains why the performance is important and, as discussed earlier, addresses the cognitive domain and can positively affect motivation and exercise compliance. For example, "You are stopping your arms at shoulder level (what you observed). That's perfect (performance standard), because it reduces the stress on the shoulder joint (rationale)." Together, this feedback increases motivation and moves the exercise participant more deeply into the autonomous stage of learning.

When participants are learning a new skill, an instructor may also need to offer corrective teaching statements, which provide the participant with the necessary information to improve performance. For example, "Joe, your knee is moving beyond your ankle during the lunge segment of class (what you observed); next time stop the knee as it approaches the point directly over your ankle (performance standard). This will reduce the amount of stress you place on your knees (rationale). A good visual cue is to look down at your knee during the exercise, and if you can see your shoelaces, you

know you have not gone too far (corrective teaching)."

A person can attend to only a few cues at any given moment. Therefore, when giving feedback, limit the number of corrections offered at any one time. Positive reinforcement is very important in the early stages of learning. Use positive **value statements** when participants make a good attempt, even if the performance is not yet correct. Appropriate feedback should always be given in a friendly manner. If several participants are performing a move incorrectly, give feedback to the entire class. However, if one person consistently performs an exercise or movement incorrectly, talk to that person privately, either when other class participants are working individually or after class.

Instructors can work with exercise participants and other fitness professionals, such as personal trainers, to periodically measure progress. If there is no access to these services, attempt to use valid tests that can be easily administered either by partners or by the participants themselves. Providing criteria cards that indicate test directions, criteria for passing, and performance levels achieved by exercisers saves valuable class time and can serve as a motivational tool for participants (see Figure 7.2).

In addition to periodic testing, an instructor should encourage participants to monitor their daily accomplishments. Most fitness facilities provide program cards or access to computer programs designed to record daily exercise participation. If these services are not provided, a simple record card can be used to keep track of daily progress (see Figure 7.3). Items such as heart rate (resting, exercise, and recovery) and the number of floor-exercise repetitions can be monitored regularly and recorded by

Teaching a Group Exercise Class

participants themselves. Criteria and record cards should be stored in an alphabetized file that is available to participants at each class meeting. Remind participants to pick up their cards, record the appropriate information, and return them to their files before leaving class.

It is important that instructors remain aware of their participants' progress toward their goals by periodically examining their record cards and through one-on-one interaction before, during, or after class. If a participant is not showing progress, it is the instructor's responsibility to help determine the problem. It may be that unrealistic goals have been set or that there has been an attendance problem. Showing genuine concern for students encourages long-term participation in a formal exercise program.

Summary

Effectively teaching a group fitness class is a challenge for every group fitness instructor. Competent instructors carefully design their programs and employ sound teaching principles; they develop effective strategies to motivate participants to continue exercising; and they remain abreast of current health, nutrition, and fitness information and trends. The extra work that is required to become an effective instructor will be repaid many times over when the instructor earns the students' respect by providing safe, fun, and well-structured group fitness classes. Demonstrating expertise in the fitness industry will provide many professional opportunities and the personal satisfaction of contributing to the overall health and well-being of numerous participants.

References

Bricker, K. (1991). Music 101. *IDEA Today,* 3, 55–57.

Copeland, C. (1991). Smooth moves. *IDEA Today,* 6, 34–38.

Fitts, P.M. & Posner, M.I. (1967). *Human Performance.* Belmont, Calif.: Brooks/Cole.

Kaess, W. & Zeaman, D. (1960). Positive and negative knowledge of results on a Pressey-type punchboard. *Journal of Experimental Psychology,* 60, 12–17.

MacLellan, M.A., Grapes, D., & Elster, D. (1987). Voice injury. In: *Aerobic Dance-Exercise Instructor Manual.* San Diego, Calif.: International Dance-Exercise Association (IDEA) Foundation.

Magill, R.A. (2000). *Motor Learning* (6th ed.). New York: McGraw-Hill.

Mosston, M. (2001). *Teaching Physical Education* (5th ed.). San Francisco: Benjamin Cummings.

Oliva, G.A. (1988). *Visual Cues for Exercise Classes.* Washington, D.C.: Gallaudet University.

Price, J. (1990). Hear today, gone tomorrow? *IDEA Today,* 5, 54–57.

Ryan, R.M. (1982). Control and information in the intrapersonal sphere: An extension of cognitive evaluation theory. *Journal of Personality and Social Psychology*, 43, 3, 450–461.

Shyba, L. (1990). Finding the elusive downbeat. *IDEA Today,* 6, 27–29.

Webb, T. (1989). Aerobic Q-Signs. *IDEA Today,* 10, 30–31.

Wlodkowski, R.J. (1998). *Enhancing Adult Motivation to Learn.* San Francisco, Calif.: Jossey-Bass.

Suggested Reading

Dishman, R.K. (1986). Exercise compliance: A new view for public health. *The Physician and Sportsmedicine,* 14, 127–143.

Fallon, D.J. & Kuchenmeister, S.A. (1977). *The Art of Ballroom Dance.* Minneapolis, Minn.: Burgess Publishing Company.

Franklin, B.A. (1986). Clinical components of a successful adult fitness program. *American Journal of Health Promotion,* 1, 6–13.

Griffith, B.R. (1992). *Dance for Fitness.* Minneapolis, Minn.: Burgess Publishing Company.

Harris, J.A., Pittman, A.M., & Waller, M.S. (1978). *Dance A While.* Minneapolis, Minn.: Burgess Publishing Company.

Institute for Aerobic Research (1988). Creative choreography with Candice Copeland. *Reebok Instructor News,* 6, 7.

Milgram, S. (1956). *Obedience to Authority: An Experimental View.* New York: Harper & Row.

Nieman, D.C. (1986). *The Sports Medicine Fitness Course.* Palo Alto, Calif.: Bull Publishing Company.

Rasch, P.J. (1989). *Kinesiology and Applied Anatomy.* Philadelphia, Pa.: Lea & Febiger.

Rogers, C. (1995). *On Becoming a Person.* Boston, Mass.: Mariner Books.

Siedentop, D. (1983). *Developing Teaching Skills in Physical Education.* Palo Alto, Calif.: Mayfield Publishing Company.

References and
Suggested Reading

Chapter Eight

Deborah Rohm Young, Ph.D., is an associate professor in the Department of Kinesiology, University of Maryland. Her research interests focus on physical-activity behavior and its association with cardiovascular-disease prevention. Dr. Young has a primary interest in developing and evaluating community-based physical-activity interventions, particularly in population subgroups that are known to be underactive. She also has expertise in evaluating determinants of physical activity and physical-activity assessment issues. Much of her research has focused on working with minority and female samples.

Abby C. King, Ph.D., professor of health research and policy and medicine at Stanford Medical School and senior scientist at the Stanford Prevention Research Center, is an expert on the behavioral determinants of physical activity. Dr. King's research interests include the applications of social cognitive theory and similar behavioral theories to achieve large-scale change in disease-prevention and health-promotion areas of relevance to adults, especially women, and mid-life and older adults; her focus has been on moving interventions that have proven effective in the laboratory to field settings.

IN THIS CHAPTER:

Adherence and Motivation

By Deborah Rohm Young and Abby C. King

Given that it is difficult to pick up a newspaper or magazine without finding an article discussing the benefits of regular physical activity, it is little wonder that most Americans know that regular physical activity is desirable. Adults are indeed aware of the health and psychological benefits associated with exercise, yet this knowledge is rarely transferred into action. Only about 30% of American adults get the recommended amount of physical activity, which is 30 minutes of moderate-intensity physical activity on most days of the week. About 40% are completely sedentary. Nearly 50% of those who start an exercise program drop out within the first six months.

Often adults do not know how to start their own physical-activity program, where to get sound advice on beginning a program, or are fearful of failing because of previous experiences with physical activity. Fitness instructors are in a fortunate situation, as they do not have to convince people to try their workout; participants have taken the first step by finding an exercise class and committing themselves to attending at least once. The instructor's challenge is to encourage continued participation.

The most common reasons given for not continuing a physical-activity program are lack of time and boredom. The time-constraint reason is intriguing; those who exercise regularly also cite lack of time as an ongoing problem for them. But these individuals fit regular exercise into their daily schedules. How do they avoid letting time pressures short-circuit their exercise programs? What "tricks" do they use to motivate themselves? Regular exercisers also report facing boredom, yet they continue with their program. How are they different from those who let boredom drive them out of aerobics classes?

Researchers who have studied physical-activity **adherence** issues have begun to formulate answers to these and other questions regarding the motivational aspects of regular physical activity. The group fitness instructor who incorporates motivational techniques into each exercise class has a unique opportunity to help participants develop positive attitudes toward, and to stay involved in, regular physical activity and exercise throughout their lives.

This chapter discusses characteristics often found in physical-activity program participants and dropouts. Knowing about the factors that influence physical-activity

adherence, and determining who are the least likely to attend regularly and who may drop out, can be crucial in the development and implementation of strategies to maximize adherence.

Numerous studies have confirmed the effectiveness of using such motivational strategies, but often these strategies are not implemented in the "real world." This chapter identifies instructor characteristics that help maintain adherence and details the strategies necessary to enhance adherence to regular class participation. Additionally, the skills needed to help participants maintain exercise programs during "high-risk" times, such as vacations, holidays, and when under pressure at work or home, are presented.

Major Factors Influencing Physical-activity Adherence

What is physical-activity adherence? Although it has been defined in a number of ways, for the purpose of this chapter it is defined as the amount of physical activity performed during a specified period of time compared to the amount recommended. The amount of physical activity can refer to the frequency, intensity, or duration, or some combination of these three dimensions. For example, if a person is taking 20-minute walks on three days each week, he or she is not adhering to current physical-activity recommendations. However, if a fitness instructor recommends 20-minute walks three days each week to that same person recovering from an injury, then he or she is adhering to recommendations.

There are a number of factors associated with physical-activity adherence. They often are categorized as personal, program, and environmental factors. This categorization scheme highlights the many different influences on physical-activity behavior.

Personal Factors

To effectively motivate participants, it is helpful to be aware of characteristics that appear to be associated with physical-activity adherence as well as dropout. Although not every person exhibiting a particular characteristic may adhere to, or drop out of, the class, understanding these characteristics may help the instructor identify those potentially at risk so that he or she can provide them with extra assistance early in the program.

Some unique characteristics exist in those who tend to adhere to physical-activity programs. One is that such individuals are more likely to have previously participated in physical-activity programs. Inquiring about prior experiences with physical activity can help the fitness instructor determine if the new participant is likely to adhere to the program. Greater adherence has also been found in individuals who have the physical and psychological/behavioral skills necessary to exercise appropriately and regularly. These include physical coordination, good time-management skills, self-efficacy (or confidence in being able to maintain an exercise habit), an ability to perceive exercise as enjoyable, and the ability to overcome typical barriers to exercise such as travel, injury, illness, competing demands on time, and high-stress periods.

Although participants will not come to a program with all of these traits and skills, some are amenable to change and can become more likely to adhere to the program. For example, by asking participants what they did and did not like about previous programs and why they discontinued

these previous programs, the group fitness instructor can adjust the current program to optimize its enjoyability for not only the new participant, but for all participants. Later in this chapter, additional ways to develop skills that participants need to maintain good exercise habits are presented in detail.

Individuals identified in the scientific literature as at increased risk for dropout include smokers, people with lower socioeconomic status, and those who are overweight. A brief interview of new participants can identify those with health habits and prior physical activity experiences that place them at risk for dropout (e.g., perceived discomfort associated with certain types of physical activity).

When a participant at increased risk for dropout is identified, extra monitoring is desirable, particularly for signs of overexertion. A high-risk participant trying to exercise at an overly vigorous pace is twice as likely to drop out. Given the strong desire to conform to the larger group, simply telling participants not to overexert may not be enough if the majority of the class is exercising at a high-intensity level. This is particularly applicable to aerobics or other classes in which the group tendency is to exercise at the same intensity as the instructor. If the class consists of participants with varying abilities, it is useful to present both a more difficult and an easier version of each routine. If possible, having a co-leader or experienced class member demonstrate a lower-intensity version of the routine at the same time that the higher-intensity version is being demonstrated gives participants a choice in intensity level. Introducing the **ratings of perceived exertion** (RPE) scale (Borg, 1998) to new participants and instructing them on how to monitor their intensity will help minimize the risk of overexertion (Figure 8.1). In general, a new participant, regardless of risk for dropout, should keep his or her RPE below 14 to 15 on the 6 to 20 scale until he or she is accustomed to the class format. Including short breaks during class also may help to maintain exercise involvement for the participant at increased risk for dropout.

It is imperative that the instructor maintain a noncondescending attitude toward all participants, including those with suboptimal health behaviors. Although it may be difficult for some fitness instructors to understand why individuals hold on to those extra pounds or continue smoking in light of overwhelming health risks, it must be remembered that every individual has unique priorities and behavior patterns in life. Rather than chastise an individual for a perceived bad habit, the instructor should praise positive behaviors and provide a good example.

Program Factors

Factors specific to the physical-activity program can also affect participant adherence. Convenience of the exercise class is often cited as a determinant of adherence. Classes should be scheduled, if possible, during times of the day when most participants potentially have free time. It is also beneficial if classes are scheduled at a variety of times so that there is an alternate class the participant can attend if unforeseen circumstances require that a participant miss a class.

To maximize adherence, classes should be no longer than 60 minutes. Programs that are longer than 60 minutes are perceived as too time-consuming by many participants.

The exercise routine itself also affects adherence. If the routine is too easy or too hard for the participant, or not varied enough to prevent boredom, chances for dropout increase. Classes that provide a well-rounded program that includes endurance, strength, flexibility, and balance components can meet the needs of all class participants. Some popular forms of group exercise, such as aerobics and kickboxing, require physical coordination that may be intimidating to new participants. Spending time with new participants to demonstrate the movements early on helps them learn the sequencing and provides the added benefit of making them feel special.

The perceived friendliness of class members can be an additional boost to adherence. When new participants feel welcome, it is easier for them to return to subsequent classes. Introducing new class participants and making a point of linking them to established members with similar interests makes participants feel welcome. It also can be used to promote a

Table 6.17
Category and Category-ratio Scales for Ratings of Perceived Exertion

RPE	Category Ratio Scale*
6	0 Nothing at all
7 Very, very light	0.5 Very, very weak
8	1 Very weak
9 Very light	2 Weak
10	3 Moderate
11 Fairly light	4 Somewhat strong
12	5 Strong
13 Somewhat hard	6
14	7 Very strong
15 Hard	8
16	9
17 Very hard	10 Very, very strong
18	* Maximal
19 Very, very hard	
20	

Source: Adapted, with permission, from American College of Sports Medicine (2006). *ACSM's Guidelines for Exercise Testing and Prescription* (7th ed.). Philadelphia: Lippincott Williams & Wilkins.

"buddy system" within the class structure. The extra accountability class participants have to each other helps foster adherence.

The intensity of the class also influences adherence. Although higher-intensity activity can result in health benefits more quickly than moderate-intensity activity, high-intensity physical activity can also lower adherence. Research studies show that moderate-intensity is preferred by many individuals for optimizing adherence, both in the short term and the long term. Over six months, Perri and colleagues (2002) found that participants assigned to moderate-intensity physical activity (45 to 55% of heart-rate reserve) completed more exercise sessions, were more likely to adhere to the recommendations, and completed more exercise in their target heart-rate zone than the participants assigned to the high-intensity program (65 to 75% of heart-rate reserve). The favorable results were, in part, attributed to fewer injuries in the moderate-intensity group. It is well-known that high-intensity physical activity results in greater risk of injury than more moderate-intensity forms of physical activity.

Environmental Factors

Environmental factors—the ambience of the exercise site, cues and reminders for exercise, weather conditions, time limitations, and the amount of support and **feedback** that is provided—can all influence whether a participant maintains the physical-activity program.

A well-lit room decorated in a pleasant motif and of sufficient size to accommodate class members, along with an adequate heating/cooling system, is preferable to a hot, dark, smelly, gym-like environment. Exercise equipment that may be used during the workout (e.g., steps, handweights, group exercise cycles) should be clean and ready for use.

It is important to start and finish classes on time; a lack of promptness disrupts everyone's daily schedule. If class must be canceled, give participants plenty of advance notice whenever possible. Setting up a "telephone tree" (where one participant has the responsibility of contacting another in an emergency-type situation) to contact class members quickly may be a worthwhile endeavor for some class situations. If classes are conducted in regions of the country that experience regular bouts of inclement weather, it is advisable to have a "bad weather" policy regarding conditions when class will be canceled. Passing out the policy at the beginning of the inclement weather season and keeping the policy posted in the exercise room will keep all participants informed of potential situations in which class will be canceled. Whenever possible, it is advisable to conduct a make-up class session soon after to keep the participants engaged.

Ongoing support by the fitness instructor and others through face-to-face, telephone, e-mail, or mail contact is particularly beneficial for adherence. Leaders can encourage long-term attendance by praising participants for daily attendance and for reaching predetermined goals. Other methods of support include reminding the participant about the progress that has been made since joining the program, and challenging the participant to set and meet physical-activity goals. Telephone and e-mail prompts can energize the wayward participant as well as remind everyone about upcoming exercise "special events," such as fitness challenges or seasonally inspired, adherence-based promotions.

In general, a telephone call or e-mail message to a participant who has missed two consecutive classes is warranted to determine reasons for nonattendance and to provide nonjudgmental support and encouragement. Newsletters that provide physical-activity tips, motivational strategies, and promotions for upcoming events are useful in building enthusiasm. With the advent of desktop publishing software, professional-looking newsletters can be achieved at minimal cost. To individualize the mail contacts, newsletters can be tailored for new participants and for those who are regular class attendees. Content for the new participants can emphasize motivational tips, ways to build support for physical activity, and how to set physical-activity goals. For the continuing exerciser, provide information about how to avoid boredom, ways to keep physical activity fun, and how to strategize or plan for high-risk situations in which disruptions in the physical-activity routine or schedule may occur.

Support from family and friends is essential for adherence. This can be accomplished by encouraging participants to talk with others about goals they have set, what has been accomplished during exercise class, and rates of progression. Ask participants to identify someone who they will ask to support them with their physical-activity program. This support can take a variety of forms; some participants may want someone to remind them to attend class, others may prefer a friend to reward them when goals are reached, and others may be interested in a buddy who also is an exerciser with whom they discuss exercise-related issues. Participants should be encouraged to share their newsletters with friends and family. They can also provide story ideas and personal anecdotes that they feel would pique the interest of others. Involving others in the exercise program or providing them with knowledge of what is going on in

class, as well as of the goals the participant has set, encourages outside support and minimizes any sabotage that might occur on the part of family members as a consequence of feeling "left out."

Characteristics of an Ideal Group Fitness Instructor

A group fitness instructor's attitudes, personality, and professional conduct are among the strongest motivating factors cited for maintaining physical-activity adherence. Although instructors are responsible for developing and administering a good class, those factors alone will not guarantee optimal adherence. Personal attributes of the fitness instructor can greatly augment his or her ability to effectively motivate participants. It is often thought that leadership is an innate trait, but leadership skills can be developed even by those not considered "born leaders." Some of the qualities of an effective, adherence-creating fitness instructor are discussed below.

Punctuality and Dependability

Instructors must assure exercise participants that each exercise class will start and end on time. A class that starts late or does not end on schedule is disruptive. Participants also want to know that their regular instructor, not a parade of substitutes, will be there to greet them. Whenever possible, absences should be planned, meaning that substitutes have been scheduled in advance and participants have been informed.

Professionalism

All participants should be treated with respect. Gossiping about other class members or staff is inappropriate and should not be tolerated. Professionalism extends to choice of exercise wear; although it is fine to be stylish, it is not professional to be dressed in a provocative manner (which can make participants feel uncomfortable).

Dedication

Part of being a professional is being dedicated to one's work. All fitness instructors should strive to obtain and maintain their group fitness instructor certification. It shows dedication to the profession. Efforts should be made on a continual basis to keep exercise classes diverse, fun, and enjoyable for participants. This means going to workshops to keep up on the latest exercise trends and finding out answers to questions participants may have on health-related topics. It is imperative to stay abreast of the latest health news and be informed of the scientific basis for health claims. Instructors should be able to discern the credible Internet sites in this area and direct participants to those sites when appropriate. Acquiring certification for newer types of exercise programming, such as Pilates, keeps the instructor informed of the latest trends and can protect against professional **burnout.**

Sensitivity to Participants' Needs

The ideal group fitness instructor recognizes that all participants are unique and come to exercise class for their own reasons. The purpose of class is not to treat all participants in the same way; instead, the instructor's responsibility is to work with the strengths of each individual participant to maximize his or her exercise session. Interacting with participants as individuals, treating them in an open, nonjudgmental manner, and expressing a willingness to listen are much appreciated.

Willingness to Plan Ahead

Participants appreciate when they are provided with advance notice of events that interfere with class, such as holiday closures, intersession breaks, or a planned vacation. They also are grateful when they are informed of upcoming events or fitness challenges that are offered in the community. If given enough advance notice, participants may want to train for a specific event. Helping participants set appropriate goals to prepare for these events and counseling them if a particular event is unrealistic demonstrates an interest in the participants and a high level of professionalism.

Recognizing the Signs of Instructor Burnout

Talking with other fitness instructors about how to prevent or work through burnout is invaluable. All exercise leaders will experience this phenomenon at some time or another, and getting another professional's advice will be useful. It is important to schedule regular vacations; it is amazing what a week or two away from work can do to improve one's attitude! Another strategy is to switch classes with another instructor for a time. Sometimes teaching a different class, using a different exercise format, or seeing different faces in the group can help alleviate burnout.

Taking Responsibility

Invariably, things will go wrong either with the exercise class itself or with the surroundings (e.g., broken air conditioning system). Taking responsibility for these problems and making sure that all efforts are made to correct the situation is appreciated by all. In addition, having backup plans

233

available when such situations arise can prove to be very useful.

Strategies That Encourage Adherence

Motivation depends on a participant's personal resources, abilities, and strengths, as well as external factors and circumstances. By assuming otherwise—that only innate personal factors influence adherence—a fitness instructor may "write off" a participant rather than try to teach skills that will help the participant develop into a regular exerciser.

Rather than placing the blame for non-adherence on the participant, the instructor must view motivation as a joint responsibility shared with the participant. It is also helpful to view the process as a dynamic one; alternative strategies may be needed for different clients at different stages in the exercise program.

Several strategies have proven successful in motivating participants to regularly attend exercise class. The following strategies can easily be integrated into any type of exercise class and will help motivate participants to become regular exercisers. (Some strategies, however, may not be applicable to a specific program, so the instructor must determine which strategies are appropriate for a given situation and subsequently apply them in an individualized manner.) After a particular strategic plan for adherence has been created, it should be reassessed often to determine its continued feasibility and effectiveness.

Formulate Reasonable Participant Expectations

Early on, determine each participant's expectations from the exercise class and help them formulate reasonable goals.

Expectations must be realistic to avoid disappointment. Although regular physical activity provides many benefits, it is not a panacea, and the participant must be informed of what benefits can be expected from the type of exercise being performed in the class. For instance, if a participant expects dramatic weight loss as a result of attending exercise class, he or she will be disappointed if this does not occur. It is preferable to advise the participant that, without a concomitant decrease in caloric intake, actual loss of body fat from physical training is likely to be negligible.

More realistic expectations would be weight loss on the order of one-half pound per week (0.23 kg/week) *if typical caloric intake is reduced,* trimmer legs or thighs over time, new friends made in class, or an increased sense of well-being or energy after completing an exercise session.

Set Exercise Goals

When an individual joins an exercise class or program, it is important to take the time to develop realistic, flexible, and individualized short-term goals with that person. This can be accomplished by setting up a brief interview with a new participant shortly after he or she joins the class. Realistic goals are important to avoid injury and maintain interest.

Participants can be taught goal-setting strategies by applying "SMART" goals. This catchy acronym includes the key components for developing effective goals. Goals should be:

S = Specific: What will you do, when, where, and with whom? Example: Not "I will go to the gym for a workout," but "I will go to SportHealth gym for cycling class on Monday, Wednesday, and Saturday at 6:30 p.m. after work."

M = Measurable: How will you know when you have reached your goals? Example: Not "I will exercise at a moderate intensity today," but "I will walk on the treadmill with my heart rate at 120 beats/minute for 2 miles." If heart rate and walking distance were achieved, then the goal was met.

A = Attainable: Can you really do this? Can you do it at this time? Example: Not "I will do 100 sit-ups without stopping Wednesday morning," but "I will do 25 sit-ups by Friday. I will work up to this by doing 16 sit-ups on Monday and 20 on Wednesday."

R = Relevant: Are your goals relevant or pertinent to your particular interests, needs, and abilities? Not "I will train to run a marathon in under three hours," but "I will increase the amount of physical activity I do by going to aerobics class twice this week."

T = Time-bound: How soon, how often, and for how long? Example: Not "I will go to boxing class twice next week," but "I will go to boxing class at 4:30 p.m. on Friday and Sunday."

Although the instructor should help in the goal-setting process, the goals should be set, as much as possible, by the participant. Short-term goals determined for each exercise session in conjunction with longer-term monthly goals allow for flexibility on a daily basis without jeopardizing the longer-term goals.

Goals can be specific to the exercise process, such as attending a certain number of classes in the coming weeks, supplementing class exercise with physical activity at home, or reaching a predetermined target heart rate during class by a certain date. They also can be related to some benefits not normally associated with physical activity, such as making new friends or developing a new social network. It is useful to encourage goals related to enjoyment and pleasure from moving and being active rather than only physical goals such as weight loss. Participants should periodically be reminded about their goals, and those who meet goals should be publicly praised. If goals are listed and displayed on a chart or are in participant files, they can easily be reviewed and evaluated regularly (e.g., twice a month). When goals are met, it is the instructor's duty to assist the participant in making new ones.

If it appears that the participant is unlikely to reach a specific goal, a more realistic goal should be encouraged. This will reduce the likelihood of disappointment or loss of interest associated with not meeting the goal, as well as the likelihood of physical injury that may occur when trying to "catch up" to reach a goal (such as performing too much exercise in too short a time). If a goal cannot be met, the fitness instructor and participant can brainstorm reasons why the goal was not met and plan more realistic goals in the future. To avoid any potential embarrassment, this should not be done publicly, but rather by talking with the participant during the warm-up or cool-down phase of the exercise class. These periods can be used to talk individually with participants and provide personalized instructions.

Formalizing the commitment to exercise with participants through written or oral contracts is another effective motivational strategy. A contract is often a written agreement signed by the participant and instructor (and others, if appropriate) that clearly itemizes the physical-activity goals and the rewards associated with achieving those goals. Contracts can increase a participant's commitment to the exercise program by defining the specific relationship

Adherence and Motivation

between exercise goals and positive out-comes contingent on meeting those goals. They also involve each participant in planning the exercise program, thereby providing a sense of ownership of the program (Figure 8.2).

Physical-activity contracts should be jointly prepared by the instructor and the participant. This can be done during a brief meeting before or after class or as part of a discussion during a warm-up or cool-down period, as previously described. The responsibilities each person has in meeting the terms of the contract can be itemized at this time. Requirements for class attendance, additional home-exercise workouts, and completion of exercise logs are often specified in contracts. Make certain that the participant has the skills necessary to meet the terms of the contract; beginning with modest goals is one way to ensure this. Precautions should be written into the contract to ensure that the participant does not engage in unhealthy practices to meet contract requirements (e.g., extended exercising over several days to meet a time-based goal or starvation tactics to meet a weight goal).

Figure 8.2 Sample Exercise Contract

This is an example of an exercise contract that can be used to formalize an individual's commitment to exercise. It specifies short-term goals, rewards to be received when goals are met, and promises of each party.

My Promises

1. To attend 10 out of 12 exercise classes during the next four weeks.

2. To exercise out of class for at least 30 minutes one time each week during the next four weeks.

3. For any exercise class I have to miss due to illness or other unavoidable reasons, I will plan to make up the session by (specify): _____

4. To reward myself at the end of each week that I meet my exercise goals by (for example, going to the movies, meeting a friend to shop, buying a new CD) (specify): _____

_____

My Group Fitness Instructor's Promises

1. To lead all classes, except when ill, unless advance notice is given.

2. To give me individual feedback regarding my progress.

3. To help me set new goals if the ones I set are unrealistic.

This contract will be evaluated on: _____
Date

_____
Participant Signature

_____
Group Fitness Instructor Signature

Strategies That
Encourage Adherence

Give Regular, Positive Feedback

As often as possible, the instructor should provide participants with ample, ongoing, positive reinforcement and individual praise. Feedback that is specific and relevant to the participant is known to be a powerful reinforcer. Specific feedback can include information regarding the number of exercise sessions attended during the month, sessions during which target exercise heart rate or RPE was met, and progress made on becoming proficient in an aerobic exercise routine. Feedback also can be oriented toward the physical-activity behavior itself, as in routine logging. A log sheet can be developed and kept at the exercise facility, where participants can keep a record of resting heart rate, exercise heart rate, RPE, and feelings before and after the exercise session each time they attend class (Figure 8.3). Recording information only takes a few minutes and can be accomplished immediately after class. Reviewing log sheets at regular intervals (perhaps monthly) provides participants with important feedback (e.g., how resting heart rate has decreased over time, how many sessions were attended during the previous month, improved sense of energy or well-being after exercise). Log sheets also provide participants with information about the intensity of their exercise sessions, letting them know if they are working too hard or need to pick up the intensity to obtain fitness benefits.

Inexpensive incentives, such as water bottles or key chains, can be provided to the participant when certain goals are met. Extrinsic rewards can be particularly important in the early stages of exercise adoption. Incentive-based goals should be set that can be realistically achieved by the majority of participants. Prizes based on attendance rather than large increases in performance are often preferred by participants and can motivate those experiencing less-than-optimal success in reaching physiological goals. Fitness "challenges" can provide rewards for different levels of participation by offering alternative prizes for a variety of achievements. It is important to be creative

Figure 8.3 Sample Exercise Log
This is an example of an exercise log in which individuals record their daily exercise. This can be kept at the exercise facility for the individual to fill out before or after class, or can be given to class members to take home and complete. Examine these records on a regular basis (e.g., once a month) to check for progress.

	Sunday	Monday	Tuesday	Wednesday	Thursday	Friday	Saturday
Date							
Type of exercise							
Number of minutes							
Resting heart rate							
Exercise heart rate							
RPE							
Feelings before class							
Feelings after class							

Adherence and Motivation

to ensure that the challenges are attractive to both the beginner and the long-term exerciser.

Public monitoring of attendance as a means of providing feedback and distributing achievement awards is useful for motivating participants. Posting attendance charts in the exercise room rewards the frequent attendee with a public display of adherence and may motivate the less-than-optimal adherer to attend class on a more regular basis. A chart with a group theme, such as "Exercise Around the World," can be devised in which daily attendance of each group member is worth a certain number of miles. When the group "reaches" predetermined countries, awards that are representative of that country can be given to all class participants. This strategy encourages group support and rewards the frequent attendee as well as the participant who attends class less often. It also may provide increased motivation to the wayward participant who receives a reward for being part of the group.

Make Exercise Sessions Interesting and Fun

As previously mentioned, aspects of the exercise session itself are related to adherence and motivational issues. The exercise routine should be easy to follow; one means of accomplishing this is to break the routine up into short segments so the participant can learn the routine and be successful.

Sure ways to guarantee dropout are to have an exercise routine that is so complicated that participants cannot follow it, or one so intense that participants are exhausted at the end of class. It is helpful to provide ample, positive reinforcement or support while participants are learning the routine. Varying the routine regularly and providing different types of music that suit the tastes of the class can be

useful. Ask participants what type of music they prefer and prepare routines to match their interests.

Participants can be regularly polled to assess the enjoyment factor of the class, perhaps through the use of the RPE scale or a simple enjoyment-assessment scale. Participants should generally be exercising in an RPE range between 11 and 15 on the "category" (6 to 20) scale. If participants are working in an RPE range that is too high, they may not be enjoying the exercise; rather, they may be working hard just to keep up with the instructor.

Exercise enjoyment also can be assessed orally during the exercise session with a six-point rating scale, with one equaling "extremely unenjoyable" and six equaling "extremely enjoyable." The instructor can determine which parts of the exercise class are most favorable to participants by asking about their enjoyment level at different points during class. Another option is to develop a brief, anonymous written survey to assess the enjoyment level of the class and satisfaction with different aspects of the exercise program. Survey responses can be saved and used as documentation of exercise-leadership skills.

If it is evident that some participants are working excessively, the intensity of the routine can be lowered until the overworkers can "catch their breath" and get back into their exercise comfort zone. As previously mentioned, if the class is of varying abilities, visually provide both a lower-intensity and higher-intensity version of the routine.

Acknowledge Exercise Discomforts

Participants should be taught how to tell the difference between the transient discomforts associated with exercise and those discomforts that are potential signs of injury or more serious problems. Newcomers to exercise may not be accustomed to the feeling of increased breathing, heart rate, and sweating associated with exercise. They must be reassured that these are normal responses and should be expected.

Participants must be informed of potential injuries that may arise and be able to recognize a symptom that warrants attention. Any sudden, sharp pain that does not dissipate or muscle soreness that does not lessen after a few days may be a sign of injury and should be examined by a health professional. Similarly, participants must know the signs and symptoms of a heart attack, particularly when the exercisers are of middle and older ages. A dull, aching discomfort in the chest, neck, jaw, or arms associated with excessive sweating or clammy skin that is not relieved with rest may be signs of a heart attack; proper medical authorities should be contacted immediately.

It is helpful to ask participants individually how they are feeling and if they are experiencing any unusual discomforts. This information is often not offered voluntarily and potential injuries may not be discovered without prompting. After learning about minor injuries, the fitness instructor can provide personal advice to take it easy for a class or two until the ache or pain lessens. Follow-up advice during successive classes lets the participant know that he or she is cared about and the instructor is looking out for the participant's best interests.

Use Exercise Reminders, Cues, and Prompts

Encourage participants to develop prompts or cues in their home or work environments that will promote regular class attendance, such as scheduling physical activity in a daily appointment book and laying out exercise gear the night before class.

Posters placed at participants' homes or work environments that depict individuals enjoying physical activity may encourage attendance. Newsletters can include clever flyers that remind participants of upcoming special events or fitness challenges. E-mail prompts are another avenue to cue participants. A variety of prompts at work, home, and the exercise location can help keep participants thinking about exercise.

Encourage an Extensive Social-support System

Develop a buddy system among participants so that they can call each other to make sure they attend class and have an additional support person to discuss progress and goals. Additional social support for exercise can be encouraged by having participants ask friends or relatives to pitch in by reminding them to attend their exercise classes. Ask participants to identify which types of support are helpful and motivating to them personally, and then ask them to identify individuals who can provide that specific type of support. Table 8.1 lists different types of support and provides examples of how they can be used to encourage exercise attendance. Support does not have to be face-to-face; telephone, e-mail, and mail contacts are additional avenues of support that can be utilized. As previously described, newsletters are a useful means for keeping participants informed of class activities, and they add to a sense of belonging. Telephone contacts initiated after one or two missed classes that let the lapsing participant know he or she was missed may encourage a return to class.

Develop Group Camaraderie

It is particularly important for class members to feel a sense of cohesiveness. Research

Adherence and Motivation

Table 8.1
Support for Exercise

There are several types of support that can help individuals adopt and maintain an exercise program. Individuals can evaluate which types of support are useful to them personally, and then identify individuals who can provide that type of support. If support is not readily available, individuals can ask friends and colleagues to support them in specific ways as they make exercise-related goals.

Types of Support	Ways Support Can Be Received	Who can provide this type of support for me? (fill in)
Emotional providers	Sympathetic to struggles with starting to exercise	
Affection providers	Comfort and reassurance when goals are not met Reward-givers when goals are met	
Challengers	Challenge to make goals and achieve them	
Listeners	Sounding board for communicating experiences associated with exercise	
Appraisers	Feedback on goal achievements	
Role models/partners	Exercise partner, set and work on goals together	
Experts	Information associated with exercise	

shows that individuals who have strong beliefs about the cohesiveness of their class attend more exercise classes, are less likely to drop out, are more likely to enjoy physical activity, and have high self-efficacy toward physical activity (Estabrooks, 2000). Group cohesion starts when participants gather around a shared task. Learning a new routine as a group or working to meet group goals will enhance this type of group cohesion. As participants become satisfied with their accomplishments, social cohesion increases. Social cohesion can be enhanced by introducing new class members and encouraging participants to share information about themselves. Providing interesting, little-known facts about each participant in a newsletter also is beneficial. The social support and reinforcement for exercise developed through group membership is powerful and should not be overlooked.

By the same token, the instructor must be aware of individual behaviors that threaten to undermine positive group dynamics. Some groups have chronic complainers or generally disruptive individuals. These individuals must be dealt with early to avoid the tendency for them to take charge of the group or monopolize class time. When dealing with a chronic complainer, the instructor should listen attentively and acknowledge understanding of the participant's complaint, then agree on a solution and follow through to make any needed changes. The participant should be informed when the issue has been resolved.

The disruptive individual should not be given too much attention (since that is probably what he or she wants). If lack of attention does not change the individual's behavior, then the instructor should speak to the individual privately to discuss the interruptions and possible reasons for the disruptive behavior.

Emphasize Positive Aspects of Exercise

Participants just starting to exercise should be encouraged to generally disregard minor exercise discomforts, recognize their own self-defeating thoughts, and counteract them with positive thoughts. Encourage participants to think "good thoughts," such as how refreshing it feels to move about freely, how encouraging other class members are, and so on, while performing the exercise routine. Comment on positive aspects of the routine throughout: "here comes the fun part," "looking great," and similar comments keep the participants focused on the positive. Martin et al. (1984) found that those who were told to attend to environmental surroundings and enjoy the outdoors during a class-based running program had greater attendance and were more likely to continue exercising after the formal program ended compared to those who concentrated on increasing their performance during the exercise sessions. Pleasant thoughts that focus on enjoyment of movement and how accomplished the participants will feel when class is over will help the time move by quickly and enjoyably. The instructor can help participants who have been exercising regularly and have specific performance goals to visualize the sense of satisfaction they will get when those goals are met. This can serve as a positive motivator when the exercise intensity necessary to meet goals may be intense and somewhat uncomfortable for the participant.

Help Participants Develop Intrinsic Rewards

Once the exercise behavior has become part of the participant's routine, it is often useful to supplement class rewards and support with a natural reward system that is provided outside of exercise class. Positive feedback on exercise habits provided by family, friends, and co-workers transfers some of the positive feedback received during exercise class to other environments, as well as providing additional avenues of social support. Encourage the participant to develop a natural reward system that focuses on increased feelings of self-esteem, a sense of accomplishment, and increased energy levels instead of merely external rewards. Natural

reinforcers add to a sense of personal identification as being an exerciser and will help participants continue to exercise even when they cannot make it to class.

Prepare Participants for Inevitable Missed Classes

It is important to realize that the participant will not be able to attend classes at some point in the program. Although the participant may be unable to make it to class during vacations, holidays, or times of increased work or family pressures, they may still be able to continue a home-based exercise program and should be encouraged to do so. Confidence about being physically active in different settings can be built by encouraging participants to add at least one day of physical activity outside of class time, preferably using a different mode of exercise (such as brisk walking, swimming, or any other type of exercise the participant enjoys). This will give participants experience with a beneficial alternative when they must miss a scheduled class. Ask participants about exercise performed outside of class and praise them when it has been accomplished. When the participant successfully exercises on his or her own, confidence for continuing exercise is being built.

Exercising with family or co-workers is ideal for out-of-class exercise sessions. If the participant cannot find someone to exercise with, encourage other class members to meet him or her in an alternative physical-activity setting. Not only does this provide an additional mode of social support for physical activity, it also provides participants with an opportunity to problem-solve any difficulties encountered with exercise. Additional days of exercise can be included in the exercise contract, and exercise logs of these sessions can be kept to document them. During times when

Adherence and Motivation

participants are extremely busy, remind them that a shorter-than-normal workout is still beneficial and will keep them exercising regularly. Three 10-minute workouts performed throughout the day are just as effective in increasing fitness levels as a single 30-minute bout. Although the instructor's primary responsibility is to encourage class attendance, supporting the concept of at least one out-of-class exercise session will ultimately help participants' overall exercise achievement.

Classes may not be offered in some instances. For example, if classes are provided as part of a university environment, there may be a break in classes due to semester breaks or holidays. By advising participants in advance, the instructor can prepare them for these breaks. It is also possible to make arrangements with other exercise classes at different locations in the community so participants can continue exercising in a similar format.

Prepare Participants for Changes in Instructors

A change in instructors is usually quite disruptive for participants. Unfortunately, typically little is done to prepare participants for this change. A planned change in leadership because of pregnancy leave, travel, or a permanent relocation can be smooth if participants are prepared for the change well ahead of time. If possible, introduce the new exercise instructor in advance. Having the regular and new instructor team-teach several exercise classes can help prevent fears of a change in format after the regular exercise instructor departs. There will undoubtedly be times of illness, so substitutes should be planned for and arranged in advance. It would be a bonus if instructors could introduce the substitutes to the partic-

ipants so that when they need to be used, participants are already familiar with them.

Train to Prevent Exercise Defeatism

Prepare participants for the eventual missed class. How slips are handled determines if they will be temporary or permanent. Let participants know that missing a class is a realistic probability. If participants can predict and prepare for lapses in their exercise program, these occurrences will likely not be as disruptive. Certain issues make class attendance unlikely (family crises, holidays, illness, and extra pressure or deadlines at work). When these can be anticipated and seen as being temporary rather than as a breakdown in the success of the physical-activity program, adherence is more likely to be maintained. Lapses should be viewed as a challenge to overcome rather than as a failure.

Participants can be made aware of the defeatist attitude that accompanies the belief that once a physical-activity program is disrupted, total relapse or dropout is inevitable. Although breaking the adherence rule does place the participant at a higher risk for dropping out, it is not inevitable. If exercise is viewed by participants as a process during which there will undoubtedly be times that they will be less active than others, they will not consider themselves nonexercisers whenever a class is missed. Rather, they will catch the next available class or exercise on their own when time permits. Participants also can be encouraged to avoid "high-risk" situations (such as going to a "happy hour" before exercise class) that test their resolve to exercise. Encourage participants to surround themselves with cues that support the physical-activity behavior. A simple telephone call or e-mail message after one or two missed sessions may bring the participant back to class if he or she understands that missing class is not a sign of failure.

Emphasize an Overall Healthy Lifestyle

Physical activity is only one of a number of lifestyle-related activities that participants engage in throughout the week. It is often assumed that those who exercise regularly also practice other healthy behaviors. Unfortunately, this is often not the case. Diets of exercisers are generally not any different from the typical American diet. The instructor has an outstanding opportunity to provide accurate information and to encourage the development of additional healthy lifestyle behaviors. Questions regarding diet, weight control, and other behaviors will undoubtedly be asked. By being well-versed in these topics, the instructor can offer sound information with a scientific basis. Displaying posters that emphasize aspects of healthy lifestyles, such as the MyPyramid Food Guidance System, can remind participants that physical activity is just one of many healthful behaviors.

Finally, the fitness instructor is viewed as a model for a healthy lifestyle and should try to live up to the participants' expectations. Encourage by example. Do not smoke or abuse alcohol, and maintain a prudent, healthy diet and an appropriate body composition.

Exercise and Body Image

Cultural norms for attractiveness are often centered on "ideal body types." In the United States, this ideal body type has, in recent times, been associated with extreme thinness, particularly in women. While this body type may photograph well for fashion magazines, it is not ideal for most women and is most likely an unattainable

and potentially unhealthy goal for many. When women perceive that their bodies are being compared to this unrealistic "ideal," many become dissatisfied with their body shape and fret over any extra pounds in undesirable places.

High levels of physical activity have been associated with a preoccupation with weight and body shape. These unhealthy attitudes may put some individuals, particularly teenage and young adult women, at risk for developing **eating disorders,** such as anorexia nervosa and bulimia, as well as **addictions** to exercise or overexercise.

By being aware of this phenomenon, the instructor can encourage participants to accept their own body shapes. Remind participants that everyone has his or her own unique body shape and no amount of exercise is going to change that basic shape. Avoid pointing out specific exercises to "fix" certain body parts, which may lead to a preoccupation or dissatisfaction with that body part. It is better for participants to focus on the enjoyment of moving and the overall good feelings associated with exercise.

While the instructor wants to encourage regular exercise participation, a small number of individuals may take the exercise habit to the extreme and exhibit signs of exercise **dependence** or addiction. Exercise dependence has been defined in a variety of ways, though a good definition is when the commitment to exercise assumes a higher priority than commitments to family, work, or interpersonal relations (Morgan, 1979).

Excessive exercise may be associated with body-image distortions or even more serious disorders, such as anorexia nervosa and bulimia, where excessive exercise is used as an additional method to lose weight or to "purge" calories that have

Adherence and Motivation

recently been consumed (Brownell & Foreyt, 1986).

Signs of exercise dependence/addiction include continuing to exercise despite injuries or illness, extreme levels of thinness, and feelings of extreme guilt, irritability, or depression when unable to exercise. If the instructor suspects a participant is exercising to excess or may have an eating disorder, the matter should be dealt with using forethought and sensitivity. Concern should be expressed over what has been observed and the participant should be asked directly about his or her exercise and eating habits. Chances are that if a disorder exists, the participant has already been confronted about the situation. Be sensitive and understanding, offering support as well as suggesting that professional guidance be sought. It is helpful if several names and telephone numbers of qualified professionals are available to the participant in need.

Summary

Dropout rates for those beginning a group fitness program can reach 50% or more after only six months. Instead of placing the blame for nonadherence on the participant, the instructor must view motivation as a shared responsibility and work with the participant to develop a successful motivational strategy. Extra assistance should be provided to the participant who has been identified as at high risk for dropout.

Motivation is a dynamic process, and by applying a variety of strategies and reviewing and refining these strategies regularly, achievement of regular exercise can be attained by most participants. Motivational techniques include structuring appropriate expectations and goals, identifying short-term benefits, providing specific feedback, teaching problem-solving skills, serving as a positive role model, and training participants to manage their own reward systems.

Additionally, the convenience and attractiveness of the exercise setting, enjoyability of the exercise class, supportiveness of the exercise environment, as well as personal factors specific to both the group fitness instructor and the participant, are factored into the exercise-adherence equation. Understanding and applying the principles of adherence and motivation described in this chapter will help the instructor become a more effective teacher and health professional.

References

Borg, G. (1998). *Borg's Perceived Exertion and Pain Scales.* Champaign, Ill.: Human Kinetics.

Brownell, K.D. & Foreyt, J.P. (Eds.) (1986). *Handbook of Eating Disorders.* New York: Basic Books, Inc.

Estabrooks, P.A. (2000). Sustaining exercise participation through group cohesion. *Exercise and Sport Sciences Reviews,* 28, 63–67.

Martin, J.E. et al. (1984). Behavioral control of exercise in sedentary adults: Studies 1 through 6. *Journal of Consulting & Clinical Psychology,* 52, 795–811.

Morgan, W.P. (1979). Negative addiction in runners. *Physician and Sportsmedicine,* 7, 57–70.

Perri, M.G. et al. (2002). Adherence to exercise prescriptions: Effects of prescribing moderate versus higher levels of intensity and frequency. *Health Psychology,* 21, 452–458.

Suggested Reading

American College of Sports Medicine (2006). *ACSM's Guidelines for Exercise Testing and Prescription* (7th ed.). Philadelphia: Lippincott Williams & Wilkins.

Marcus, B.H. & Forsyth, L.H. (2003). *Motivating People to Be Physically Active.* Champaign, Ill.: Human Kinetics.

Trost, S.G. et al. (2002). Correlates of adults' participation in physical activity: Review and update. *Medicine & Science in Sports & Exercise,* 34, 1996–2001.

Sallis, J.F. & Owen, N. (1998). *Physical Activity and Behavioral Medicine.* Thousand Oaks, Calif.: Sage.

U.S. Department of Health and Human Services (1996). *Physical Activity and Health: A Report of the Surgeon General.* Atlanta, Ga.: U.S. Department of Health and Human Services, Centers for Disease Control and Prevention, National Center for Chronic Disease Prevention and Health Promotion.

References and
Suggested Reading

Chapter Nine

James H. Rimmer, Ph.D., is a professor in the Department of Disability and Human Development and adjunct professor in the Department of Movement Sciences and the School of Public Health at the University of Illinois at Chicago. He also is an adjunct professor in the Department of Physical Medicine and Rehabilitation at Northwestern University, which is affiliated with the Rehabilitation Institute of Chicago. For the past 25 years, Dr. Rimmer has been developing and directing physical-activity and health-promotion programs for people with disabilities. He has published more than 85 peer-reviewed journal articles and book chapters on various topics related to physical activity, health promotion, secondary conditions, and disability. He is director of two federally funded centers, the National Center on Physical Activity and Disability (www.ncpad.org) and the Rehabilitation Engineering Research Center on Recreational Technologies and Exercise Physiology Benefiting People with Disabilities (www.rercrectech.org). Dr. Rimmer has published standardized measurement instruments that can be used to evaluate the accessibility of fitness and recreation facilities for people with disabilities, and was recently funded by NIH to develop a health empowerment zone for people with disabilities in and around the UIC medical campus.

Jennifer L. Rowland, Ph.D., M.P.H., P.T., is a research assistant professor in the Department of Disability and Human Development and has an adjunct faculty appointment in the School of Public Health at the University of Illinois at Chicago, where she is working with Dr. Rimmer as project director for a grant from the National Institutes of Health to examine environmental effects on obesity for people with disabilities. Dr. Rowland has 11 years of experience as a physical therapist working in rehabilitation centers, long-term care facilities, and home health settings, developing and implementing exercise programs for people with disabilities. She has also performed research evaluating Internet-based feedback mechanisms for preventing secondary conditions among people with newly diagnosed spinal cord injuries. Dr. Rowland is a member of the executive committee for Disability Forum, a special interest group within the American Public Health Association, and is a federal grant reviewer for the National Institute on Disability and Rehabilitation Research.

Disabilities and Health Limitations

By James H. Rimmer and Jennifer L. Rowland

Until recently, many fitness professionals considered the words health and disability to be on opposite ends of the spectrum. How could a person be considered healthy if he or she already had a disability? That viewpoint is slowly changing, and the benefits of physical activity touted by fitness organizations and policymakers for the general population are now being directed at persons with chronic diseases and disabilities.

Disabilities and Health Limitations

Joining a fitness center is a viable way for persons with disabilities and health limitations to maintain their physical function after rehabilitation, and offers them the opportunity to improve their overall health in a supervised setting where, if necessary, they can get immediate assistance from a fitness professional. People with disabilities are often faced with a higher incidence of secondary conditions (e.g., obesity, pressure sores, infections, osteoporosis), which cause further disability, and in many cases a loss of physical independence. This loss of independence often leads to depression, which causes further disease and disability (Rimmer, 1999). This downward spiral takes a heavy physical and psychological toll on people with disabilities and often creates a life of permanent dependence on others for daily care (Figure 9.1).

People with disabilities are slowly becoming aware of the importance of maintaining an active lifestyle. They are starting to realize that as they age, exercise becomes more and more important in preserving, and in some cases restoring, their physical independence. Whereas a few years ago joining a local fitness center to maintain one's health was not even a thought among the millions of people with disabilities, particularly those with severe disabilities, today's new generation is starting to feel more comfortable using fitness centers to improve their health. The **Americans with Disabilities Act** has shed new light on the importance of making fitness facilities architecturally and programmatically accessible to persons with disabilities, and has raised a new awareness in the fitness community that persons with disabilities have a right to equal access to their facilities.

Fitness professionals now have an exciting opportunity to reach out to people with disabilities. As managed-care organizations continue their cost-saving strategies by downsizing the rehabilitation industry, there is a window of opportunity for fitness professionals to become part of the paradigm for

Figure 9.1
Downward spiral of disability and dependence

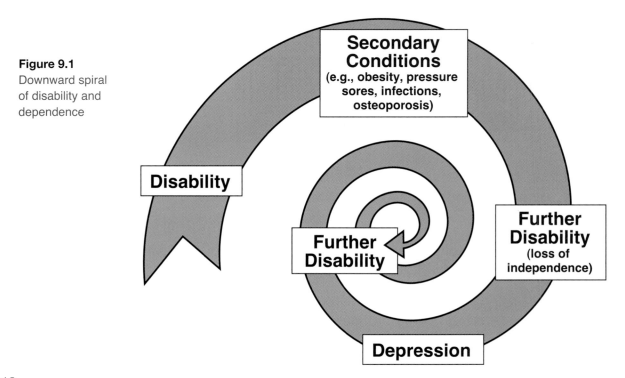

improving the health of people with disabilities who will need community-based settings to restore, maintain, and improve their overall function. What better place to do this than in a local fitness center a few blocks from home? The purpose of this chapter is to provide an overview of the major disabilities and health limitations that require modified exercise programs.

Metabolic Disorders

Obesity

The most prevalent health disorder in American society is obesity, and the number of people affected by obesity has increased markedly in the past 20 years (Hedley et al., 2004). According to information reported in the *Journal of the American Medical Association* that was gathered as part of the National Health and Nutrition Examination Survey (NHANES) from 1999–2002, 30.4% of adults over the age of 20 were obese. The same survey found that 31% of children ages six to 19 were at risk for being overweight or were already overweight (Hedley et al., 2004). Another study examining the prevalence of overweight, obesity, and extreme obesity in a predominantly minority group of adults with disabilities found that extreme obesity was approximately four times higher among people with disabilities than the general population (Rimmer & Wang, 2005).

In large-scale studies consisting of thousands of people, **body mass index (BMI)** is used to calculate the number of Americans who are **overweight.** The formula for computing BMI is weight (kg)/height^2 (m)* (see Tables 6.7 and 6.8, page 166). An adult who has a BMI between 25 and 29.9 is considered to be overweight, and an adult with a

* 1 kg is equal to 2.2 lb, and 1 m is equal to 39.37 in.

BMI of 30 or higher is considered to be obese (Expert Panel, 1998). Obesity is associated with many other medical conditions, including hypertension, **type 2 diabetes, osteoarthritis,** heart disease, and **low-back pain** (Han et al., 1997; Rice et al., 1993). Excess weight is considered a major risk factor for premature mortality, **cardiovascular disease,** type 2 diabetes, osteoarthritis, certain cancers, and a multitude of other medical conditions, and accounts for more than 280,000 deaths annually in the U.S. (Flegal et al., 2002; Rimmer & Braddock, 1997).

Exercise is one of the three major cornerstones of treatment for obesity. The other two components, which are not discussed in this chapter, are diet and behavior modification (Rimmer, 1994). Since diet alone results in a loss of lean muscle tissue, the only long-term mechanism for maintaining weight loss is to increase daily energy expenditure.

Exercise Guidelines for People Who Are Obese

• A major strategy for getting persons who are excessively overweight to develop lifelong exercise habits is to make the activity as enjoyable and pain-free as possible. Exercising with an excess amount of body fat presents a major challenge because of the additional stress on joints and muscles, particularly in participants who are severely overweight. Additionally, these participants are often in extremely poor condition. The key to a successful program is to identify the right combination of activities that do not lead to pain or discomfort. Finding the appropriate comfort level must be done on an individual basis. Do not assume that participants that come to you with suggested activities know what is best for their body types.

- The number-one priority with obese participants is to keep the activity at an intensity level that does not cause pain and soreness. Many persons who are severely overweight already have joint pain from simply performing daily activities. By using a variety of activities that involve the arms and legs together, the stress load on the joints will be displaced over four limbs as opposed to two. Do not place heavy emphasis on the intensity level of the activity. Emphasize low-intensity, high-duration activities. It is more important for the participant to move more and enjoy the feeling of being physically active.

- Since weight maintenance is a lifelong process, participants should understand the caloric balance equation: energy input = energy output. If this balance tilts toward the energy-input side, there will be an excess of calories taken in and those not used will be stored as fat. Therefore, a daily dose of physical activity is needed to offset the calories being consumed. This does not necessarily mean that they have to go to the fitness center seven days a week, but it does suggest they should be physically active every day. A daily dose of physical activity can be performed at home or at work by using a variety of activities that can include housework and gardening.

- Since arthritis is a highly prevalent condition among persons who are overweight (Rimmer, 1994), protecting the joints is paramount. Cross-training programs should be employed that involve various types of exercise routines for 10 minutes or less. More and more products are coming on the market that require a lower load on the knee and hip joints. The elliptical trainer, stationary bike, and recumbent stepper (performed in a sitting position) are very popular among severely overweight participants. Some participants may perform 10-minute sessions on two or three different machines. Additionally, water-based activities are excellent for obese participants who also have arthritis because of the reduced weightbearing effects of the water. Many participants, however, will not want to join an aquatics program because of their reluctance to wear a swimsuit.

- One of the areas often forgotten when developing exercise programs for individuals who are overweight is seat comfort. Many bicycle seats are too small or have too hard of a surface for obese participants. In some cases, it may be necessary to construct a special seat for severely overweight participants [300 lb (136 kg) or more]. It is also important to make sure that the seat position is adjusted in such a way that a person's stomach does not impair his or her ability to pedal the bike. Some overweight participants prefer to have their seat adjusted a little higher than normal to prevent their midsection from getting in the way of the pedaling motion. This position usually requires the knee to be in full extension to pedal without obstruction.

- Resistance training should be performed for 10 to 15 minutes a day, three days a week. This can be done with weights or elastic bands. Weight training improves body image and increases lean body mass, which makes this activity a nice complement to the cardiovascular-training component and adds variety to the program. Additionally, resistance training improves strength and makes activities of daily living such as walking up a flight of steps easier to manage.

Diabetes

Diabetes is one of the most debilitating conditions affecting the U.S. population and is often linked to a number of chronic diseases and disabilities, including heart disease, stroke, amputations, blindness, kidney failure, autonomic neuropathy [affects heart rate (HR)], and peripheral **neuropathy** (affects sensation in distal extremities) (National Institutes of Health, 2006). There are two types of diabetes: type 1 and type 2. **Type 1 diabetes** is caused by a destruction of the pancreatic cells that produce the body's **insulin** (Tsai et al., 2006). Type 2 diabetes results from insulin resistance combined with defective insulin secretion (Parchman, Romero, & Pugh, 2006).

Diabetes is a broadly applied term used to denote a complex group of syndromes that result in a disturbance in the utilization of glucose. Type 1 diabetes is a more serious condition and can result in death if not properly treated. A person with this condition must take regular amounts of insulin to sustain a safe amount of glucose in the blood. When insulin is not taken, blood glucose, which normally ranges between 80 and 120 mg/dL, can reach 1,000 mg/dL or higher, and cause the person to go into a diabetic coma or die.

Type 2 diabetes is the most common form of diabetes, affecting 90% of all individuals with diabetes. It typically occurs in adults who are overweight and is characterized by insulin resistance, a reduced sensitivity of insulin target cells to available insulin. Insulin resistance, a condition in which the body is unable to use its own insulin efficiently, affects approximately 60 million people in the United States, one in four of whom will develop type 2 diabetes. Unfortunately, increasing numbers of children are being diagnosed with type 2 diabetes, making the term "adult-onset diabetes" obsolete. Some people with type 2 diabetes never exhibit any of the classic symptoms of diabetes. Treatment usually includes diet modification, medication, and exercise therapy.

Exercise can have a significant effect on lowering blood glucose and is an essential component of treatment for persons with type 1 and type 2 diabetes. However, because glucose is needed to perform exercise, persons with diabetes can easily run into trouble if their baseline blood glucose level is too high or too low.

Exercise Guidelines for Persons With Diabetes

Important considerations when creating exercise programs for people with diabetes include:

- Knowledge of the type of medication they may be taking to lower blood glucose (insulin or oral hypoglycemic agents)
- Timing of medication administration
- Blood glucose level prior to exercise
- Timing, amount, and type of previous food intake
- Presence and severity of diabetic complications
- Use of other medication secondary to diabetic complications
- Intensity, duration, and type of exercise (Albright, 2003)

According to recommendations from *ACSM's Exercise Management for Persons with Chronic Diseases and Disabilities* (Albright, 2003), people with type 2 diabetes can especially benefit from exercise in addition to medication and dietary factors that will work together to improve blood glucose control. Exercise can also be important in type 2 diabetes prevention. However, the same source indicates that those with type 1 diabetes may not encounter the same blood glucose-lowering advantages. People with type 1 and type 2 diabetes are encouraged to exercise, however, to gain other benefits, such as reduction in body fat, cardiovascular improvement, and stress reduction, all of which improve overall health and well-being. The following are general exercise training guidelines for people with either type of diabetes.

- The most important aspects of the exercise program for persons with diabetes is maintaining the proper balance of food and insulin dosage and reducing heart-disease risk. If too many calories are ingested before exercise or too little insulin is taken, blood glucose can reach a high enough level where exercise will actually cause a further increase in blood glucose levels because of the breakdown of fatty acids and glycogen (the storage form of glucose).

- Physicians will usually instruct their patients to check their blood glucose level before and after exercise. Exercise should be curtailed if pre-exercise blood glucose is below 100 mg/dL. With additional carbohydrate consumption, exercise may be allowed to take place. Exercise should also be curtailed if pre-exercise blood glucose is greater than 300 mg/dL or greater than 240 mg/dL with urinary ketone bodies. In the latter scenario, exercise would need to be postponed until the participant's blood sugar is under control. Your participants with diabetes should have specific guidelines to follow in these situations. These guidelines will depend upon a participant's clinical status and medical history with respect to blood glucose control.

- Persons with diabetes should carry a portable **glucometer** with them. This device is inexpensive and can be used to check blood glucose before and after exercise. Persons with diabetes should check

their blood glucose level a few minutes before exercising and follow the guidelines regarding exercise.

- Another common problem in persons with diabetes is a condition known as **hypoglycemia,** which is defined as a blood glucose level lower than 60 mg/dL, and occurs when there is not enough glucose in the bloodstream. Most experts agree that this is an even more dangerous situation than **hyperglycemia** (high blood glucose) because it can happen very quickly and can lead to an **insulin reaction.** This is often a greater problem in persons who have type 1 diabetes. If some form of food (preferably carbohydrate) is not ingested immediately, the person could go into **insulin shock** and die. Table 9.1 lists the early and late symptoms of an insulin reaction and details how to treat one if it does occur. Fitness professionals should keep rapidly absorbed carbohydrates on site (e.g., orange juice or other fruit drinks) in case of an emergency.

- Blood glucose should also be measured after exercise to make sure the participant does not become hypoglycemic. In persons with recently diagnosed diabetes, it will take a few sessions to learn how to maintain a normal balance of glucose and insulin before and after exercise.

- Fitness professionals should know if participants with diabetes have secondary conditions that must be considered in the exercise program (e.g., foot ulcers, visual or kidney problems, hypertension). For example, if a participant has a foot ulcer, high-impact or weightbearing exercise is contraindicated. If a person has diabetic retinopathy (damage to the retina) or hypertension, heavy resistance training is unsafe. It is important to know the complete medical history of the participant and develop the exercise program based on individual needs and limitations.

- Aerobic exercise that involves repetitive submaximal contractions of major muscle groups, such as swimming, cycling, and brisk walking, are recommended for persons with diabetes. These activities are less jarring than jogging, racquet sports, basketball, and high-impact aerobics.

- The intensity, frequency, and duration of exercise should be based on the age, fitness medical status, and motivational level of the participant. For example, consider a participant with type 2 diabetes who wants to run on a treadmill. In doing so, she elevates her heart rate to over 85% of her age-predicted maximum heart rate. Since she has other secondary conditions of concern (e.g., hypertension, retinopathy, kidney complications), she is only permitted to exercise at 50 to 65% of her target heart rate as prescribed by her physician.

- Since it is difficult to maintain an optimal balance of glucose and insulin, exercise should be performed daily. This does not necessarily mean that the participant has to come to the fitness center on a daily basis. There are many other activities that can be done at home. Having the "best of both worlds" may involve a three-day-a-week structured program in the fitness center and a four-day-a-week program of general activity, including walking, gardening, or stationary cycling. The key is to get a regular "dose" of daily activity, preferably at the same time each day for better control.

- The duration of activity will also depend on the participant's comfort level, with a goal of 30 to 60 minutes. Individuals with a higher tolerance for exercise, and who are more motivated, will generally prefer to exercise for 45 to 60 minutes.

- Avoid exercise in the late evening. A person can have a nocturnal insulin reaction (i.e., an insulin reaction during sleep) if he or she exercises too close to bedtime and is low in carbohydrates. Since the person is unaware of the insulin reaction, he or she could go into a coma and die.

- People with diabetes need to take very good care of their feet, which should be regularly checked for any cuts, blisters, or signs of infection. Good quality exercise shoes also are very important.

General guidelines and safety tips for persons with diabetes are listed in Table 9.2.

Table 9.1
Symptoms and Treatment of
Insulin Reaction (Hypoglycemia)

Early Symptoms	*Late Symptoms*
Anxiety, uneasiness	Double vision
Irritability	Sweating, palpitations
Extreme hunger	Nausea
Confusion	Loss of motor coordination
Headaches	Pale, moist skin
Insomnia	Strong, rapid pulse
	Convulsions
	Loss of consciousness
	Coma

Treating a Participant Who Is Having an Insulin Reaction

1. Stop the activity immediately.
2. Have the person sit down and check his or her blood glucose level.
3. Have the participant drink orange juice or some other rapidly absorbing carbohydrate.
4. Allow the client to sit quietly and wait for a response.
5. When the client feels better, check the blood glucose level again.
6. If the blood glucose level is above 100 mg/dL and the participant feels better, resume activity.
7. Check blood glucose level after 15 to 30 minutes to reassure that levels are within a safe range.
8. Do not allow the participant to leave the facility until blood glucose levels are within a normal range.
9. If the participant does not improve, seek medical attention immediately.

Rimmer, J.H. (1994). *Fitness and Rehabilitation Programs for Special Populations.* Dubuque, Iowa: WCB McGraw-Hill.

Disabilities and Health Limitations

Table 9.2
General Guidelines and Safety Tips for Persons with Diabetes

1. Regulating blood glucose levels requires optimal timing of exercise periods in relation to meals and insulin dosage.
2. Aim to keep blood glucose levels between 100 and 200 mg/dL one to two hours after a meal.
3. Exercise can have a significant effect on insulin reduction (American Diabetes Association, 2006). Some experts note that insulin may need to be reduced by 10 to 50% when starting an exercise program (Wallberg-Henriksson, 1992).*
4. If blood glucose levels are lower than 100 mg/dL, have the person consume a rapidly absorbing carbohydrate to increase blood glucose.
5. If blood glucose is greater than 300 mg/dL before exercise (some doctors may recommend that exercise not be initiated at blood glucose levels greater than 250 mg/dL), make sure that insulin or the oral hypoglycemic agent has been taken. In some circumstances, participants with a high blood glucose level (>300 mg/dL) may lower it to a safe enough level to exercise by drinking water.
6. No participant should be allowed to exercise if his or her blood glucose level does not fall to a safe range before exercise.
7. Teach participants to check their feet periodically to avoid foot ulcers. If an ulcer is found, have the person consult with his or her physician immediately for proper treatment. Foot ulcers can worsen and cause major problems if left untreated.
8. Check blood glucose at the end of the exercise session to make sure that the person does not become hypoglycemic. This could happen very quickly, particularly after high-intensity or long-duration activities or when the person is not accustomed to understanding how the body reacts to exercise.
9. Make sure the participant is well hydrated and drinking water frequently during the exercise class.

Note: A change in insulin or oral hypoglycemic medication should only be made on the recommendation of a participant's physician.

Respiratory and Pulmonary Disorders

Asthma

Chronic obstructive pulmonary disease (COPD) is the fourth leading cause of death in the United States and is projected to be the third leading cause of death by the year 2020 (U.S. Dept. of Health and Human Services, 2003). The three major types of COPD are **asthma, chronic bronchitis,** and **emphysema.**

Asthma is the leading cause of respiratory problems in the U.S., affecting up to 15 million Americans, or roughly 6.4% of the population. Of those diagnosed with asthma, 4.8 million are children (Centers for Disease Control and Prevention, 1999). It is considered a multifactorial disease because it is linked to several potential causes, which include heredity, infections, allergies, socioeconomic status (incidence is higher in low-income groups), and psychosocial and environmental factors.

The majority of persons with asthma have a reduction in breathing capacity during and, more commonly, after exercise (Rimmer, 1994). This is called **exercise-induced asthma (EIA)**, which is characterized by transient airway obstruction usually five to 15 minutes following physical exertion (Clark, 2003). In addition to EIA, other conditions that may trigger an asthma attack are cold temperatures, stress, and air pollution (Blumenthal, 1996). Exercise is beneficial for persons with asthma, provided the program is tailored to the individual's needs (Emtner, Herala, & Stalenheim, 1996). Most doctors recommend exercise to child and adult asthma sufferers because of the physiological and psychological benefits derived from physical activity.

Exercise Guidelines for Persons With Asthma

- It is important to make sure that the exercise program is coordinated with the timing of the asthma medication. Based on input from the participant's physician, the instructor must know when the medicine has to be taken to avoid an asthma episode during exercise. This will depend on the type of medication that is taken. Medicines used in inhalers work within a few minutes, while medicines taken in oral form may take up to 30 minutes to reach full capacity.

- Encourage the participant to use a **peak flow meter** to monitor the flow of air through the lungs. This simple plastic device can often determine if an asthma attack will occur or is occurring during or after exercise. The person simply blows into the meter and records the score. When peak flow drops more than 20% from normal values, activity should be reduced on that day. Peak flow meters can be purchased at any pharmacy for approximately $20 to $30. Steps for managing an asthma attack are shown in Table 9.3.

- Light warm-ups may be very helpful in reducing the risk of an asthma attack. The participant should perform a light cardiovascular activity at 40 to 50% of target heart rate for five to 10 minutes. This will help prepare the pulmonary system for more vigorous activity.

- Short bouts of exercise may reduce the incidence of an asthma attack in persons with severe asthma as noted by their physician. For example, three sets of four- to six-minute aerobic exercise routines with a five-minute rest interval between sets will allow the respiratory system to gradually adjust to the workload.

- Exercise intensity should lie within the participant's comfort zone. Young individuals with asthma may be able to exercise at very high intensity levels provided they take their medication before exercise. However, older individuals may have greater difficulty exercising at moderately high intensity levels (60 to 75% of target heart-rate range). This will depend on the participant's functional capacity and the severity of the asthma. Use the ratings of perceived exertion (RPE) scale (see Figure 8.1, page 230) and peak flow readings along with heart rate to monitor the intensity of the exercise. A sample exercise program for persons with asthma is shown in Table 9.4.

- Persons with exercise-induced asthma should always carry their inhalers with them. If an asthma episode occurs, a **beta-adrenergic stimulating agent** (found in inhalers) is the only way to reverse the symptoms of a full-blown attack. Make sure that the inhaler is with the person at all times.

- Since cold air is a major trigger of asthma attacks, when exercising outdoors the participant may be advised to wear a scarf or surgical mask over the nose and mouth to warm the inspired air and reduce heat loss.

- After a cold or flu, persons with asthma are more susceptible to breathing problems during exercise. The participant should be monitored closely after an illness and should be encouraged to return to physical activity very slowly by reducing the duration and intensity of the exercise.

Table 9.3
Steps for Managing an Asthma Attack

The time to treat an asthma episode is when the symptoms (e.g., coughing, wheezing, chest tightness, difficulty breathing) first appear.

Attack-management Steps

1. Have the person rest and relax.
2. Have the person use medicines (inhaler) prescribed for an attack.
3. Have the person drink warm liquids.

Rest and Relax

- At the first sign of breathing difficulties, the person should STOP and rest for at least 10 minutes.
- Make the person feel comfortable and relaxed.

Take Medication

- Make sure the prescribed medicine is available and that the person understands how to correctly take the medicine (inhalers require practice).

Drink Warm Liquid

- Have the person drink slowly.
- Do not allow the person to ingest cold drinks.

Emergency Care

- If you have any doubts about the severity of the attack, get medical help immediately.
- If the person's lips or fingernails are turning blue or if he or she exhibits shallow breathing and is focusing all attention on breathing, get medical help immediately.

Disabilities and Health Limitations

Table 9.4
A Sample Exercise Program for Persons with Asthma

Duration	*Intensity*	*Frequency*	*Modality*
In the early stages of the program, some individuals will respond more positively to short workouts with brief rest intervals.	Begin at a low intensity and gradually increase as the person's fitness level improves.	Frequency should range between three and seven days a week, depending on the interest and motivational level of the participant.	Swimming is highly recommended for persons with asthma because the temperature and humidity of the air above the water seem to protect the person from an asthma episode. The one exception is with individuals who are allergic to chlorine and other chemicals that are used in pools.
At certain times of the year (e.g., cold weather, high pollution), duration may have to be reduced to avoid an asthma episode.	Intensity should fall between 50 and 75% of age-predicted maximum heart rate (MHR).		
	If using interval-training techniques, the rest period should be short enough or long enough, depending on the individual's fitness level, to lower the heart rate to 40 to 50% of age-predicted MHR before initiating the next exercise bout.		Stationary cycling, brisk walking (performed indoors on high-pollution, high-pollen, or cold days), and circuit training (with adequate rest intervals) should be safe activities.
	Always check peak expiratory flow rate (PEFR) before starting the exercise session. If PEFR drops below 20% of normal values, reduce the intensity level and monitor the participant carefully for dyspnea and fatigue.		Anaerobic activities such as weight training and softball should not cause problems.
			High-intensity activities such as running, soccer, and basketball may cause the most problems.

Bronchitis and Emphysema

In the U.S., cigarette smoking is the primary risk factor for developing bronchitis and emphysema, which accounted for approximately 119,000 adult deaths in 2000 (U.S. Dept. of Health and Human Services, 2003). Both conditions cause severe problems in breathing capacity. Damaged lung tissue reduces the delivery of oxygen to working muscles. As pulmonary function declines, breathlessness and exercise intolerance become hallmark symptoms of these diseases.

Exercise is considered to be an essential component of treatment for persons with bronchitis and emphysema. The primary aim of the exercise program is to reduce breathlessness and improve exercise tolerance. Exercise intensity should be based on RPE, which seems to be a more reliable indicator than heart rate in these participants (O'Donnell, Webb, & McGuire, 1993). Individuals who are in the advanced stages of the disease may require supplemental oxygen during exercise. If you do not feel comfortable working with this population, a respiratory therapist or physical therapist should be consulted.

Exercise Guidelines for Persons With Bronchitis and Emphysema

- The more impaired a participant with COPD is, the greater the emphasis on interval-training techniques. In some participants with very low exercise-tolerance levels, it may be necessary to exercise for 30 to 60 seconds and then rest for 30 to 60 seconds. As the person improves his or her fitness level, these numbers can be altered to accommodate a higher intensity level. For example, as the person's conditioning improves, the instructor might increase exercise time to two minutes with a 30-second rest interval.

- The exercise program should address the interest level and capabilities of the participant with prescribed endurance activities that vary little in oxygen cost. A relatively constant intensity may help prevent **dyspnea** (difficulty breathing), which is the number-one problem with exercise. Examples of low-variability exercises include walking, recumbent stepping, and stationary cycling. High-variability exercises include walking up and down inclines, calisthenics, dancing, and sports such as basketball and racquet sports.

- Low-intensity weight training is relatively safe for persons with COPD. The person should feel comfortable lifting the weight and should not hyperventilate or become breathless. Avoid spikes in breathing rate by making sure that the weight is not too heavy and the person is not holding his or her breath.

- Although warm-up and cool-down activities are important components of an exercise program for all individuals, they are particularly important for persons with COPD. The goal of the exercise program is to gradually increase heart rate so that the lungs can slowly adjust to the increased workload. If strenuous exercise is started too quickly, there is a higher likelihood of respiratory distress. In addition, make sure the cool-down includes exercises of decreasing intensity

(e.g., walking or cycling at a progressively slower rate).

- Teach participants to decrease their breathing frequency and to increase the amount of air they take into their lungs with each breath. Many participants with COPD take shallow breaths and do not get enough oxygen into the pulmonary system, which ultimately leads to dyspnea and fatigue. **Diaphragmatic breathing** and pursed-lip breathing can be used to help patients improve their breathing capacity. Table 9.5 explains the technique for teaching and performing these two very important techniques.

Table 9.5
Diaphragmatic and Pursed-lip Breathing Techniques

Diaphragmatic Breathing
1. Have the participant lie down on his or her back.
2. Have the participant place one hand on the abdomen and one hand on the chest.
3. Teach the participant to inspire with maximal outward movement of the abdomen.
4. Once the participant is comfortable in the supine position, he or she can perform the technique in sitting and standing positions.

Pursed-lip Breathing
1. This can be performed separately or during diaphragmatic-breathing exercises.
2. Teach the participant to slowly exhale against a slight resistance created by lightly pursing the lips. The resistance has the potential to increase oxygen saturation.

Joint and Bone Disorders

As the average lifespan approaches 80 years of age, joint and bone disorders will become pandemic in American society. Baby boomers that are starting to enter older adulthood will, in a few short years, dramatically increase the number of people who have arthritis and/or osteoporosis. Fitness professionals will have to be integrally involved in finding ways to develop exercise programs that will allow

Disabilities and Health Limitations

individuals with these conditions to continue to maintain an active lifestyle.

Arthritis

The two major types of arthritis are **osteoarthritis** and **rheumatoid arthritis (RA).** Osteoarthritis is a degenerative joint disease characterized by cartilage deterioration that results in pain and loss of movement as bone surfaces interface (American Academy of Physical Medicine and Rehabilitation, 2006). Rheumatoid arthritis is a systemic autoimmune disease in which membranes lining the joints become inflamed, causing pain, warmth, redness, and movement-limiting swelling (American Academy of Physical Medicine and Rehabilitation, 2006). Both arthritis types have the same joint-destroying properties and similar treatment strategies, which include exercise.

One disease associated with arthritis because of primary associated arthritic symptoms is **systemic lupus erythematosus (SLE).** SLE is an autoimmune disease that affects connective tissues and results in painful joints and arthritis. Some sources state that SLE mimics RA, and in addition to the joint symptoms can include skin lesions, temporal-frontal hair loss, oral and nasal mucosal lesions, and in some cases there may be associated renal disease (Merck Manual, 2006c). Severe cases can result in death, with nearly 1,500 fatalities per year attributed to this condition (Centers for Disease Control and Prevention, 2002). For the purposes of providing general guidelines for exercise programs appropriate for people with arthritis, SLE will be included in this category.

Most persons with arthritis experience some degree of pain. While some participants will be able to tolerate high levels of pain, others will be unwilling to perform any exercise that causes discomfort. The exercise program must be tailored to the individual's pain threshold if he or she is likely to continue with the program.

Exercise Guidelines for Persons With Arthritis

- Most persons with arthritis can benefit from an exercise program (Ettinger et al., 1997). The fitness program must not place excessive loads around damaged joints. For persons who have been sedentary for a long time, starting slowly is very important.
- The immediate goal of exercise is to increase muscle strength to maintain or improve joint stability. By strengthening muscles around damaged joints, there is a greater displacement of the stress load away from the joint and onto the muscle.
- Swimming is an ideal activity because of the lower stress loads on the joints due to the buoyancy of the water. However, many older adults are adverse to the time and energy that it takes to prepare for an aquatics class, particularly if it is difficult to dress and undress because of joint stiffness and pain. Others may not know how to swim or may feel self-conscious in a swimsuit.
- The emphasis of the exercise program for persons with arthritis is to mitigate pain during activity. Low-impact, nonweightbearing activities are recommended. The participant must understand that he or she will probably have to learn to tolerate some amount of pain or discomfort with any movement, but as long as the pain does not linger for longer than two hours after exercise or return 24 to 48 hours after exercise, it is considered an acceptable activity. Pain can be minimized in a number of ways, including using braces or straps, ice and/or heat before and after exercise, isolating the dam-

aged joint during exercise, using water-based exercises, and not overusing the damaged joint. Consult with a physical therapist to learn more about pain management during activity.

- Exercise machines that allow the person to use all four limbs simultaneously seem to have the most benefit for persons with arthritis because the stress load is evenly distributed to all the limbs. Machines that require the use of all four limbs include some recumbent steppers and stationary bikes, which are utilized while sitting, and elliptical machines and cross-country ski machines, which are utilized while standing (this last machine may require some practice time to perform correctly).

- In circumstances where the participant is unable to use a certain leg or arm because of pain, the person can exercise with two or three limbs while resting the damaged joint. If both legs are affected, the person can use just the arms to perform a cardiovascular workout.

- One machine that may be too difficult to use or cause too much pain for some participants with arthritis is the stairclimber. This machine can place somewhat uncomfortable loads on the knees, hip joints, and spine and often results in pain in persons with arthritis. Other weightbearing activities that may cause pain include treadmill running and high-impact aerobics classes. Individuals with arthritis are advised to avoid these activities. General exercise guidelines for persons with arthritis are listed in Table 9.6.

Fibromyalgia

Fibromyalgia is defined as a group of common nonarticular disorders characterized by achy pain, tenderness, and stiffness of mus-

Table 9.6
Exercise Guidelines for
Persons With Arthritis

1. Any exercise that causes pain during exercise, two hours after exercise, or 24 to 48 hours after exercise should be discontinued.

2. Find alternative ways to exercise muscles around painful joints. For example, straight-leg exercises are a good way to strengthen the leg muscles around a painful knee.

3. Warm-up and cool-down segments are essential components of most exercise programs, but are especially important for persons with arthritis due to joint stiffness.

4. Resistance-training activities should be conducted, but exercises that cause pain to a particular joint should be replaced with isometric strength exercises.

5. If conducting pool exercise, try to maintain a water temperature between 85° and 90° F (29° and 32° C).

6. Use smooth, repetitive motions in all activities.

7. Keep the exercise intensity level below the discomfort threshold.

8. Be aware that acute flare-ups can occur in persons with rheumatoid arthritis. Exercise may not be advisable until the flare-up subsides.

9. Participants with osteoarthritis often perform better in the morning, while participants with rheumatoid arthritis may be better off exercising several hours after waking.

cles, areas of tendon insertions, and adjacent soft-tissue structures (Merck Manual, 2006a). This condition is thought to increase in severity when stress, poor sleep patterns, trauma, damp and cold conditions, or systemic infections are present (Merck Manual, 2006a). Approximately 6 million people in the U.S. have been diagnosed with fibromyalgia, 80% of whom are females between the ages of 20 and 55 (Meyer & Lemley, 2003).

Exercise Guidelines for
Persons With Fibromyalgia

Potential benefits of exercise training for people with fibromyalgia include (Meyer & Lemley, 2003):

- Reduced number of tender points and decreased pain at tender points
- Decreased general pain
- Improved sleep and reduced fatigue
- Fewer feelings of helplessness and hopelessness
- More frequent and meaningful social interactions
- Lessened impact of the disease on daily activities

Generally recommended exercises for this population, provided there are no symptoms of pain or soreness 24 to 48 hours after exercise, are as follows:

- Aerobic training: Guidelines include achievement of 50 to 60% of maximal heart rate for 20 to 40 minutes, two to three days per week, favoring duration over intensity. Cycling may be appropriate (using a ramp or staged protocol, depending on the individual's tolerance level). Treadmill walking may be appropriate (increasing time and incline from 15 to 20 minutes to 40 minutes, depending on the individual's tolerance level).
- Flexibility training: Sit and reach activities may be used to increase range of motion, especially in the shoulders, hips, knees, and ankles, as well as decrease the risk of injury.
- Functional training: Exercises associated with household tasks may be appropriate, such as carrying laundry, vacuuming, and performing activities of daily living.

Osteoporosis

It is estimated that 10 million people in the U.S. have osteoporosis, which drains the bones of their mineral content and increases their susceptibility to fractures (American Academy of Physical Medicine and Rehabilitation, 2006; National Osteoporosis Foundation, 2006). In the later stages of the disease, bones often become brittle enough to fracture at the slightest tap of the wrist, or a rib could fracture from a cough or sneeze. In severe cases, the vertebra can become as thin as eggshells, leading to compression fractures and resulting in a stooped posture.

Osteoporosis is often referred to as the silent disease because in the majority of cases there are no signs of the disease until the person fractures a hip and complications ensue. However, as a person reaches his or her 60s and 70s, signs of osteoporosis may develop. As the bones in the spine lose their mineral content, the spine begins to curve forward at the top, which is referred to as **kyphosis** or **dowager's hump.** This is often accompanied by pain and psychological distress (Rimmer, 1999).

Reduced weightbearing due to disuse or immobilization leads to progressive thinning of the bone and eventual loss of bone mineral. Studies on astronauts found significant bone loss from being suspended in a gravity-free environment (Kaplan, 1995). Likewise, studies have demonstrated that individuals who were confined to bed for several weeks at a time were also shown to have accelerated bone loss.

Exercise Guidelines for Persons With Osteoporosis

- Before developing the exercise program, the instructor must know if any of the older male participants (over 65) or post-menopausal women have been diagnosed with osteoporosis. Since the vast majority of older individuals have never been tested for osteoporosis, it is important for the instructor to go through the following checklist to determine if a participant should be screened by their physician.

– Is there a family history of osteoporosis?

– Did the person go through early menopause?

– Has the person had a hysterectomy?

– Does he or she smoke or have excessive alcohol intake?

– Does he or she have a low calcium intake?

– Are there any signs of osteoporosis (previous fracture, stooped posture)?

– Does the person have a thin, small build?

– Is he or she taking any medication that may increase bone loss (e.g., prednisone)?

If the participant answers yes to any of these questions, it is suggested that the person be screened by his or her physician for osteoporosis. By knowing that a participant may be at risk for osteoporosis, the instructor ensures that the exercise program will be tailored to the individual's needs and that the program will be as safe as possible.

• For participants who have been diagnosed with osteoporosis and/or have signs of the disease, resistance exercises should be approved by their physician. For safety reasons, it is always best to progress slowly, using light weights for the first month of the program. As his or her strength increases, progress to heavier weights if there is no pain in the area being strengthened. Begin with six to 12 repetitions and perform one to three sets, depending on the participant's comfort level. For participants with advanced osteoporosis (as noted by their physician), use elastic bands in the early stages of the program. Some weight machines start at too high a resistance and are difficult to get into and out of for some older, frail participants. After two to three months, progress to heavier bands or light weights. An individual with advanced osteoporosis will require more time to adapt to a

resistance-training program and must progress at a much slower rate than a healthy older adult to avoid injury.

• Resistance exercises should be performed two to three days a week. Avoid exercises near or over the spine if pain is present. If pain is not present, target the muscles around the spine by performing shoulder-retraction exercises and shoulder raises. Make sure the movements are performed slowly and do not cause pain. These exercises will also help improve posture (many older adults become round-shouldered as they age), and will potentially "load" the vertebra enough to increase or maintain their density.

• In younger individuals (<50 years) who do not have advanced osteoporosis, it is acceptable to use plyometric-type exercises to improve bone density. This may be the most effective way to increase bone mass. Many experts have noted that bones must be stressed to a minimal threshold value to attain significant gains in bone mass (Frost, 1997). If the stress threshold is not high enough, the potential for bone development is greatly reduced. One study found that exercises such as step aerobics and jumping down from a box or platform approximately 12 to 15 inches high significantly increased bone mineral density in healthy sedentary women between the ages of 35 and 45 years (Heinonen, 1996). However, one very important caveat is that there is a higher risk of injury when performing these types of exercises. Older persons and postmenopausal women interested in participating in a high-impact group fitness class should ideally obtain medical clearance, progress slowly, and be asked to sign a waiver that explains the risk of injury when performing these types of exercises.

• When developing plyometric step exercises, start with one step and gradually add steps as the person becomes more conditioned. Emphasize to the participants that they should limit these classes to two to three days a week because of their high stress load and potential for injury. Monitor participants very closely to make sure there is no soreness or pain after each class.

- Although most of the studies on exercise and osteoporosis have indicated that resistance training and plyometric-type exercises have achieved the greatest results in bone density, older persons with osteoporosis often become deconditioned from a lack of activity. This deconditioned state often leads to higher levels of inactivity and spirals the person into further disease and disability. If a person is in the advanced stages of osteoporosis (as noted by their physician), it is best to perform cardiovascular exercises from a seated position for part of the class time. A recumbent stepper is an excellent machine that allows frail participants to perform safe cardiovascular exercise. The person sits in a large seat and moves the arms and legs simultaneously. Many older adults prefer this machine over a stationary bike or standing machine (e.g., treadmill) because it is relatively easy to use and has a comfortable seat.

- Older persons with osteoporosis may have difficulty performing repetitive exercises that use the same muscle groups for extended periods of time. Therefore, circuit-training programs that require short periods of work using various muscle groups are recommended.

- In addition to circuit-training programs, interval-training activities that require brief periods of work followed by a rest interval may also be beneficial for deconditioned participants with advanced osteoporosis. For example, riding a stationary bike for one minute fol-

lowed by a 30-second rest interval may delay fatigue and allow the person to sustain longer periods of activity. Other cardiovascular activities can be used to improve functional performance, provided that they do not incur pain or result in premature fatigue. Although swimming and aquatic exercises are excellent modalities for improving cardiovascular endurance, they are not recommended for improving bone density. Water is a nongravity environment and does not seem to place enough of a stress load on bone tissue to increase its mass (Bravo et al., 1997). General safety guidelines for developing an exercise program for persons with osteoporosis are shown in Table 9.7.

Table 9.7
Safety Concerns When Developing an Exercise Program for Persons With Osteoporosis

---

- Always obtain physician consent before developing the exercise program.
- Screen the participant before developing the program. Consult with his or her physician on developing resistance exercises at the site where a fracture may have occurred.
- Avoid jarring or high-load exercises in persons with advanced osteoporosis.
- Avoid back exercises in participants who have localized pain in this region and show signs of kyphosis.
- When performing standing exercises with older participants who have a high risk of injury from a fall or fracture, or who have fallen previously, make sure there is something to hold onto at all times (e.g., ballet barre, parallel bars, chair).
- Reevaluate the program if there are any signs of pain or fatigue during or after an exercise session in the osteoporosis zones (hip, back, and wrist).

Low-back Pain

Approximately 50% of persons over the age of 60 complain of low-back pain, making it a common occurrence associated with aging (Cassidy et al., 2005). Many factors may influence the occurrence and severity of low-back pain. Sleep deficiency, physical deconditioning, psychosocial difficulties, and generalized fatigue are all contributors to this condition (Merck Manual, 2006b). Low-back pain can present clinically as an acute ligamentous sprain, a muscular strain, or as a chronic condition related to fibromuscular disorders, osteoarthritis, and ankylosing spondylosis (Merck Manual, 2006b).

Exercise Guidelines for Persons With Low-back Pain

Exercise programs for persons with low-back pain will be limited by the severity of pain and the degree to which the individual is able to tolerate different types of activity. With this in mind, it's important to determine the location of the pain, to receive a diagnosis from a physician to determine the cause (etiology) of the pain, and to determine whether the pain is exacerbated by certain movements or exercise positions. An exercise program recommended by ACSM (Simmonds & Dreisinger, 2003) for persons with lower-back pain syndrome are as follows:

- Strength program: Resistance-based abdominal strengthening may be used to increase abdominal strength and lumbar-extensor strength. Recommendations vary from eight to 15 repetitions, two to four times per week, depending on individual tolerance.
- Flexibility program: Flexibility exercises must be performed gently so as to not increase the low-back pain, and may include gentle forward stretches while sitting, or pendulum exercises in which the arms gently rotate as the individual flexes at the hips and shoulders. The goal of these stretches is to increase trunk and hip flexor and extensor range of motion.
- Functional-exercise program: The goal of this type of program is to increase the ability to perform activities of daily living (ADL)

and to maintain maximum function during episodes of low-back pain. Activities may include short walks to increase aerobic conditioning (starting at 15 minutes and increasing gradually until the individual is able to return to his or her previous level of functional activity and exercise). Other exercises may include performing sit-to-stand activities from a chair and increasing repetitions and altering the level of the starting surface to increase lower-extremity and abdominal strength. It is important when performing this activity to instruct the individual to maintain a straight back, and to flex and extend at the hips when sitting and standing. This technique will prevent additional injury.

Medications and modalities used to treat low-back pain vary from nonsteroidal anti-inflammatory drugs (NSAIDs) such as aspirin, ibuprofen, indomethacin, and nabumetone to non-narcotic analgesics such as acetaminophen (Simmonds & Dreisinger, 2003). Ice or heat applied to the area are standard modalities shown to be effective in treating low-back pain. Other modalities known to be effective for some individuals include ultrasound, electrical stimulation, or a TENs unit. It should be noted that these treatments can only be administered by a properly licensed professional.

Autoimmune Diseases

Multiple Sclerosis

Multiple sclerosis (MS) is one of the most common neuromuscular disorders, affecting approximately 400,000 people in the U.S. Diagnosed more often in Caucasians and women (National MS Society Sourcebook, 2006), multiple sclerosis is classified as a progressive disease, which means that the symptoms have a tendency to worsen as

263

the person ages. A wide variety of complications can occur from multiple sclerosis, including gait disturbances and bladder and bowel problems. The disease often consists of flare-ups (called exacerbations) and periods of stability (remission). In the usual course of the disease, exacerbations occur every few years. The progression of the disease varies from person to person.

Exercise Guidelines for Persons With Multiple Sclerosis

- Be aware that the symptoms of multiple sclerosis may get progressively worse over time. The treatment strategy aims to slow the progression of the disease. People with multiple sclerosis should make exercise an integral part of their daily regimen. As long as activities are not too strenuous, exercise should not be harmful.
- Balance is often compromised in persons with multiple sclerosis. Take every precaution to make the exercise setting as safe as possible to minimize the risk of falling. Provide chairs or a portable ballet barre that the person can hold onto for stability while performing exercises in the standing position.
- As balance worsens, the risk of falls increases. When and if balance worsens, develop activities that can be performed in a sitting position. Change from free weights to machines to eliminate the risk of a weight being dropped on a participant's foot. Stationary bikes, recumbent steppers, and upper-arm ergometers can be used to enhance cardiovascular fitness in a seated position. When balance is very poor, use a recumbent bike for further stability.
- Because participants with multiple sclerosis often experience a great deal of spas-

ticity (tightness) as their condition progresses, make sure that flexibility exercises are a major component of the program.
- Because participants with multiple sclerosis often have difficulty initiating a movement in the advanced stages of the disease, allow them the extra time to begin and complete each movement.
- Swimming is one of the best activities for participants with multiple sclerosis, provided the water temperature remains below 80° F (27° C). Warm water will cause premature fatigue in this population.
- Since overheating can cause a temporary loss of function, make sure the facility is well-ventilated and the room temperature is at a comfortable level. Exercise should be discouraged in warm, humid environments.
- Individuals with multiple sclerosis often lose control of their bladder in the later stages of the disease. Make sure the bladder is voided before and after exercise. Be prepared for possible accidents by having the appropriate cleaning materials available (e.g., bleach), and make sure that the participant understands that you are aware that a possible accident can occur.

Cardiac Diseases

Coronary Heart Disease

Coronary heart disease (CHD) is the leading cause of death in the U.S. for both males and females, accounting for one of every five deaths in 2003 (American Heart Association, 2006). CHD is a multifaceted disorder that varies greatly from person to person. Since the purpose of this chapter is to discuss conditions that fitness professionals will be exposed to in the workplace, patients with advanced coronary heart disease will not be discussed, as they would not be advised to exercise in these settings. It would be more appropriate to recommend an outpatient cardiac rehabilitation program. General exercise guidelines for participants with known coronary heart disease are shown in Table 9.8.

Table 9.8
General Exercise Guidelines for Participants With Known Coronary Heart Disease

---

1. Avoid extremes of heat and cold that can place a greater stress on the heart.

2. Use heart-rate monitors to regulate exercise intensity, and avoid activities that cause large fluctuations in heart rate.

3. Stay within the blood-pressure and target heart-rate zones established by the participant's physician.

4. Report all symptoms, especially light-headedness, chest pain, or dizziness, to the participant's physician.

5. Make sure that heart rate and blood pressure return to resting levels before the participant leaves the exercise setting.

6. If a participant complains of chest pain before, during, or after exercise, contact emergency medical services.

Exercise Guidelines for Persons
With Coronary Heart Disease

• If a participant has been approved by a physician to exercise in a less-supervised setting such as a fitness center, the major goal is to avoid high-intensity exercise that has a greater likelihood of precipitating a coronary event. The exercise program for persons with known coronary heart disease should include an advanced warm-up that consists of low-intensity exercise such as light walking or riding a stationary bike with little or no resistance; several different stretching exercises, particularly in the chest region if a person has had open-heart surgery; and some mild breathing exercises that could be part of a yoga or postural relaxation class. An advanced warm-up session may determine if any chest discom-

fort or dizziness is present before initiating higher-intensity exercise.

• RPE should be taught to participants with known coronary heart disease. Some participants may have a pacemaker or be on **beta adrenergic blocking agents,** which blunt the heart-rate response and will not give an accurate indication of exercise intensity. Try to associate a certain RPE value with the person's heart rate. Although the heart rate will be lower in persons who are on beta blockers, the RPE value should correlate fairly well with heart rate.

• Persons who have had a stroke or cerebrovascular accident (CVA) often suffer from coronary heart disease as well (Warden-Tamparo & Lewis, 1989). Strokes are caused by years of living with high blood pressure and high cholesterol, often precipitated by an unhealthy lifestyle (e.g., poor eating habits, lack of physical activity, obesity). The term brain attack has been used to associate the circumstances of having a stroke with a heart attack.

• The two major types of stroke are **hemorrhagic** and **ischemic.** Hemorrhagic strokes (a ruptured blood vessel in the brain) are usually more life-threatening than ischemic strokes. Ischemic strokes are much more common and involve a reduced blood supply to the brain.

• Since stroke is sometimes accompanied by memory loss, it is important to make sure the participant has taken his or her medication before exercising. Participants should carry their medication with them at all times in case they forget to take it before leaving home. This will allow them to take their medicine while at the fitness center and not have to miss a day of exercise. Since many people with strokes have

Disabilities and Health Limitations

hypertension, exercise should be postponed until blood pressure is under good control.

- As a precautionary measure, the participant should complete a detailed evaluation of how he or she feels before each exercise session. This includes whether or not they have taken their medication, generally feel good, have no signs of fatigue or chest discomfort, have had a good night's sleep, have eaten a light breakfast or meal earlier in the day, have a resting blood pressure within their normal range, and have consumed adequate amounts of fluid, especially participants who are taking diuretics to control blood pressure. If all of these responses are positive, the participant can begin the workout. At the end of the exercise session, the participant should have his or her blood pressure and heart rate checked before leaving the exercise setting to make sure that resting values have been restored.

Hypertension

More than 50 million Americans have high blood pressure requiring some form of medical treatment (Burt et al., 1995). Hypertension is an important risk factor for cardiac insufficiency, myocardial infarction, stroke, and sudden death. For adults over age 50, systolic blood pressure greater than 140 mmHg is a more important cardiovascular disease (CVD) risk factor than diastolic blood pressure. Specifically, beginning at 115/75 mmHg, CVD risk doubles for each increment of 20/10 mmHg, according to findings from The Seventh Report of the Joint National Committee on Prevention, Detection, Evaluation, and Treatment of High Blood Pressure (Chobanian et al., 2003) (Table 9.9).

Table 9.9
Classification of Blood Pressure for Adults Age 18 and Older*

Category	Systolic (mmHg)		Diastolic (mmHg)
Normal[†]	<120	and	<80
Prehypertension	120–139	or	80–89
Hypertension[‡]			
Stage 1	140–159	or	90–99
Stage 2	≥160	or	≥100

* Not taking antihypertensive drugs and not acutely ill. When systolic and diastolic blood pressures fall into different categories, the higher category should be selected to classify the individual's blood pressure status. For example, 140/82 mmHg should be classified as stage 1 hypertension, and 154/102 mmHg should be classified as stage 2 hypertension. In addition to classifying stages of hypertension on the basis of average blood pressure levels, clinicians should specify presence or absence of target organ disease and additional risk factors. This specificity is important for risk classification and treatment.

[†] Normal blood pressure with respect to cardiovascular risk is below 120/80 mmHg. However, unusually low readings should be evaluated for clinical significance.

[‡] Based on the average of two or more readings taken at each of two or more visits after an initial screening.

Source: Chobanian, A.V. et al. (2003). Seventh report of the joint national committee on prevention, detection, evaluation, and treatment of high blood pressure. *Journal of the American Medical Association, 289,* 2560–2572.

Exercise Guidelines for Persons With Hypertension

It's important to remember that exercise is one component of hypertension management. Other healthy-lifestyle components for managing this disease include: (1) consuming a diet rich in fruits, vegetables, and low-fat dairy products; (2) reducing dietary sodium to no more than 2.4 g daily; and (3) limiting alcohol consumption to no more than two drinks per day for males and one drink per day for women (American Heart Association, 2006).

In addition to these lifestyle recommendations, the American Heart Association also recommends:

- Maintaining normal body weight (BMI of 18.5–24.9 kg/m²)
- Engaging in regular aerobic activity such as brisk walking (at least 30 minutes per day, most days of the week)

Regular exercise for persons with hypertension can create a decrease in blood pressure that may last from four to 10 hours after exercise, with some reports indicating effects lasting up to 22 hours. These effects can translate into 15 mmHg systolic and 4 mmHg diastolic blood-pressure drops (Pescatello et al., 2004).

Exercise programs recommended by ACSM (Durstine & Moore, 2003) are as follows:

- Aerobic training: Large-muscle activities with goals to increase $\dot{V}O_2$max and ventilatory threshold; increase peak work endurance; increase caloric expenditure; and control blood pressure. Frequency of exercise is three to seven days per week for 30 to 60 minutes per session, RPE of 11 to 14 (on the 6 to 20 scale), 40 to 70% $\dot{V}O_2$max or maximal heart-rate reserve, 50 to 80% peak heart rate
- Strength training: Circuit training with the goal to increase muscular fitness, incorporating high repetitions and low resistance

Before placing a person with hypertension in an exercise program, it's important to note medications that may affect their response to exercise (Appendix C). Medications may include beta blockers, which can attenuate heart rate by approximately 30 contractions per minute. Alpha blockers, calcium channel blockers, and vasodilators may cause postexertional hypotension. It's important not to have the individual exercise if his or her resting systolic blood pressure is >200 mmHg or if his or her diastolic blood pressure is >115 mmHg.

Human Development and Aging

Children

This section identifies exercise guidelines and considerations for children, whose needs differ from adults in that their growth status is an indicator of health. For children with disabilities who may be restricted by exacerbations of illness, exercise may be difficult at certain stages in the child's life. Although children without disabilities may not have the periods of restriction imposed by a chronic condition or illness, lack of regular exercise could impact functional development and skeletal and muscular growth. In addition, inactive lifestyles could lead to obesity, which has become an epidemic among today's youth (Riner & Sabath, 2003). A report to the President of the United States from the Secretary of Health and Human Services and the Secretary of Education stated that "Our nation's young people are, in large measure, inactive, unfit, and increasingly overweight" (Centers for Disease Control and Prevention, 2000). Sadly, this trend has only worsened in the years since this report, increasing the importance of the role of health professionals in designing and implementing effective exercise and activity programs for youth.

Exercise Guidelines for Children

Recommendations to increase physical activity and fitness for youth put forth in the 2000 presidential report include (Centers for Disease Control and Prevention, 2000):

- Promoting physical activity within families who model and support participation in enjoyable physical activity
- Engaging children in physical education, health education, recess, and extracurricular activities in the context of school programs that promote these behaviors

- Involving children in youth sports and recreation programs for developmentally appropriate activities that are accessible to all children
- Involving children in community activities such as riding bicycles and walking to physical-activity facilities

Physical-activity promotion for children can have lasting effects on the health and healthy-lifestyle behaviors for their entire lives. For example, physical-activity programs for children can (1) help strengthen and maintain healthy joints, muscles, and bones; (2) control weight, build lean muscle, and reduce fat; (3) prevent or delay high blood pressure or reduce hypertension in youth; (4) prevent the development of type 2 diabetes; and (5) reduce feelings of depression and anxiety.

General exercise recommendations for children include the following:

- The CDC recommends that children and adolescents participate in at least 60 minutes and up to several hours of moderate-intensity physical activity most days of the week, preferably daily.
- Some of the exercise should occur in several bouts of moderate to vigorous physical activity lasting 10 to 15 minutes or longer each day (Centers for Disease Control and Prevention, 2000).
- Children should start out slowly with an exercise program that is interesting and fun to them. By beginning a program gradually, children can decrease the risk of injury and lowered self-esteem that could result from unrealistic goals.
- Be aware that children sweat less than adults during heat-related exercise and therefore have a more difficult time acclimating to exercising in the heat. Take special precautions to gradually expose children to exercising in high-heat conditions and

encourage them to drink fluids every 15 to 20 minutes.
- For children, maximal heart rate is much higher than in the adult population, and is generally 200 to 205 contractions per minute (Riner & Sabath, 2003).
- . Resting breathing rate also differs between children and adults. As children age, their resting breathing rate decreases progressively, as does maximal breathing frequency (Riner & Sabath, 2003).
- Blood pressure responses during exercise are similar among children and adults, although systolic blood pressure changes during exercise tend to be lower in children. For young children, a 2 to 3 mmHg rise may occur per MET, while adolescents may experience a 4 to 6 mmHg per MET increase in exercise intensity (Riner & Sabath, 2003).
- Ratings of perceived exertion (RPE) may be a way to measure exercise intensity for children over age eight, but young children may not have the cognitive skills to use the RPE accurately and consistently.
- For children, muscle-mass increases occurring during growth lead to increased muscular strength. There are marked differences among males and females during this growth process, particularly in terms of upper-body strength. Before the onset of puberty, muscular strength can be improved similarly in both males and females through the use of resistance training, whereas during the onset of puberty, maturation and testosterone levels increase muscle size and strength more significantly among males (Riner & Sabath, 2003).

Older Adults

As discussed previously in this chapter, older adults face many debilitating health problems that affect them physically, psychologically, and socially. A fitness professional can motivate older adults to perform exercises as a way of improving function, but also as a means of improving the ability to live an emotionally satisfying life.

Among the health problems associated with aging are cardiovascular disorders such as heart disease, coronary artery disease, and hypertension; respiratory disorders such as asthma, bronchitis, and emphysema; and the two primary types of arthritis (osteoarthritis and rheumatoid arthritis).

When recommending exercise programs for older adult populations, consider their medical history, and also assess their fitness level, mobility limitations, motivation to participate, self-efficacy, willingness to commit time to a program, and their goals and interests. By incorporating all of these variables into a program, an instructor will be able to identify the best approach for maximizing participants' ability and willingness to commit to a long-term exercise program.

Exercise Guidelines for Older Adults

General exercise recommendations for older adult populations include the following:

• Design interventions that participants can replicate on their own at home or elsewhere once formal training ends.

• Tailor the intervention to participants' perceived performance needs and goals, as well as their health and cognitive conditions.

• Provide systematic reinforcement regarding participants' ability to improve their exercise performance over time.

• Key components of physical-activity programs for older adults include endurance, strength, flexibility, and balance activities.

– Endurance activities include physical activity with continuous movement that involves large muscle groups and is sustained for a minimum of 10 minutes. Examples include biking, swimming, and walking.

– Strength activities increase muscle strength by moving or lifting some type of resistance such as weights or elastic bands at a level requiring physical effort. Examples include biceps curls, triceps extensions, hip abduction or adduction against resistance of an elastic band, and squats while holding hand weights.

– Flexibility activities facilitate greater range of motion around the joint. They should be performed a minimum of two days per week in addition to a formal physical-activity program. Examples include arm circles or pendulum exercises that involve suspending the arms while flexed at the hips and performing circles with gravity eliminated.

– Balance activities promote the ability to maintain control of the body over its base of support. Static-balance activities include performing standing exercises while decreasing the base of support and progressing to single-leg support. Dynamic-balance activities involve movement, and examples include decreasing the base of support while walking or altering a normal walking pattern around set obstacles such as cones or blocks laid out on the gym floor.

Summary

There are 54 million Americans with disabilities, and their numbers are expected to increase substantially as the baby boomers reach retirement age. In the new millennium, persons with disabilities will have a better understanding of the

Summary

importance of maintaining a physically active lifestyle, and will want, perhaps even demand, the same quantity and quality of programs afforded to the nondisabled community. Fitness professionals must be knowledgeable of the specific exercise guidelines for the various disabling conditions. The key to a successful program is for the group fitness instructor to understand what types of modifications need to be made to accommodate each participant's specific limitations in movement and function. A competent fitness professional must possess the skills requisite for adapting and modifying exercise programs to meet the unique needs of each individual participant, regardless of age or disability.

References

Albright, A.L. (2003). Diabetes. In Durstine, J.L. and Moore, G.E. (Eds.). *ACSM's Exercise Management for Persons with Chronic Diseases and Disabilities* (2nd ed.). Champaign, Ill.: Human Kinetics.

American Academy of Physical Medicine and Rehabilitation (2006). http://www.aapmr.org/condtreat/pain/arthritis.htm.; http://www.aapmr.org/condtreat/other/osteorisk.htm. Topics: Arthritis, Osteoporosis.

American Diabetes Association (2006). *Complete Guide to Diabetes* (4th ed.). New York: Bantam Press.

American Heart Association (2006). Heart disease and stroke statistics—2006 update: A report from the American Heart Association Statistics Committee and Stroke Statistics Subcommittee. *Circulation,* http://circ.ahajournals.org.

Blumenthal, M.N. (1996). Sports-aggravated allergies: How to treat and prevent the symptoms. *The Physician & Sportsmedicine,* 18, 12, 52–66.

Bravo, G. et al. (1997). A weight-bearing, water-based exercise program for osteopenic women: Its impact on bone, functional fitness, and well-being. *Archives of Physical Medicine & Rehabilitation,* 78, 1375–1380.

Burt, V.L. et al. (1995). Prevalence of hypertension in the US adult population: Results from the Third National Health and Nutrition Examination Survey, 1988–1991. *Hypertension,* 25, 305–313.

Cassidy, J.D. et al. (2005). Incidence and course of low back pain episodes in the general population. *Spine,* 30, 2817–2823.

Centers for Disease Control and Prevention (1999). *Vital health statistics: Current estimates from the National Health Interview Survey, 1996.* Hyattsville, Md.: U.S. Department of Health and Human Services, CDC.

Centers for Disease Control and Prevention (2000). *A Report to the President from the Secretary of Health and Human Services and the Secretary of Education.* Atlanta GA: Centers for Disease Control and Prevention.

Centers for Disease Control and Prevention (2002). Trends in deaths from systemic lupus erythematosus—United States, 1979–1998. *Morbidity and Mortality Weekly Report,* 17, 371–373.

Chobanian, A.V. et al. (2003). Seventh report of the joint national committee on prevention, detection, evaluation, and treatment of high blood pressure. *Journal of the American Medical Association,* 289, 2560–2572.

Clark, C.J. (2003). Asthma. In Durstine, J.L. and Moore, G.E. (Eds.) *ACSM's Exercise Management for Persons with Chronic Diseases and Disabilities* (2nd ed.). Champaign, Ill.: Human Kinetics.

Durstine, J.L. & Moore, G.E. (Eds.) (2003). *ACSM's Exercise Management for Persons with Chronic Diseases and Disabilities* (2nd ed.). Champaign, Ill.: Human Kinetics.

Emtner, M., Herala, M., & Stalenheim, G. (1996). High-intensity physical training in adults with asthma. A 10-week rehabilitation program. *Chest,* 109, 323–330.

Ettinger, W.H. et al. (1997). A randomized trial comparing aerobic exercise and resistance exercise with a health education program in older adults with knee osteoarthritis. *Journal of the American Medical Association,* 277, 1, 25–31.

Expert Panel (1998). Executive summary of the clinical guidelines on the identification, evaluation, and treatment of overweight and obesity in adults. *Archives of Internal Medicine,* 158, 1855–1867.

Flegal K.M. et al. (2002). Prevalence and trends in obesity among US adults 1999–2000. *Journal of the American Medical Association,* 288, 1723–1727.

Frost, H.M. (1997). Why do marathon runners have less bone than weight lifters? A vital biomechanical view and explanation. *Bone,* 20, 183–189.

Han, T.S. et al. (1997). The prevalence of low back pain and associations with body fatness, fat distribution and height. *International Journal of Obesity,* 21, 600–607.

Hedley, A.A. et al. (2004). Prevalence of overweight and obesity among US children, adolescents, and adults, 1999–2002. *Journal of the American Medical Association,* 23, 2847–2850.

Heinonen, A. (1996). Randomised controlled trial of effect of high-impact exercise on selected risk factors for osteoporotic fractures. *Lancet,* 348, 1343–1347.

Kaplan, F.S. (1995). Prevention and management of osteoporosis. *Clinical Symposia,* 47, 1–32.

Merck Manual (2006a). Fibromyalgia. Section 5, Musculoskeletal and Connective Tissue Disorders, Chapter 59: Nonarticular Rheumatism, http://www.merck.com/mrkshared/mmanual/section5/chapter59/.

Merck Manual (2006b). Low Back Pain. Section 5, Musculoskeletal and Connective Tissue Disorders, Chapter 59: Nonarticular Rheumatism, http://www.merck.com/mrkshared/mmanual/section5/chapter59/.

Merck Manual (2006c). Rheumatoid Arthritis. Section 5, Musculoskeletal and Connective Tissue Disorders, Chapter 50: Diffusive Connective Tissue Disorders, http://www.merck.com/mrkshared/ mmanual/section5/chapter50/.

Meyer, B. & Lemley, K. (2003). Fibromyalgia. In Durstine, J.L. and Moore, G.E. (Eds.) *ACSM's Exercise Management for Persons with Chronic Diseases and Disabilities* (2nd ed.). Champaign, Ill.: Human Kinetics.

References

References and Suggested Reading

National Institutes of Health (2006). National diabetes statistics; National Diabetes Information Clearinghouse. National Institute of Diabetes and Digestive and Kidney Diseases (NIDDK), http://diabetes.niddk.nih.gov/dm/pubs/statistics/index.htm

National Osteoporosis Foundation (2006). http:/www.nof.org

National MS Society Sourcebook: Epidemiology (2006). Library and Literature, http://www.nationalmssociety.org/Sourcebook-Epidemiology.asp.

O'Donnell, D.E., Webb, K.A., & McGuire, M.A. (1993). Older patients with COPD: Benefits of exercise training. *Geriatrics,* 48, 1, 59–66.

Parchman, M.L., Romero, R.L., & Pugh, J.A. (2006). Encounters by patients with type 2 diabetes—complex and demanding: An observational study. *Annals of Family Medicine,* 4, 40–45.

Pescatello, L.S. et al. (2004). American College of Sports Medicine position stand: Exercise and hypertension. *Medicine and Science in Sports and Exercise,* 36, 3, 533–553.

Rice, T. et al. (1993). Segregation analysis of fat mass and other body composition measures derived from underwater weighing. *American Journal of Human Genetics,* 52, 967–973.

Rimmer, J.H. (1999). Programming for participants with osteoporosis. *IDEA Health and Fitness Source,* 17, 6, 46–55.

Rimmer, J.H. (1994). *Fitness and Rehabilitation Programs for Special Populations.* Dubuque, Iowa: WCB McGraw-Hill.

Rimmer, J.H. & Braddock, D. (1997). Physical activity, disability, and cardiovascular health. In: A. Leon (Ed.) *Physical Activity and Cardiovascular Health: A National Consensus* (pp. 236–244). Champaign, Ill.: Human Kinetics.

Rimmer, J.H. & Wang, E.W. (2005). Obesity prevalence among a group of Chicago residents with disabilities. *Archives of Physical Medicine and Rehabilitation,* 86, 1461–1464.

Riner, W.F. & Sabath, R.J. (2003). Considerations regarding physical activity for children and youth. In Durstine, J.L. and Moore, G.E. (Eds.). *ACSM's Exercise Management for Persons with Chronic Diseases and Disabilities* (2nd ed.). Champaign, Ill.: Human Kinetics.

Simmonds, M.J. & Dreisinger, T.E. (2003). Lower back pain syndrome. In Durstine, J.L. and Moore, G.E. (Eds.). *ACSM's Exercise Management for Persons with Chronic Diseases and Disabilities* (2nd ed.). Champaign, Ill.: Human Kinetics.

Tsai, E.B. et al. (2006). The rise and fall of insulin secretion in type 1 diabetes mellitus. *Diabetologia,* 49, 21–270.

U.S. Department of Health and Human Services, National Institutes of Health, National Heart, Lung, and Blood Institute (2003). *Chronic Obstructive Pulmonary Disease, Data Fact Sheet,* NIH Publication No. 03-5229.

Wallberg-Henriksson, H. (1992). Exercise and diabetes mellitus. In Holloszy, J.O. (Ed.), *Exercise & Sport Sciences Reviews,* Vol. 20, 339–368. Baltimore, Md.: Williams & Wilkins.

Warden-Tamparo, C. & Lewis, M.A. (1989). *Diseases of the Human Body.* Philadelphia: F. A. Davis.

Suggested Reading

Bryant, C.X. & Franklin, B. A. (2007) *ACE's Guide to Exercise Testing and Program Design: A Fitness Professional's Handbook* (2nd ed.). Monterey, Calif.: Healthy Learning.

Franklin, B.A., Gordon, S., & Timmis, G.C. (1989). *Exercise in Modern Medicine.* Baltimore, Md.: Williams & Wilkins.

Gordon, N.F. (2003). Hypertension. In Durstine, J.L. and Moore, G.E. (Eds.) *ACSM's Exercise Management for Persons with Chronic Diseases and Disabilities* (2nd ed.). Champaign, Ill.: Human Kinetics.

Kavanagh, T. (1994). Cardiac rehabilitation. In Goldberg, L. & Elliot, D.L. (Eds.), *Exercise for Prevention and Treatment of Illness* (pp. 41–79). Philadelphia: F. A. Davis.

McNeil, J.M. (1997). *Americans with Disabilities: 1994–95.* U.S. Bureau of the Census. (Current Population Reports, P70-61). Washington, D.C.: U. S. Government Printing Office.

Miller, P.D. (1995). *Fitness Programming and Physical Disability.* Champaign, Ill.: Human Kinetics.

Rimmer, J.H. (1997). Programming for participants with disabilities: Exercise guidelines for special medical populations. *IDEA Today,* 15, 5, 26–35.

Rimmer, J.H. (2005). Common health challenges faced by older adults. In Bryant, C.X. (Ed.), *Exercise for Older Adults: ACE's Guide for Fitness Professionals.* San Diego, Calif.: American Council on Exercise.

Rimmer, J.H. (1999). Health promotion for persons with disabilities: The emerging paradigm shift from disability prevention to prevention of secondary conditions in persons with disabilities. *Physical Therapy,* 79, 5, 495–502.

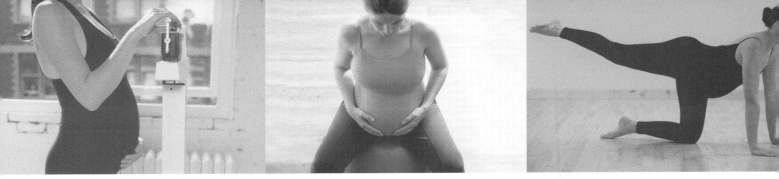

Chapter Ten

Lenita Anthony, M.A., is a clinical exercise physiologist and exercise specialist with 25 years of experience in group exercise and personal training. As a Reebok Master Trainer and Program Development team member for Reebok University, she is a well-known presenter, author, and trainer of trainers. She is also the National Coach for Reebok Women's Triathlon Series.

Camilla Callaway, M.Ed., owns and operates a personal training facility in Columbus, Georgia. Working with Denver's Swedish Medical Center and Katie Beck's "Mothers in Motion," Callaway has trained instructors, taught prenatal classes, educated moms-to-be throughout the Colorado region, and facilitated classes at the IDEA International Convention. She has been a volunteer with various committees with the American Council on Exercise and serves as an ACE media spokesperson.

Exercise and Pregnancy

By Lenita Anthony and Camilla Callaway

The number of women who exercise during their pregnancy has increased steadily in recent years. Cross-sectional surveys have reported that the percentage is as high as 42% (Zhang & Savitz, 1996). An increased focus on health during pregnancy means that more pregnant women will be seeking the instruction of knowledgeable fitness professionals. These participants will need sound information and guidance regarding exercise, and instructors need to be aware of the unique physical and physiological changes that occur during pregnancy.

Exercise and Pregnancy

These adaptations require continual exercise modifications to ensure exercise effectiveness and safety. Each woman enters pregnancy with different abilities and different goals and attitudes toward exercise. While broad, general guidelines apply to the pregnant population as a whole, they do not take into account the specific needs of every individual.

Research on exercise and pregnancy over the last several years has demonstrated that the "right" exercise program for a pregnant woman should be based on many factors, pregnancy being only one of them. Equally important are the pregnant exerciser's goals, experience, state of training, apprehensions, expectations, and motivation. In other words, "one size" will not fit all when it comes to prenatal exercise programs.

The objective of the American Council on Exercise is for group fitness instructors to be knowledgeable about the special needs of pregnant women and to provide classes that are well-designed, effective, challenging, and, above all, safe. Accordingly, the main purpose of this chapter is to enable instructors to develop such exercise programs for pregnant participants and educate instructors on important issues regarding exercise and prenatal conditions.

Benefits and Risks of Exercise During Pregnancy

The ACOG Guidelines: Clearing Up the Confusion

The American College of Obstetricians and Gynecologists (ACOG) first published recommendations on exercise and pregnancy in 1985. This information was widely disseminated to physicians, fitness professionals, and concerned women, who were eager to hear the long-awaited answers to their questions. Due to the limited scientific evidence and lack of outcome data on the topic at that time, the 1985 guidelines were written from a perspective of "first do no harm" and thus were extremely conservative. Specifically, restrictions were placed on the type of exercises performed, duration, and intensity.

However, the guidelines were soon challenged by individuals in the exercise science and fitness communities, as well as by women who had continued to exercise vigorously through their pregnancies with no ill effects. A number of research studies using human subjects were published over the ensuing years, leading to the need for substantial revisions to the original document. In 1994, ACOG published a second set of guidelines. The specific application of these guidelines for prenatal exercise, as well as of the 2002 ACOG guidelines, is discussed later in this chapter.

Although most of the restrictions outlined in the 1985 ACOG guidelines became "outdated" with the publication of the 1994 guidelines, the use of the earlier document is still widespread among physicians and fitness professionals. Instructors must understand the differences that exist among the three sets of recommendations and the confusion surrounding them. It is likely that, in some cases, pregnant women will have been given information based on the original guidelines published in 1985 that is outdated and unnecessarily restrictive.

While much more research is available on the effects of exercise and pregnancy than existed in 1985, there are still areas in which the literature is limited. For example, most of the current research involves the effects of cardiovascular exercise, with little data on the effects of strength training during pregnancy.

Exercise and Pregnancy

Additionally, current studies using human subjects have utilized a rather homogeneous subject group; the effects on a more diverse sample may impact future results and conclusions. It is important that fitness professionals working with this population keep an eye toward ongoing research developments and how this information applies to pregnant exercisers.

Benefits of Prenatal Exercise

Benefits During Pregnancy

The potential benefits of a well-designed prenatal exercise program are numerous. Pregnant women who exercise can maintain or even increase their cardiovascular fitness, muscular strength, and flexibility. Research has shown that women who exercise during pregnancy experience fewer common prenatal discomforts such as constipation, swollen extremities, leg cramps, nausea, varicose veins, insomnia, fatigue, back pain, and other orthopedic conditions (Clapp & Little, 1995; Artal, 1992). Exercise can assist in controlling gestational diabetes and help prevent urinary incontinence, pregnancy-induced hypertension, diastasis recti, and deep vein thrombosis (Hall & Brody, 1999; Yeo et al., 2000). Additionally, exercise can improve posture and body mechanics, facilitate circulation, reduce pelvic and rectal pressure, and increase energy levels (Sternfeld, Sidney, & Eskenazi, 1992). While even very fit women will experience fatigue at some point during their pregnancy, their energy reserve and fatigue "threshold" remain consistently higher than in unfit women. Fit pregnant women also retain a lower resting heart rate, a higher stroke volume, and higher $\dot{V}O_2$max throughout pregnancy and during the **postpartum** period.

Pregnant women who exercise have a lower incidence of excessive weight gain and are more likely to stay within the range recommended by ACOG. Exercise also helps to stabilize mood states during pregnancy. Active women have been shown to experience fewer feelings of stress, anxiety, insomnia, and depression—negative emotions that are commonly experienced during pregnancy (American College of Sports Medicine, 2006; Goodwin, Astbury, & McKeeken, 2000). In general, exercise appears to enhance women's psychological well-being, increase confidence in their changing body image, and decrease feelings of apprehension about labor and delivery.

Pregnancy is one of the critical "windows" of time in the female lifespan during which positive health-behavior changes are more readily accepted. During pregnancy, many women sense an increased responsibility toward their personal health as they become aware of how their behaviors and actions impact the health and well-being of their unborn child. There is frequently an increased motivation to eat more healthfully, stop smoking, and become more physically active. By seizing this opportunity to help pregnant women acquire an exercise "habit," and to realize the benefits this provides, instructors can set the stage for their activity patterns for the rest of their lives.

Benefits During Labor and Delivery

There are mixed reports on the effects of exercise during pregnancy on the course or outcome of labor and delivery. Some studies show exercise has no effect, yet others show exercise causes either shorter or longer labors. These variances may have been due to differences in exercise programs, data collection, or other methodological

Exercise and Pregnancy

discrepancies. A study conducted by Clapp (1998) compared the labors of women who continued performing vigorous, weightbearing exercise throughout pregnancy to "physically active" controls. The women who continued weightbearing exercise throughout gestation experienced less problematic deliveries, including a 75% decrease in the need for forceps or Caesarean section, a 75% decrease in maternal exhaustion, a 50% decrease in the need for oxytocin (Pitocin—a labor-inducing drug), and a 50% decrease in the need to intervene due to fetal heart-rate abnormalities. Clapp also found exercising women had a significantly higher rate of uncomplicated, spontaneous deliveries and an active labor that was 30% shorter than the controls (Figure 10.1). However, the women who discontinued exercise midpregnancy did not experience these benefits and did not differ significantly from the controls. Another study on exercise and the type of delivery found non-exercising women to be four-and-a-half times more likely to have Caesarean section (Bungum et al., 2000). It appears that for labor and delivery benefits, it is important to encourage pregnant women to continue exercising regularly until they are as near term

as possible (barring any medical reasons to the contrary).

Benefits During Recovery

Exercise during pregnancy appears to promote a faster recovery from labor. Women who exercise throughout their pregnancies return to activities of normal daily life 40% faster than less-active controls (Clapp, 1998). It stands to reason that women with higher functional capacities going into the marathon of labor and delivery would be taxed to a lesser degree than women with low functional capacities. Fit women recover faster than unfit women because of their greater energy reserves. Others have reported that exercisers retain less weight and score higher on measures of maternal adaptation (Sampselle & Seng, 1999). Exercising women also experience fewer incidences of postpartum depression. Additionally, women who have made exercise part of their lifestyle during pregnancy are more likely to continue exercising after the baby is born than those who did not (Devine, Bov, & Olson, 2000).

Ultimately, a healthy **placenta** that can adequately support the needs of the growing **fetus** is perhaps the most critical determinant of the advisability and benefits of exercise. Emphasis should be placed on early prenatal care, healthy lifestyle habits, and optimal prenatal nutrition to help ensure the growth of a healthy placenta. If the placenta is not functioning optimally, the potential exists for exercise to place excess and even unhealthy stress on maternal and fetal systems.

Contraindications and Risk Factors

Research indicates that healthy women with uncomplicated pregnancies do not need to limit their exercise for fear of adverse effects. There are no reported increases in the

Figure 10.1
Regular exercise shortens labor by approximately one-third on average.

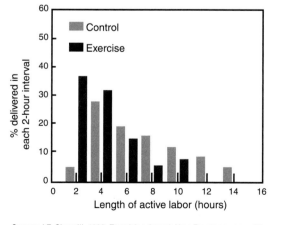

Source: J.F. Clapp III, 1998, Exercising through Your Pregnancy, page 94, figure 6.6. © 1998 by James F. Clapp III. Reprinted with permission from Human Kinetics (Champaign, IL).

rate of spontaneous abortion or rupture, incidence of preterm labor, fetal distress, or birth abnormalities (American College of Sports Medicine, 2006). Conversely, "extreme" training such as that involved with marathons, triathlons, adventure racing, and competitive athletics is not encouraged. While no known adverse effects have been documented in pregnant women participating in competitive athletics, potential risks of fatigue, **dehydration,** and under-nutrition make them poor candidates for such vigorous activity.

It is important to recognize that ACOG has established that there are some women for whom exercise during pregnancy is absolutely contraindicated, and others for whom the potential benefits associated with exercising may outweigh the risks (American College of Obstetricians and Gynecologists, 2002). It is outside the scope of practice of a group fitness instructor to attempt to diagnose any of the **contraindications** outlined by ACOG (Tables 10.1 and 10.2). Therefore, it is imperative that an instructor perform routine health screening on all participants and that instructors require a physician's clearance before any pregnant or postpartum woman begins an exercise program. Should an instructor become aware of any of these conditions, exercise should be stopped immediately until the postpartum period, unless the participant obtains written permission from a physician to resume. Additionally, it is recommended that instructors secure an informed consent or waiver of liability prior to participation.

Encourage participants to give regular feedback on how they are feeling during and after exercise, and remind them to alert an instructor to the presence of any unusual symptoms. Instructors should familiarize themselves and their participants with specific signs or symptoms that may indicate a problem, including the

Table 10.1
Absolute Contraindications to
Aerobic Exercise During Pregnancy

• Hemodynamically significant heart disease
• Restrictive lung disease
• Incompetent cervix/cerclage
• Multiple gestation at risk for premature labor
• Persistent second- or third-trimester bleeding
• Placenta previa after 26 weeks of gestation
• Premature labor during the current pregnancy
• Ruptured membranes
• Preeclampsia/pregnancy-induced hypertension

Exercise during pregnancy and the postpartum period. ACOG Committee Opinion No. 267. American College of Obstetricians and Gynecologists. Obstetrics and Gynecology, 2002; 99, 171–173.

Table 10.2
Relative Contraindications to
Aerobic Exercise During Pregnancy

• Severe anemia
• Unevaluated maternal cardiac arrhythmia
• Chronic bronchitis
• Poorly controlled type 1 diabetes
• Extreme morbid obesity
• Extreme underweight (BMI <12)
• History of extremely sedentary lifestyle
• Intrauterine growth restriction in current pregnancy
• Poorly controlled hypertension
• Orthopedic limitations
• Poorly controlled seizure disorder
• Poorly controlled hyperthyroidism
• Heavy smoker

Exercise during pregnancy and the postpartum period. ACOG Committee Opinion No. 267. American College of Obstetricians and Gynecologists. Obstetrics and Gynecology, 2002; 99, 171–173.

items listed in Tables 10.3 and 10.4. Refer women with any of these complaints to their physician for evaluation before continuing any exercise program.

High-risk Exercise

Women can continue most activities during their prenatal period by using common sense and making appropriate modifications. However, they should avoid any activity that has a potential for impact that may cause abdominal trauma. Additionally, exercises

Exercise and Pregnancy

Table 10.3
Reasons to Discontinue
Exercise and Seek Medical Advice

- Any sign of bloody discharge from the vagina
- Any "gush" of fluid from the vagina (premature rupture of membranes)
- Sudden swelling of the ankles, hands, or face (possible preeclampsia)
- Persistent, severe headaches and/or visual disturbances (possible hypertension)
- Unexplained spell of faintness or dizziness
- Swelling, pain, and redness in the calf of one leg (possible phlebitis)
- Elevation of pulse rate or blood pressure that persists after exercise
- Excessive fatigue, palpitations, or chest pain
- Persistent contractions (more than six to eight per hour) that may suggest onset of premature labor
- Unexplained abdominal pain
- Insufficient weight gain [less than 1 kg/month (2.2 lb/month) during last two trimesters]

Source: American College of Sports Medicine (2006). ACSM's Guidelines for Exercise Testing and Prescription, 7th ed. Philadelphia: Lippincott, Williams & Wilkins.

Table 10.4
Warning Signs to Cease
Exercise While Pregnant

- Vaginal bleeding
- Dyspnea prior to exertion
- Dizziness
- Headache
- Chest pain
- Muscle weakness
- Calf pain or swelling (need to rule out thrombophlebitis)
- Preterm labor
- Decreased fetal movement
- Amniotic fluid leakage

Exercise during pregnancy and the postpartum period. ACOG Committee Opinion No. 267. American College of Obstetricians and Gynecologists. Obstetrics and Gynecology, 2002; 99, 171–173.

Table 10.5
High-risk Exercises

- Snow- and waterskiing
- Rock climbing
- Snowboarding
- Diving
- Scuba diving
- Bungee jumping
- Horseback riding
- Ice skating/hockey
- Road or mountain cycling
- Vigorous exercise at altitude (nonacclimated women)

Note: Risk of activities requiring balance is relative to maternal weight gain and morphologic changes; some activities may be acceptable early in pregnancy but risky later on.

---

involving a high degree of balance or agility (e.g., gymnastics, rock climbing, downhill skiing) are not recommended during pregnancy (Table 10.5). This is particularly important in the latter trimesters, when changes in a woman's center of gravity put her at increased risk of falling. Women who are not accustomed to exercising at high altitude (e.g., cross-country skiing, hiking) should use caution and exercise at lower-than-normal intensities, as well as ensure adequate oxygenation to avoid undue complications.

Physiological Adaptations to Pregnancy

Of the myriad physiological changes that occur during pregnancy, perhaps those that have the most impact on exercise-program design are those related to the cardiovascular system, the respiratory system, and the musculoskeletal system. While the adaptations listed below are by no means the only ones, a group fitness instructor who understands them will have a foundation of knowledge that allows more effective work with this special group.

Cardiovascular System

When instructors prepare beginner participants for group fitness classes, they often inform them of the short-term effects of exercise. They discuss how the body will heat up and feel hotter, that their breathing rate will increase because they are using more oxygen, and that their heart rate will rise to help move the much-needed oxygen and nutrients to the working muscles via the blood or circulatory system. This simplistic statement could also describe the body's response to pregnancy; pregnancy and exercise elicit many similar physiological responses. During an exercise session, heart rate, respiratory rate, oxygen consumption, metabolic rate, cardiac output, stroke volume, and body temperature all increase; pregnancy mimics these responses. A pregnant woman's body is in a constant state of work; the acute physiological responses of a low level of exercise are constantly present. It is not an exaggeration to say that the pregnant woman is performing a certain amount of exercise, even when she is at rest.

The cardiovascular system, the respiratory system, and the reproductive system must each adapt to the level of function required to grow a new life in 40 weeks. These adaptations include a gradual climb in resting heart rate, which reaches a peak of 15 beats per minute (bpm) over prepregnancy rates near the third trimester. Left ventricular volume and stroke volume increase 40%. Resting cardiac output and blood volume are 40% higher by the third trimester (Artal, 1992; Clapp, 1998). Resting oxygen consumption also climbs and reaches a level near term approximately 20 to 30% above prepregnancy levels (Wolfe et al., 1989; Artal, 1992).

These physiological changes have implications for the exercise program. Because the heart is already working at a higher capacity to pump the increased blood volume throughout the body, there is a decrease in **cardiac reserve**. The oxygen cost of weightbearing activity is also greater, due to increases in body weight. All of these factors combine to decrease maximum work capacity as pregnancy advances. Prenatal exercisers should gradually yet progressively reduce the volume

of work done during exercise so as to complement the increased work load under which their body is functioning as they advance through their pregnancy.

Respiratory System

Pregnant women ventilate 50% more air per minute than nonpregnant women. This occurs through a 40 to 50% increase in tidal volume, or the amount of air in each breath. Although many pregnant women feel that it is difficult to get a deep breath, maximum breathing capacity is actually maintained or increased over prepregnancy values. Respiratory rate does not change significantly. As the baby grows, the uterus pushes the diaphragm farther up into the chest cavity. The pregnant woman has to use more oxygen during inspiration as the diaphragm contracts to push the uterus downward. This increase in the oxygen cost of breathing also means less oxygen is available to the working muscles. The rib cage often flares and widens to help compensate for the decrease in lung space caused by the growing fetus.

Musculoskeletal System

To facilitate the expansion of the uterine cavity, increased amounts of the hormones **relaxin** and **progesterone** are released during the first trimester. These hormones act to soften the ligaments surrounding the joints of the pelvis (hips and lumbosacral spine), thereby increasing mobility and joint laxity. A gentle but effective expansion occurs, providing the necessary space. This effect continues through the postpartum lactating period, when relaxin levels have been reduced.

The by-product of this hormonally induced joint laxity is a decrease in joint stability, which may leave the affected joints more susceptible to injury. Whether or not joint laxity occurs in

Exercise and Pregnancy

the neck, shoulders, and peripheral joints is still controversial. If it does, the pregnant woman may have a greater chance of injuries resulting from overstretching, ligamentous tears, or sprains. However, research does not demonstrate an increased incidence of exercise-related joint injury among pregnant women (Clapp, 1998; Karzel & Friedman, 1991; Schauberger et al., 1996). Researchers speculate that this is because pregnant women take greater precautions and are more careful during exercise. Whether or not relaxin has any effect on joints like the knees, common sense indicates that the increased mechanical stress of a 25- to 40-pound weight gain is cause to use caution with high-impact activities.

As weight is gained and hormonal influences on the hips and low back deepen, postural alignment is altered. The pelvis tilts anteriorly, changing the center of gravity and increasing the lordotic curve of the lumbar spine. The upper back is also realigned due to the increased weight of the breast tissue. The chest and shoulders are pulled forward and inward, increasing the kyphotic curve of the thoracic spine. A forward neck often accompanies these postural deviations and an extreme exaggeration of the vertebral column's normal "S" curve results. This is known as a kyphotic lordotic postural alignment and is further explained in Chapter 3 (Artal et al., 1990; Jacobson, 1991). Postural realignments induced by the anterior weight gain of pregnancy, and the attendant muscular imbalances created, could predispose women to upper- or lower-back pain. These conditions are addressed more fully later in this chapter.

Additional Concerns

Blood returning to the heart from the body is known as venous return. Due to the increase in

blood volume and sensitivities to postural positions, venous return may be impaired or disturbed during pregnancy. **Supine hypotension** is an example of such a disturbance. In the supine position (lying on the back), the weight of the uterus presses against blood vessels, especially the inferior vena cava. This pressure occludes the vessels, causing a restriction in blood flow, which may, in turn, cause a reduction in cardiac output, blood pressure, and blood flow to the fetus. If the fetus is subjected to repeated periods of **hypoxia** due to prolonged and/or repetitive supine exercise, there is the potential for developmental disorders to occur. Participants should be advised to avoid exercise in the supine position after the first trimester (American College of Obstetricians and Gynecologists, 2002; 1994).

Instructors often have to remind pregnant women that they are supposed to gain weight during pregnancy. Exercise should not be used as a means to prevent a healthy, normal weight gain during pregnancy. Average pregnancy weight gains are between about 27 and 34 pounds; body fat increases by an average of 4 to 5% (Artal, 1992; Clark, 1992). Prevention of normal weight gain may be detrimental since weight gains are predictive of fetal birth weight. Nutritional diets should be encouraged to provide for the baby's growth and development and appropriate weight gains.

Fetal Risks Associated With Exercise

Available research includes no evidence to show that regular exercise during a normal, healthy pregnancy is associated with any adverse fetal outcomes. However, there are several areas of theoretical concern of which you should be aware. These include the effects of exercise on uterine-placental blood flow, carbohydrate utilization, and **thermoregulation**. This section addresses the basis for these concerns and the practical application for the group exercise setting.

The first concern is the potential conflict between the circulatory demands of exercise and those of pregnancy. During exercise, the oxygen transport system analyzes the actions taking place and reacts to provide for the higher level of activity. Blood flow is preferentially redistributed to the heart, skin, and working muscles and shunted away from the renal, gastrointestinal, and reproductive organs. The concern is that this may result in a decreased oxygen supply (hypoxia) and/or decreased nutrient supply to the fetus. If the fetus is subjected to repetitive, sustained bouts of hypoxia brought on by exercise, developmental abnormalities could occur.

Research has shown that the fetus can adjust safely to reductions of blood flow resulting from moderate exercise bouts (Uzendoski et al., 1989; American College of Sports Medicine, 2000). Several adaptations have been identified that protect the fetus and compensate for the decrease in visceral blood flow during exercise. These adaptations include a significant increase in maternal **hematocrit,** which occurs with exercise. This adjustment decreases plasma volume and increases the oxygen-carrying capacity of the blood. Also, cardiac output in the fetus is redistributed to favor vital organs such as the heart, brain, and adrenal gland. Women who exercise regularly in early to midpregnancy experience a more rapid growth of the placenta and have improved placental function. At any rate of uterine blood flow, oxygen and nutrient delivery to the baby will be higher in a woman who exercises than in one who does not

(Clapp 1998; Wolfe, Brenner, & Mottola, 1994). And finally, an inverse relationship exists between blood flow and oxygen extraction in which the arterio-venous oxygen (a-$\bar{v}O_2$) difference increases as flow decreases. As a result of these compensatory adjustments, oxygen delivery to the fetus does not appear to be compromised during maternal exercise (Sternfeld, 1997).

The second area of concern is that of carbohydrate utilization. Maternal blood glucose is the fetus' primary energy source. Several studies have shown maternal blood glucose to drop significantly following vigorous exercise in late gestation. This has been cause for concern, since low maternal blood glucose could compromise fetal energy supply. If this scenario were repeated regularly (as with physical conditioning), intrauterine growth retardation, lower birth weight, or other developmental problems might result. Several studies have reported lower birth weights in women who continued heavy exercise through pregnancy. This weight discrepancy was primarily attributed to a decrease in subcutaneous fat in the newborn (Clapp & Capeless, 1990). Intrauterine growth retardation, or other short- or long-term effects on newborns of this decreased fat, has not been documented (American College of Obstetricians and Gynecologists, 2002; 1994; Clapp, Lopez, & Harcar-Sevcik, 1999).

Other studies have found no difference in birth weight among exercising mothers, particularly when the mothers received nutritional counseling. Clapp and Rizk (1992) studied placental weight in recreational athletes and found that it was significantly greater than the controls at 16, 20, and 24 weeks. The athletes who remained active but decreased or modified their activities in late pregnancy had the highest birth weight and placental weight, while the athletes who maintained or increased their exercise in late pregnancy had birth weights lower than the controls. This study suggests that exercise through midpregnancy may stimulate placental growth, allowing for better delivery of oxygen and nutrients to the baby. However, high-volume exercise in late pregnancy, when fetal and maternal energy requirements are high, may reduce fetal and placental weight (Clapp et al., 1992).

A group fitness instructor working with prenatal exercisers should be aware of the nutritional demands of pregnancy and reinforce good dietary habits. The metabolic needs of pregnancy add approximately 300 kcal/day. The energy requirements of exercise must be factored in as well. Pregnant women have lower fasting blood glucose levels than nonpregnant women and also utilize carbohydrate during exercise at a greater rate (American College of Obstetricians and Gynecologists, 2002; 1994). They are therefore more likely to become **hypoglycemic**, both during exercise and at rest. Pregnant women should be reminded to have a pre-exercise snack and to eat frequent small meals throughout the day. Help pregnant participants recognize the signs of hypoglycemia, such as weakness, dizziness, fatigue, and nausea. Suggest to those performing high levels of exercise that their exercise volume should start to taper from mid- to late-pregnancy. Finally, maternal weight gain and fetal growth (measured by her doctor at regular prenatal visits) should be within normal limits.

The third area of concern is that of fetal **hyperthermia** (overheating). Hyperthermia is known to be **teratogenic** (that is, capable of causing birth defects) (McMurray & Katz, 1990). Febrile illness in the first trimester has been associated with neural tube defects. Retrospective studies searching for a common factor in neural development defects found that heat (such as would be seen in fetal hyperthermia) was a major cause. However, there is no demonstrated increase in neural tube defects or other birth defects in women who participate in even vigorous exercise during early pregnancy (American College of Obstetricians and Gynecologists, 2002; 1994; Clapp & Little, 1995).

Normal fetal temperature is slightly higher than that of the mother. Fetal temperature is contingent on maternal temperature, fetal metabolic rate, and uterine blood flow, with the greatest effect stemming from maternal temperature. Fetal thermoregulation depends on the mother's ability to cool herself. Very high-intensity exercise, or exercise in a hot, humid environment, has the potential to raise maternal core temperature above the baby's and reverse the temperature gradient. This could cause the baby to take on heat from the mother.

Maternal resting core temperatures are slightly higher than prepregnancy levels, but exercise temperatures in pregnant women do not mirror this increase. Peak rectal temperature in pregnant women after exercise at 64% of $\dot{V}O_2$max has been shown to decrease by 0.3° C by eight weeks and continues to drop at a rate of 0.1° C per month through the 37th week (Clapp, 1991; American College of Obstetricians and Gynecologists, 2002; 1994).

It appears that pregnant women have physiological adaptations that enhance thermoregulation during exercise. These adaptations include a downward shift in the sweating threshold (allowing evaporative heat loss at a lower body temperature), better skin-to-environment heat transfer due to increased skin blood flow during pregnancy, and increased heat loss through the respiratory tract due to increased ventilation in pregnancy.

While these compensatory mechanisms serve to protect the fetus from heat stress, caution should nevertheless be taken to avoid overheating when working with this population. Remember that early pregnancy (the first trimester) is the most critical phase regarding heat sensitivity and fetal development. Participants should be advised to (1) exercise in a cool, well-ventilated, low-humidity environment, (2) drink plenty of cool water to avoid dehydration, and (3) avoid very high-intensity activities.

Musculoskeletal System Imbalances and Dysfunctions

An understanding of alterations to the musculoskeletal system will enable instructors to wisely choose and modify various exercises for the benefit of their pregnant participants. The following are some of the most commonly encountered complaints among prenatal exercisers.

Muscle Imbalances

When posture is not in the ideal alignment, muscle imbalances are likely to arise. The common muscle imbalances identified in pregnancy are either "tight" (scapula protractors, levator scapula, thoracolumbar area, hip flexors, tensor fascia latae, piriformis, hamstrings, adductors, and calves) or "weak" (scapula retractors, low lumbar paravertebral, gluteus maximus and medius, abdominals, and quadriceps) (Wilder, 1988).

Muscle imbalances must be considered when an instructor is choosing exercises for class. Prenatal classes should be designed to reduce these muscle imbalances. The reduction will, in turn, help reduce the postural devi-

ations. When dealing with muscle imbalances, it is more effective to first relax the tightened muscles through stretches and mobility exercises and then follow with strengthening exercises for the weaker muscle groups.

When participants are unable to perform certain exercises because of discomfort or irritation, the instructor should react to the short-term situation by modifying exercises to reduce such difficulties. When discomfort or irritations persist, the participant must realize that she may need to cease the activity to rest the area and prevent further aggravation. In all cases, the participant should communicate concerns to her physician. In severe cases in which discomfort becomes chronic, consulting a physical therapist specializing in prenatal care should be considered.

Dysfunctions and Irritations

This section provides a summary of common dysfunctions and irritations, including backache, **pelvic floor** weakness, **diastasis recti,** ligament strain, pubic pain, sacroiliac joint dysfunction, **sciatica**, nerve compression syndromes, overuse syndromes, and muscle cramps. While suggestions for exercise modifications are touched on in this section, detailed exercises are found later in this chapter.

Backache

The most frequent complaint during pregnancy is backache. About half of all pregnant women develop pain in the low-back area. Proper body mechanics, exercise, massage, relaxation, and physical therapy can help reduce and, in some cases, prevent low-back pain.

As noted previously, postural realignments during pregnancy contribute heavily to the incidence of backache. An exaggeratedly curved lower back, rounded upper back, and a forward head characterize the typical posture of a pregnant woman.

Exercises appropriate for this situation should focus on reducing the improper alignment. Mobility and stretching exercises should emphasize relaxing and lengthening the back extensors, hip flexors, shoulder protractors, shoulder internal rotators, and neck flexors. Strengthening exercises focused on the abdominals, gluteals, and scapula retractors will reinforce their ability to support proper alignment.

Gentle reminders to participants are helpful in maintaining proper alignment throughout each section of class. To practice maintaining a neutral pelvis, participants can strengthen the muscles that tilt the pelvis posteriorly (i.e., the abdominal and gluteal muscle groups). The gluteal muscles should be pulled downward and together with an upward pull of the abdominals. This motion should reduce the anterior pelvic tilt position.

Various cues, such as heads up, shoulders back, buttocks tight, belly buttons up, or abdominals hugging the baby, may communicate alignment to participants. Even a simple question such as, "How does that low back feel?" may stimulate better posture. Posture breaks during class for pelvic tilts and other back exercises can increase comfort.

Aside from postural alterations that bring on back pain, other factors that may contribute to the condition are increases in relaxin, hypermobility of the sacroiliac joint, improper body mechanics, **vascular disturbances** (a particular cause of nighttime back pain), **transient osteoporosis** from dietary calcium deficiency, and psychosocial stress (Hummel-Berry, 1990).

Pelvic Floor Weakness

The five layers of muscle and fascia attached to the bony ring of the pelvis are commonly referred to as the pelvic floor. From superficial to deep layers, they are as follows: the superficial outlet muscles, urogenital triangle, pelvic diaphragm or levator ani muscles, smooth muscle diaphragm, and endopelvic diaphragm. They support the pelvic organs like a sling to withstand all the increases in pressure that occur in the abdominal and pelvic cavity and provide **sphincter** control for the three **perineal** openings (Noble, 1995).

There are fascial connections between the levator ani muscles, the sacroiliac ligaments, the hip rotator muscles, and the hamstrings. These connections allow weaknesses of the pelvic floor muscles to refer stress to these areas. Pelvic floor weaknesses can cause the pelvic alignment to falter and thus irritate the sacroiliac joint and the hip joint (Wilder, 1988). It is crucial that these muscles function competently. In addition, prolapse of the bladder, uterus, or rectum may develop if muscles become too weak to support the pelvic organs. Finally, urinary **incontinence** can often be initiated during pregnancy because of pelvic floor weakness.

Kegel exercises are designed to strengthen the pelvic floor and ensure its proficient function. The benefits of strengthening the pelvic floor include providing support for the heavy pelvic organs; preventing prolapse of the bladder, uterus, and rectum; supporting pelvic alignment; reinforcing sphincter control; enhancing circulation through a congested area of the vascular system; and providing a healthy environment for the healing process after labor and delivery (Dunbar, 1992).

Diastasis Recti

This is the partial or complete separation of the rectus abdominis muscle. Diastasis recti occurs as the linea alba widens and finally gives way to the mechanical stress of an advancing pregnancy (Wilder, 1988). The linea alba, a tendinous fiber that merges the abdominal muscles with the fascia, extends from the xiphoid process to the **symphysis pubis.** Some separation is a normal part of every pregnancy.

Proficient prenatal instructors may test for diastasis recti. The most common test is performed by placing two fingers horizontally on the suspected location of the diastasis recti while the participant lies supine with knees bent. Have her perform a curl-up. If the fingers are able to penetrate at the location, there is probably a split. The abdominal muscles can be felt to the side of the split. The degree of separation is measured according to the number of fingerwidths of the split. One to two fingerwidths is considered normal. If the separation is greater than three fingerwidths, avoid exercises that place direct stress on this area (Noble, 1995). Focus on abdominal compression exercises and using the abdominals to help maintain neutral spinal alignment with all activities. Abdominal curl-ups can be performed in a semirecumbent position rather than supine.

Diastasis recti is most common during the third trimester and immediately postpartum and is attributed to the following influences:

• *Maternal hormones.* Relaxin, **estrogen,** and progesterone encourage the connective tissue to become less supportive. There is a loosening effect on the abdominal fascia and a reduction of the cohesion between the collagen fibers.

• *Mechanical stress within the abdominal cavity.* This varies according to fetus size and number, placenta size, the amount of amniotic fluid, the number of previous pregnancies, and the amount of weight gain. The abdominal musculature is designed to shorten and lengthen in a vertical direction, but pregnancy demands that the abdominal wall expand horizontally, and it is not normally elastic in the transverse direction. This situation causes mechanical stress that can end in functional failure for the abdominal wall. After a slow deformation of the soft tissue, the separation is often caused by a sudden action made with improper body mechanics.

• *Weak abdominal muscles.* A correlation exists between diastasis recti and weak abdominal muscles. Women with strong abdominal musculature are considered more prepared to resist this condition (Boissonnault & Blaschak, 1988). Other predisposing factors include heredity, obesity, multiple-birth pregnancy, a large baby, excess uterine fluid, and a lax abdominal wall from former pregnancies.

Abdominal exercises that may introduce susceptibility in people prone to diastasis are those that put direct pressure on the linea alba from within due to uterine resistance, and from without due to gravitational resistance.

Round, Inguinal, and Broad Ligament Irritations

The round, inguinal, and **broad ligaments** are the ligaments most commonly irritated or strained during pregnancy. The **inguinal ligament** is formed as the fascia of the internal oblique, the external oblique, and transverse abdominis muscles blend together at their lower margin. It runs between the pubic tubercle and the anterior superior iliac spine. As the abdominal wall expands, the inguinal ligament is also stretched. It continues to be stretched throughout the pregnancy, slowly adapting with the abdominal wall expansion. This constant state of tension can easily turn into a spasm with an increase in abdominal

287

Exercise and Pregnancy

pressure such as that which results from a cough, sneeze, or laugh.

Workouts must be attuned to the current state of ligamentous tension. On days when the participant feels vulnerable, the intensity of the workout and strain put on the ligament should be reduced. Sensitivity is common with abdominal exercises and inner- and outer-thigh exercises. When performing abdominal exercises, try to relieve the tension by keeping the knee and hip joints bent and the curling height low. With hip abduction and adduction, the knee and hip joints should again be slightly bent. This places the inguinal ligament in a more relaxed position and reduces the leverage of the leg. Avoid quick shifts of body position, especially changing from right to left side-lying positions. Prepare the body to change positions by warming joints with pelvic tilts, maintaining proper alignment, and using the arms to help lift the body from the floor.

The round and broad ligaments directly support the uterus within the pelvic cavity. The **round ligament** connects to both sides of the uterine fundus and extends forward through the inguinal canal and terminates in the labia majora (Figure 10.2). The round ligament may be irritated with extreme stretches above the head, rapid twisting movements, or jackknifing off the floor or bed. The use of proper mechanics for lying down and rising will also prevent strain on the round ligament (Figure 10.3). In the exercise arena, women may experience

Figure 10.2
Round and broad ligaments

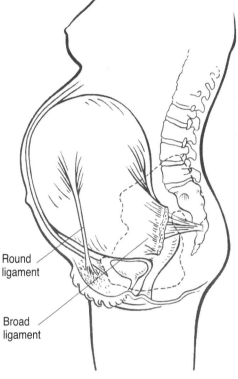

Round ligament

Broad ligament

Figure 10.3a-c
Proper body mechanics for rising from the side-lying position to the sitting position

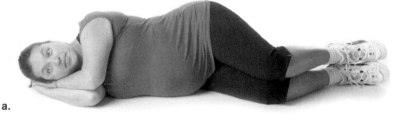

a.

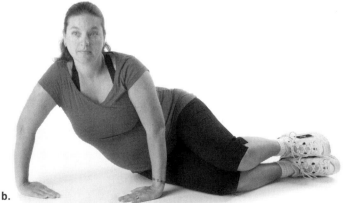

b.

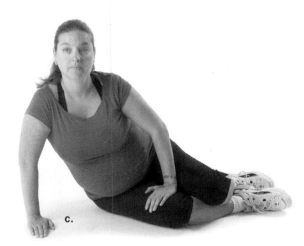

c.

discomfort when the round ligament is jostled from jogging or jumping. A unilateral, standing hip hike held for five seconds and repeated for several repetitions can decrease the discomfort of, or even prevent, round ligament pain. To perform this exercise, have the participant elevate one illiac crest by shifting the weight to one leg, thereby unloading the other leg and lifting it slightly off the floor. The knee should be straight. Adequate warm-up for the inguinal ligament, the round ligament, and the abdominal wall may also include torso range-of-motion activities, pelvic tilts, and an effleurage massage. (An effleurage massage is a very light, stroking movement, done in this case by placing the fingertips on the pubis and sliding them upward along the linea alba, then sliding them down both sides of the abdominal wall near the round ligament, gently rubbing along the inguinal ligament, and meeting at the pubis to begin the circular motion again.)

The largest ligament supporting the ovaries, as well as the uterine tubes, uterus, and vagina, is the broad ligament. It connects the lateral margins of the uterus to the posterior pelvic walls. The pull it receives from the enlarged uterus can cause a severely arched and aching low back. Relaxation of this ligament can be aided with performance of pelvic tilts, the cat stretch, trunk flexion exercises, self-massage of the low back, and torso range-of-motion movements, all of which help to relieve tension in the broad ligament as well as in the extensor muscles of the back. Encourage participants to avoid exaggerating the arch of the low back, maintain good postural alignment, and use good body mechanics.

Pubic Pain

As the growth of the fetus demands more space, the pelvis accommodates by expanding. The loosened ligaments that allow this necessary expansion also allow increased motion. The irritation of the pubic symphysis caused by the increased motion at the joint is called **symphysitis** (Wilder, 1988). This irritation may be worsened by exercise. Ice may be used to relieve immediate irritation (see Chapter 11 for RICE guidelines). A physician consultation is advised and physical therapy

Figure 10.3d-f
Proper body mechanics for getting up from the floor

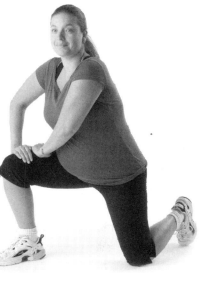

d.

e.

f.

Exercise and Pregnancy

may be ordered. Pelvic belts, which compress the pelvis and minimize motion in the symphysis pubis and sacroiliac joint, may be prescribed. Partial symphyseal separations and complete dislocations are possible during pregnancy, as are pubic stress fractures. They usually result from delivery and, therefore, are a greater concern for postnatal participants.

When pubic pain occurs, efforts to alleviate irritation will determine the choice of activity and exercise. Exercises using hip adduction and abduction and, to a lesser extent, hip extension can cause further irritation of the pubis. The relationship of the tendons to the hip joints during hip abduction, adduction, and extension may cause excessive movement of the pubis, which intensifies the pain. Appropriate modifications include reducing hip joint exercises to a level of tolerance or to avoid pain completely. Perform standing hip abduction and extension exercises to reduce symphysis pubis irritation. Reduce the impact and weightbearing aspects of aerobic activities and suggest aqua aerobics, swimming, or stationary biking as alternative exercises. Shoe quality is important to mention to these participants; walking or jogging in worn-out shoes can worsen joint irritations.

Sacroiliac Joint Dysfunction

According to Hummel-Berry (1990), 50% of all back pain is related to lumbosacral pain. During pregnancy, the sacroiliac joint functions to resist the anterior pelvic tilt that is accentuated by the increase in lumbar lordosis caused by the uterine growth and weight gain. To facilitate the passage of the fetus through the pelvis, relaxin is released and softens the normally rigid ligaments of the sacroiliac joint and symphysis pubis. Postural adjustments, which pull the pelvis anteriorly, in conjunction with the hormonal relaxation

effect, ultimately combine to force the sacroiliac ligaments to give, stretch, and, possibly, become hypermobile (Daly et al., 1991).

Symptoms of sacroiliac dysfunction include pain during the following activities: prolonged sitting, standing, or walking; climbing stairs; standing with weight on one leg; and twisting (Lile & Hagar, 1991). The pain is usually unilateral (on one side) and in some cases radiates to the buttocks, lower abdomen, anterior medial thigh, groin, or posterior thigh (Daly et al., 1991). Participants may complain of having pain in the sacroiliac area when they stand up out of a chair or when they get out of bed. The pain is felt at the sacroiliac joint and radiates into the buttocks, but it does not radiate down the leg, as is characteristic of sciatica.

Exercises should be chosen to add strength and support to the sacroiliac area and to facilitate pelvic stability. If the lumbosacral angle (the angle between the lumbar vertebrae and the sacrum) is reduced, pain will usually be reduced. The gluteal muscles add the most direct support, but endurance exercises for the abdominals are also helpful. Abdominal endurance assists in preventing the anterior pelvic tilt that is straining the sacroiliac joint and ligament. Suggestions for class include accentuating proper postural alignment, using abdominal compression exercises throughout class, and using standing hip extension and abduction exercises. All of the preceding actions should incorporate pelvic stability (refer to the hip exercises in the floor-work section of this chapter). Participants with severe cases of sacroiliac dysfunction should be advised to see their physician.

Sciatica

Pressure placed on the sciatic nerve due to the position of the fetus or postural structures can produce nerve irritation that is extremely painful. A woman experiencing pain that radiates from her buttocks down to her legs is probably experiencing sciatic nerve irritation. Exercise can do little to relieve this situation. Participants should be advised to note the activities that preceded the irritation and either avoid those activities in the future or review the body mechanics used during the aggravating activity. Pelvic tilts may offer some immediate relief by shifting the irritating pressure away from the nerve. After experiencing a sciatic nerve irritation, the gluteal muscles and hamstrings will respond by tightening. Gently stretching these muscles can help to relax them out of this protective response.

Nerve Compression Syndromes

More than 80% of pregnant women have some degree of swelling during their pregnancy. Soft-tissue swelling may decrease the available space in relatively constrained anatomical areas. The result of this constriction and fluid retention can be nerve compression syndromes or, less commonly, compartment syndromes. Nerve compression syndrome is possible in many areas that have a compressed nerve compartment.

The most prevalent nerve problem during pregnancy is carpal tunnel syndrome. It results from compression of the median nerve within the wrist. Complaints of numbness and tingling sensations in the thumb and index and middle fingers are characteristic. Avoid loading the wrists in hyperextension, grasping objects tightly, and repetitive flexion/extension of the wrist. Keep the wrist joint in its neutral position as much as possible.

A related nerve compression syndrome, tarsal tunnel syndrome, involves cramping and compression of the posterior tibial nerve. The characteristic complaint is numbness from the inside of the ankle to the medial plantar aspect

of the foot. Thoracic outlet syndrome results from compression and aggravation of the brachial plexus. Tingling and numbing sensations may be felt down the arms and hands. Postural deviations with internally rotated shoulders can aggravate the situation. Exercises to encourage external rotation of the shoulder and stretches to reduce internal rotation of the shoulder should be added to the workout regimen to balance the muscles. A bra that supports the weight of the breast tissue may help to reduce upper-back strain.

Encourage participants to avoid long periods of standing and sitting throughout their day. Taking short breaks at work to walk around and sitting with the feet elevated can help to improve circulation and reduce swelling. Prolonged standing should be avoided, as it can cause significant reductions in venous return and cardiac output. Advise participants to lie whenever possible on their left side with the feet slightly elevated. An example of this position involves side-lying on a sofa with the feet elevated on the sofa arm. This position is the most efficient at facilitating venous return and reducing fluid retention. Drinking plenty of water and reducing salt intake may also prevent excessive fluid retention. Severe swelling and fluid retention can indicate other medical conditions related to pregnancy, in addition to contributing to nerve compression, and should be reported immediately to the primary physician.

Overuse Syndromes

Weight gain, postural changes, and hormonal influences create a perfect environment for producing overuse syndromes. Many common overuse syndromes associated with exercise are intensified by these adaptations of pregnancy. Chondromalacia, a gradual

Exercise and Pregnancy

degeneration of the articular cartilage that lines the back surface of the patella, can become irritated and inflamed because of the stress placed on the knee joint due to poor alignment. Pain can become incapacitating. Classes should include strengthening exercises for the quadriceps muscles to add support to the knee joints, and extra attention should be given to maintaining proper knee alignment during these exercises. Hyperflexion of the knee when bearing weight can accentuate the aggravation. Alignment is an especially important issue in stepping activities because the repetitive motion can easily result in improper alignment as the participant becomes fatigued.

The feet often become flatter and more pronated during pregnancy due to weight gain. When the feet are not striking properly, further alignment deviations in the hips and knees can result. Plantar fasciitis, which is an inflammation of the plantar fascia, the broad band of connective tissue running along the sole of the foot, may result from improper foot placement. Advise participants to avoid wearing worn or unsupportive shoes.

Muscle Cramps

Awakening abruptly to a muscle cramp can be very painful and frustrating. This is not an uncommon experience for pregnant women, who often do not know how to relieve cramps. Advise participants to avoid extreme pointing of the toes (plantarflexion) and wearing high heels and tight shoes, as these actions may stimulate muscle cramping. To relieve a muscle cramp, put the muscle in a stretched position and hold it there until the sensation subsides. For example, straighten the knee to alleviate a hamstring cramp, straighten the knee and dorsiflex the foot to relieve a calf cramp, and dorsiflex the foot and spread the toes to relieve a foot cramp.

Exercise Classes and Programs for Pregnant Women
Cardiovascular Exercise

Research on pregnancy and exercise has advanced significantly since ACOG published the first guidelines on the topic in 1985. At that time, most of the research was limited to animal subjects. The initial guidelines were justifiably conservative, reflecting the lack of information available at that time. Since 1985, studies involving the use of human subjects have provided much more information on the physiological responses (both maternal and fetal) to exercise during pregnancy. Both the 2002 and 1994 ACOG guidelines reflect this increase in the body of scientific knowledge and include significant changes from the original recommendations. Notably, the recommendation to use heart rate as a means of monitoring exercise intensity has been removed (the original recommendation was to limit heart rate to 140 bpm or less). The heart-rate response to exercise among pregnant women is variable. Blunted, exaggerated, and normal linear responses may all be seen at different stages during the same pregnancy. It is important to realize that these changes are not due to exercise itself but rather to the other physiological influences of pregnancy. Ratings of perceived exertion (RPE) has been shown to correlate much more closely than heart rate to actual measured oxygen consumption during exercise in pregnancy. RPE is a simple yet effective way to cue intensity. Since it is a subjective rating, it allows for the large variances in exercise capacity that exist in a typical class setting. The "category" RPE scale (6–20) or the "category-ratio" Borg scale (0–10) may be used. The numbers corresponding to "fairly light" to "somewhat hard" are the recommended range during pregnancy (Pivarnik et al., 1991; Clapp, Lopez, & Harcar-Sevcik 1999).

The 1994 ACOG guidelines state: "There are no data to indicate that pregnant women should limit exercise intensity and lower target heart rates because of potential adverse effects." However, you must keep in mind that there may be other reasons to limit exercise intensity. The 1994 ACOG recommendations also removed specific limitations on exercise duration, reflecting the tremendous individual differences that exist in pregnant women's abilities. ACOG recommends "mild to moderate" exercise, but adds that highly trained women may be able to maintain higher intensities in the earlier part of pregnancy. ACOG further states that consistent exercise (three days per week or more) is preferable to intermittent activity. It is essential that the instructor knows the participants and their exercise histories and cues pregnant women regarding the effort appropriate for the individual. The exercise intensity and duration selected should not result in fatigue or exhaustion. Maternal symptoms are the basis for changes and modifications to the program (American College of Obstetricians and Gynecologists, 2002; 1994). ACOG's recommendations are the standard of care for exercise during pregnancy.

It takes a thoughtful and purposeful plan to teach an effective fitness class. The challenge is to design and choose exercises that will allow success, comfort, and safety for the pregnant participant.

Whether a pregnant exercise participant wishes to be integrated into an exercise class of nonpregnant women—perhaps a class she has already been in—or joins a prenatal class, it is the instructor's responsibility to be aware of any pregnant woman's new physical status and to make appropriate individualized adjustments for that participant.

For instructors with large classes, the greatest challenge may be just knowing who, if anyone, is pregnant in the class. Many women well into their second trimester may not "show." While pre-exercise screening will identify the newcomer to exercise, it does not help the instructor identify a new pregnancy in a regular class participant. Therefore, unless an instructor actually mentions to the class from time to time the need to know about pregnancies, he or she may not find out about pregnancies for quite a while.

Specialized classes for pregnant women have several benefits over integrated classes. Individual participants can be better monitored for such things as strain, discomfort, and fatigue. In addition, the prenatal exercise class forms a natural support group, with discussions of many pregnancy-related issues and help in maintaining stress control, self-esteem, and body confidence.

However, the experienced or highly fit pregnant woman may wish to continue to exercise in a nonspecialized group fitness environment, especially when her favorite exercise mode is not taught specifically for pregnant women. This situation may arise in early pregnancy or if it is not the participant's first baby. While this should not be discouraged, the instructor will need to give additional attention and guidance to the pregnant participant in an integrated class.

In both specialized and integrated classes, there should be communication between the instructor and pregnant participants on a range of subjects, including sufficiency of warm-up time, needed modifications of exercises, intensity of movements, perceived exertion, weight gain, and comfort and pain levels.

Always be mindful of conditions such as hyperthermia, hypoxia, hypoglycemia, and

293

Exercise and Pregnancy

musculoskeletal injuries. An exercise activity should be stopped and alternatives immediately given if the participant finds it awkward to perform or if it causes discomfort, pain, or embarrassment.

The aerobic exercise warm-up should gradually increase muscle temperature through general body movement and joint range-of-motion activity. Give special emphasis to stimulating those areas under mechanical stress from pregnancy—the abdomen, pelvis, back, and hips.

Conditioning Exercises

All exercises should be performed with smooth and controlled speed and a range of motion that allows the exerciser to maintain proper alignment and comfort. If any exercise stimulates discomfort it should be immediately discontinued. Special attention should be given to teaching proper body mechanics when moving to a seated position or rising from the floor (see Figure 10.3).

Neck

Neck range-of-motion activities help to reduce tension. After muscles are warmed, stretch the sternocleidomastoid, levator scapulae, and upper trapezius to further relieve tension and reduce the forward-head position associated with poor postural alignment. During this segment, it is important to keep some movement in the legs to facilitate circulation. Complete the neck stretches with an examination of proper head and neck alignment (refer to discussions related to spinal alignment in Chapter 3).

Shoulder Girdle

To correct suspected muscle imbalances, begin with a warm-up and stretch of the scapula levators, scapula protractors, and

shoulder internal rotators. Balance this with scapula retraction exercises of the rhomboids, middle trapezius, and lower trapezius. Correct body placement during scapula retraction exercises can reduce the chance of low-back extension; a slight lunge such as used when stretching the calf muscles is a perfect adjustment. The abdominals and gluteals function as pelvic stabilizers and need to be incorporated into this workout to prevent hyperextension of the lower back. Shoulder external rotation exercises improve postural alignment by widening and opening the chest area. They also reduce constriction of the brachial plexus, a negative element associated with thoracic outlet syndrome.

Shoulder and Elbow Joints

The workout of the anterior, middle, and posterior deltoids, pectoralis major, and the latissimus dorsi may proceed as usual. Work on the biceps and triceps also does not need extensive modification. Maintaining functional ranges of motion during exercises, especially when weights are being used, will help prevent overlengthening muscles, tendons, and ligaments associated with vulnerably loose joints. The body placement and positioning chosen for various exercises should facilitate circulation and promote proper alignment. Many arm exercises can be performed in combination with other exercises, such as standing legwork or stretches. If exercises are performed in a sitting position, back alignment may be facilitated by placing a towel roll just under the tailbone, which will tilt the pelvis slightly anteriorly and adjust for the rounded back (Figure 10.4). Sitting on the edge of a bench may be another comfortable sitting position when working on the shoulder and elbow joint muscles.

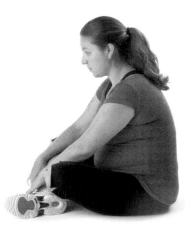

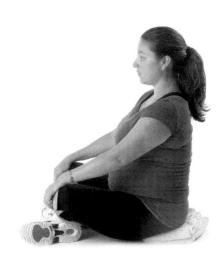

Figure 10.4
Back alignment may
be facilitated by
placing a towel roll just
under the tailbone to
slightly tilt the pelvis
anteriorly.

Wrist Joint

A small amount of time should be allocated to wrist range of motion to promote circulation in a tight compartment area. Finger motion may also be performed to reduce swelling of this stagnant peripheral circulatory area. These movements can be used during arm exercises or choreographed into the aerobic segment.

Low Back

These muscles are often tight and strained from the weight of the uterus pulling the abdominal wall and pelvis forward, resulting in the exaggerated lumbar lordosis posture. The class goal for this area is to relax these muscles to improve posture and decrease possible back pain. Range-of-motion exercises may be used to warm these muscles, followed by stretches to encourage them to lengthen and relax. Back range of motion consists of flexion, extension, lateral flexion, and rotation. The many possible exercises and stretches for the low back include side bends, twists, standing back rolls, pelvic tilts, pelvic rotations, pelvic side lifts, cat stretches (Figure 10.5), lateral rolls, tail wags, modified press-ups, cross backs, knee-to-chest stretches, and knee rolls. Please refer to the ACE fitness guide, *Pre- and Post-Natal Fitness,* for a more complete collection of photo illustrations of various exercises and stretches.

Abdominal Wall

The abdominal wall seems to be of particular concern to instructors. The concern is probably derived from attempting to maintain

Figure 10.5
The cat stretch

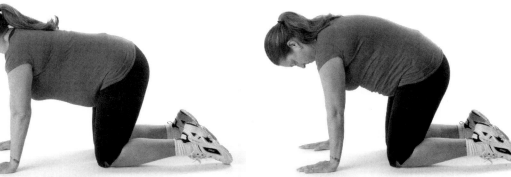

Exercise and Pregnancy

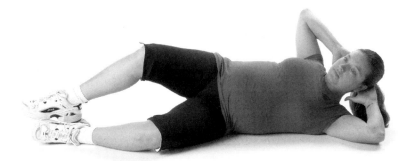

Figure 10.6
The semirecumbent position easily replaces the supine position for many abdominal exercises.

abdominal strength while avoiding supine hypotension and diastasis recti. Concern is definitely warranted, since most abdominal workouts are performed in the supine position. Exercising in the supine position may induce supine hypotension syndrome and place excessive mechanical stress on the abdominal wall along the linea alba, especially in mid- to late-pregnancy. Positioning participants in a semirecumbent position removes the constricting uterine pressure from the inferior vena cava and aorta and reduces the direct gravitational strain on the linea alba. Many conventional abdominal exercises may be easily modified for the semirecumbent position (Figure 10.6). For additional support to the linea alba, the abdominal wall may be splinted with crossed arms and hands (Noble, 1995). Stress to the inguinal ligament is reduced when the hip and knee joints remain flexed and rolled to the side, as in the semirecumbent position. Besides the usual curl-up abdominal exercises, experiment with various pelvic tilt and abdominal compression exercises. This group of exercises is essential for maintaining postural alignment and pelvic stability. They may be performed in a variety of positions, from standing to the all-fours position. Abdominal compression should be combined with other exercises throughout class to help maintain proper pelvic alignment.

Pelvic Floor

The introduction of Kegel exercises to participants is essential. There are numerous routines for performing Kegel exercises. For example, have participants begin with an isometric contraction of the pelvic floor, feel the muscles lift and tighten, hold it for a slow count of 10, then relax the muscles for another count of 10 and repeat. Most participants will have difficulty identifying and isolating these muscles if they have not performed Kegels before. Since it is impossible for an instructor to know if participants are performing them correctly, effective cues are essential. Asking participants to contract the muscles they would use to stop urinary flow improves awareness and control of these muscles (Noble, 1995). Another technique is to imagine an elevator going up and down as the pelvic floor is lifted. Stopping the elevator on each floor is a variation that requires more muscle control (Noble, 1995).

Kegel exercises can be placed in class along with abdominal and gluteal exercises. For example, initiate a semirecumbent curl-up, lift for two counts, hold for two counts, incorporate a Kegel during the hold for two counts, then lower for two counts and repeat the sequence again. Suggest that each participant choose a cue to remind herself to Kegel outside of class; when they brush their teeth, talk on the phone, cough, sneeze, or laugh, they can be cued to Kegel. A suggested workout program includes four daily sets of 10 initially, working up to four daily sets of 25.

Hip Flexors

The hip flexor muscles are often tight as a result of the prenatal posture. The fact that people tend to spend a large part of their day sitting causes them to shorten. Therefore, the emphasis in class is to stretch and relax them. Care should be taken not to hyperextend the low back when performing hip flexor stretches in the standing, kneeling, or side-lying positions.

Hip Extensors

The role of the hip extensors is to oppose the hip flexors' pull of the pelvis anteriorly and to assist the abdominals in their role of tilting the pelvis posteriorly. In assisting with the posterior pelvic tilt, the hip extensors also help alleviate the strain placed on the sacroiliac joint. Standing may be a more comfortable position for gluteus maximus workouts, since it seems to place less stress on vulnerable areas. The common all-fours and side-lying positions often place strain on the symphysis pubis, inguinal ligament, sacroiliac joint, and the lumbar spine and, therefore, may be replaced with the standing position. To facilitate support for the sacroiliac joint, hip extension exercises are used to strengthen the gluteal muscles. To recruit more muscle fibers from the gluteal muscle group, perform hip extensions while the hip joint is abducted, adducted, or externally rotated (Figure 10.7). Abdominal compression should be included in the exercises to assist in maintaining pelvic stability.

Hip Abduction

To promote more fiber recruitment of the gluteal muscles, perform hip abduction while the hip is extended and/or externally rotated, in addition to in the neutral position. Participants should be encouraged to

Figure 10.7
Standing hip exercises should be performed in conjunction with a posterior tilt of the pelvis triggered by abdominal and gluteal contractions.

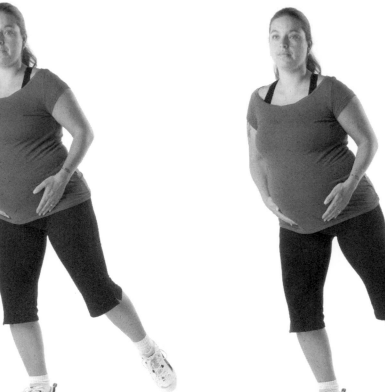

Standing hip extension   Standing hip extension while hip is abducted and externally rotated

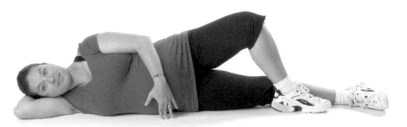

Figure 10.8
A towel roll or the exerciser's arm may be used to support the neck and facilitate proper alignment.

perform this exercise in a standing position, as with the hip extensors. This is another exercise that offers indirect muscle support to the sacroiliac joint. Incorporating abdominal compression will assist in maintaining a stable pelvis. A towel roll may be used to support the neck and the abdominal wall, and thus maintain body alignment when lying sideways (Figure 10.8). If the inguinal ligament or the symphysis pubis is sensitive, the hip and knee joints should be flexed during hip abduction. This reposition-

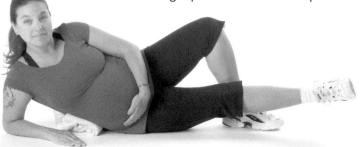

Figure 10.9
Hip adduction is performed with both the knee and hip joints bent to reduce the leverage of the leg.
Note: A towel roll can be used to support the abdominal wall.

Figure 10.10
The butterfly sitting position for hip adduction

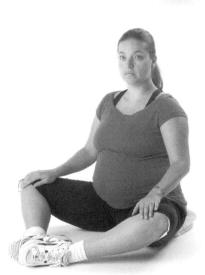

ing reduces the leverage weight and puts the inguinal ligament in a more relaxed position. If irritation still occurs, then the exercise should be deleted from the workout.

Hip Adductors
Because of the anterior tilt position of the pelvis, the tendons of the hip joint muscles are pulled slightly forward. The hip adductors may become tensed and strained in this new alignment. During hip adduction exercises, strain may occur in nearby vulnerable areas, such as the symphysis pubis, the groin area, or the inguinal ligament. If exercises cause a significant amount of stress on these areas, the participant may complain of discomfort during or after class. Modifications for hip adductor work may relieve the stress. Side-lying hip adductor exercises may be conducted with minute variations, such as use of a towel roll to promote body alignment (Figure 10.9). In addition, bending the hip and knee joints reduces the amount of stress placed on the inguinal ligament, symphysis pubis, and hip joint because the leverage of the leg is reduced in this more relaxed position (Figure 10.10). If irritation becomes chronic or if the exercise feels uncomfortable, then adductor exercises should be deleted from the workout. Lateral movement such as slide training is best avoided because of the decreased stability of the pelvis during pregnancy.

Quadriceps/Knee Extension
An important muscle group to strengthen is the quadriceps. Strength in this muscle group better equips the participant for the squatting and bending necessary in her daily activities. Activities such as getting out of a chair take on new dimensions with the pregnant body. The abdominal wall may limit the ability to lean for-

ward and stand, and so the legs and arms must assist more in rising. Exercises that incorporate daily activities are most helpful. They not only train the muscles, but also educate participants on proper body mechanics when performing simple activities with a sometimes awkward pregnant body. Pretending to be picking up a two-year-old child, taking groceries out of the car, opening lower drawers, vacuuming, or any other daily scenario may be utilized. Safety for the knee joint is the same as with all populations, but remember that a greater weight is being carried. Deep knee bends or squats past 90 degrees of flexion should be avoided. Participants should remain around a comfortable 45 degrees of flexion. Avoid hyperflexion of the knee while bearing weight because of the extreme pressure this places on the knee joint.

Hamstrings/Hip Extensors and Knee Flexors

The hamstrings may be tighter during pregnancy due to postural adaptations, such as the anteriorly tilted pelvis. Range-of-motion activities and stretches may be implemented to reduce tightness. The common supine hamstring stretch may be replaced with a standing or side-lying hamstring stretch to avoid discomfort and supine hypotension.

Ankle Joint

The main goals for this joint are to facilitate circulation and maintain flexibility. Warm-ups should include stimulation of the calf muscles and the anterior lower-leg muscles. Ankle range-of-motion activities may help reduce swelling in the ankles by promoting venous return. Avoid extreme plantarflexion or pointing of the toes in all exercises, as this can easily initiate a calf muscle cramp, which may be relieved by dorsiflexing the ankle to stretch the calf muscles. A pleasant activity for cool-

down or relaxation is a self-foot massage. The pregnant woman's feet are overloaded with her natural weight gain, and a massage can be very soothing.

Aquatic Exercise

The favorite exercise modality for many pregnant women is water activities. In the water, body temperatures appear to rise less and dissipate sooner, which can help minimize the risk of hyperthermia (McMurray & Katz, 1990). However, water temperatures should feel cool or these benefits may be negated. If the water feels like bath water, it is probably too warm (Karsenec & Grimes, 1984). Because of the hydrostatic effects of water, submaximal exercise in water is associated with a smaller plasma volume decrease than exercise on land, which may result in better maintenance of uterine and placental blood flow (Watson et al., 1991).

The pressure of water appears to lessen fluid retention and swelling, two common discomforts of pregnancy. The prone position in swimming actually facilitates optimum blood flow to the uterus by redistributing the weight of the uterus away from the inferior vena cava and the aorta. Another positive attribute of water classes is the buoyant effect of water, which increases comfort by supporting body weight and eliminating trouble with balance. This wonderful weightless feeling can be a major relief to the pregnant woman. Water exercises are easy on the musculoskeletal system, due to the reduced stress placed on the weightbearing joints and ligaments. This nonweightbearing position gives relief to those muscles bearing extra mechanical stress and pressure from the pregnancy.

Pregnant swimmers should use caution with forceful frog or whip kicks, as they may place undue stress on the unstable pubic joint. Additionally, traditional use of a kickboard may amplify the exaggerated lumbar lordosis of pregnancy and should therefore be used judiciously.

Indoor Cycling

Because cycling is nonweightbearing, many women find it a comfortable activity even in the later trimesters, when activities like walking can become awkward and difficult. As with other forms of exercise, there are some modifications and precautions that should be kept in mind when pregnant women participate in studio cycling classes. Crosscurrent convective cooling (fans) and adequate hydration are musts, as the potential to overheat or dehydrate is great. Fluids should be taken frequently, with a goal of drinking 7–10 ounces for every 10–20 minutes of exercise. Workload (cadence, resistance, or both) should be decreased to achieve the same relative cardiovascular overload as pregnancy progresses. The tendency to overexert in these classes may be high, and, therefore, specific, individualized instruction should be given to the pregnant rider. Morphologic changes will affect cycling mechanics; the hips gradually externally rotate to accommodate the enlarging uterus. Increased weight on the saddle may necessitate wider, padded saddles or seat covers, in addition to padded shorts. The anterior weight gain of pregnancy, coupled with the laws of gravity, makes maintaining neutral lumbar alignment while hinging at the hip to reach the bars difficult and fatiguing; adjust the handlebars to the most upright position and give pregnant riders frequent postural breaks. Be aware that toward the later trimesters, anterior weight gain will tend to

pull a pregnant rider further forward over the pedals during out-of-the-saddle drills, putting the knees in a position susceptible to injury. Edema (swelling) in the feet can make tight toe straps uncomfortable; cleated shoes eliminate this problem.

Strength Training

Strength training is a beneficial and safe activity during a normal, uncomplicated pregnancy if the standard safety rules of weightlifting are adhered to. Safety suggestions include staying in control of the weights, moving through a functional range of motion, using slow, appropriate speeds for the exercise, and avoiding the Valsalva maneuver and the supine position (Work, 1989; Sinclair, 1992). Problems could arise if the participant tends to jerk, swing, perform the exercise too quickly, or use poor control when she is lifting. Functional range of motion should match (not exceed) the prepregnancy range to protect the joints from injury. Exercises done in the supine position should be modified after the first trimester; a semirecumbent position is often an acceptable modification. Overhead lifting should be avoided to prevent irritation or injury to the low back due to the decreased ability of the weakened abdominals to stabilize the torso against the pull of the belly (Artal, 1992).

Functional strength training is recommended for pregnant participants. Exercises should be selected based on the physical demands a new mom will face. Extended periods of time spent carrying, lifting, nursing, and holding an infant place the postpartum participant at risk for upper- and lower-back strain and injury. The emphasis during prenatal training is to develop the muscular strength and endurance necessary to ward off the chronic aches and pains common in new moms. Regular strength training will also help to reduce the time needed to resume normal activities of daily life without undue fatigue.

Repetitions and load will be determined based on the individual's exercise history, state of pregnancy, motivation, and other variables. Repetitions in the range of 10 to 15 would be appropriate for the pregnant woman who is new to strength training, while a woman who has been lifting regularly and is in the early prenatal stages may safely perform eight to 12 repetitions and make very few changes, if any, to her current program. Instructors teaching group strength training classes will need to pay close and constant attention to the pregnant participants' technique, biomechanics, and exercise choice, giving modifications as necessary.

Mind-Body Classes

Classes like tai chi, yoga, and Pilates, among others, are seeing more pregnant participants as well. The mind-body orientation of these classes is known to facilitate relaxation and reduce stress. Most women feel that although pregnancy is a happy, exciting time for them, it is also a stressful time. Any major change in one's life, good or bad, can create stress—and a new baby certainly changes one's life. Classes such as these can be a great opportunity for effective management of stress. Other relaxation techniques, such as progressive relaxation, visualization, and breathing techniques, can easily be incorporated into the cooldown/stretch portion of any group exercise class, and will especially benefit the pre- or postnatal woman. Participants should be cautioned to stretch or perform exercise

movements in an average to normal range of motion to protect potentially hypermobile joints. Additionally, the instructor can reassure the pregnant participant that the stress or anxiety she feels is a normal part of pregnancy, and help equip her with tools she can use once the baby arrives.

Programming Suggestions and Modifications

The following suggestions and modifications may be implemented as needed to further individualize programming for the prenatal exerciser.

- Design longer warm-ups to soothe vulnerable areas, such as the inguinal, round, and broad ligaments.
- Demonstrate and emphasize proper alignment to be used throughout class.
- Keep legs moving while standing to stimulate sluggish venous return.
- Choose positions to give the participant the best workout within her comfort zone while maintaining proper body alignment.
- Replace supine positions with semirecumbent positions, and replace prone positions with an all-fours position or an elbows-and-knees position.

Many positions may be easier with the use of towel rolls or pillows to help maintain body alignment. Changing positions often in class may facilitate circulation, but be aware that simply moving from the left side to the right side can be a strain if good body mechanics are not used. There are an infinite number of exercises for each muscle of the body. Use creativity to discover exercises to train muscles without causing discomfort for the pregnant participant. Experiment with methods to challenge participants appropriately.

The prenatal exerciser presents many interesting challenges to a fitness instructor.

Exercise and Pregnancy

From the initial warm-up through the final cool-down, numerous factors must be considered to make an exercise program both safe and effective for the pregnant exerciser. Table 10.6 summarizes an entire prenatal class format in the form of substitute instructor guidelines.

Postnatal Exercise

Returning to exercise after delivery is like going backward through pregnancy. The situation is similar to the relationship between a warm-up and cool-down; they mirror each other, but in reverse. All of the things a woman does to prepare for and endure pregnancy continue to be done in the postpartum period to slowly return to prepregnancy status.

The first priority after delivery is to bond with one's baby. The second priority is to resume Kegel exercises as soon as possible. The pelvic floor has been traumatized during delivery by severe stretching and possibly episiotomy or tears. Kegels after delivery may be a little scary, since the incision may be felt. Postoperative nurses should assure patients that Kegels will help the healing process of the pelvic floor. Before intense abdominal exercises can be considered, the pelvic floor should be rehabilitated.

Postpartum Return to Exercise

The suggested time for returning to group exercise activities is after the participant's postpartum doctor appointment, or six weeks after delivery. Factors that may determine postpartum return include complications of labor and delivery, uterine involution, pelvic floor healing, prepregnancy fitness levels, and self-motivation. Before this appointment, gentle walking can be resumed and gradually progressed if the participant desires.

Walking will help tone and strengthen the muscles of the lower body and, to some extent, the torso. During labor and delivery, the muscles of the pelvic floor undergo considerable stress and become relaxed and weakened. Temporary urinary stress incontinence is a common problem and may make exercise like running or aerobics difficult. The low-impact nature of walking helps to minimize this problem. Additionally, it has been shown that women who exercise during their pregnancy and in the early postpartum months have a shorter duration of urinary stress incontinence than those who do not (Clapp, 1998). Focusing on good spinal alignment and form while walking will allow the body to strengthen important postural muscles in the torso that have become weakened by the shift in center of gravity created by the increased size of the uterus during pregnancy.

When a participant returns to group exercise classes, advise her to gradually build back up to prepregnancy exercise levels. Remind her to listen to her body, exercise comfortably hard, but not to overdo it. Goals at this time are often unrealistic. A return to prepregnancy body weight and composition will take six months to one year in most cases. An instructor can help set realistic goals and create an environment that discourages weight loss as the sole reason to exercise.

As the postpartum participant rejoins the group exercise class, remember that caring for an infant is a 24-hours-a-day, seven-days-a-week commitment. Personal time often disappears, sleep is diminished, and a feeling of being overwhelmed coupled with fatigue may cause increased tension and

Table 10.6
Prenatal Class Format (Substitute Instructor Guidelines)

Carefully observe each individual student for signs of stress, strain, discomfort, and/or fatigue. Always be prepared to show modifications of exercises to meet each student's personal needs. The instructor must ask her if she need modifications.

Warm-up	General movements to increase muscle temperature	
	Normal joint range of motion (ROM): Neck, shoulders, wrist, pelvis, hips, knees, and ankles	
	Emphasis on back, pelvis, and hip joints	
	Stimulate postural alignment	
	Keep movements slow, controlled, and comfortable	
	Gradually increase ROM	
Nonimpact Aerobics	Intensity	Perceived exertion, fairly light to somewhat hard
		Breathing rate, conversational
	Duration	Depends on each participant's fitness level and state of pregnancy
	Mode	Nonbouncy, nonjerky, and rhythmical
		Contract–relax, smooth, and flowing
		Large, controlled ROM of arms and legs
		Maximize traveling; minimize standing in place
		Avoid quick changes of direction
Cool-down I	Easy, pumping leg movement to facilitate circulation (ankle ROM, anterior lower leg stimulated)	
	Stretches—easy positions, not to maximum ROM or tension	
Body Work	Positions	Varied to promote circulation (standing, sitting, or side-lying)
	Upper body	Deltoids, triceps, pectorals, biceps, middle and lower traps (stimulate scapular retraction and posture here and throughout class)
(Muscular strength, endurance, and flexibility)	Lower body	Quadriceps, hips (extension, abduction, and adduction in controlled repetitions; keep knees and hips slightly bent to eliminate strain to commonly irritated areas)
	Abdominals	Avoid or limit time in the supine position in those past the first trimester
		Slow repetitions, smaller ROM, low lift, knees and hips bent, predominately from side
		Alternative: use stability ball as an incline
		Abdominal compression exercises
		Pelvic tilts with emphasis on lower abdominals
		Attention to posture with all standing activity
	Additional	Exhale during contraction; inhale as relaxing
		Remember modifications for those with diastasis recti
		Pelvic tilts as well as back ROM exercise (e.g., cat stretch) are welcomed throughout class whether standing, sitting, or lying
Cool-down II	Final stretching; low-back stretch	
	Relaxation, visualizations, and deep breathing	
	Neck ROM and stretches	
	Normalize circulation for standing	

Exercise and Pregnancy

anxiety. This can affect not only the new mom's health and well-being, but also her relationship to the baby and other family members. One out of four first-time moms experience these feelings to such a degree that postpartum depression occurs. Help new moms learn to recognize this "overwhelmed" feeling in the early stages and encourage them to create some time for self-care. This time can help them to master the necessary coping skills. Exercise has been shown to help reduce stress and create significant gains in general psychological well-being. Studies have indicated that women who engage in regular exercise programs before, during, and after pregnancy have higher levels of self-esteem, which has been linked to a reduction in symptoms of postpartum depression.

Postpartum Musculoskeletal Conditions

Many women find that the back pain they experienced during pregnancy is relieved once the baby is born. However, attention should still be placed on low-back health. The weight of the uterus is no longer pressing against the abdominal wall, but the abdominal wall is now loose and nonsupportive to the low back. The use of good body mechanics is crucial during this hectic, new period. Poor body mechanics and postural adjustments, in combination with the fatigue experienced by a new mother, can easily predispose her to back pain unless these muscles are retrained and are again able to effectively stabilize the spine.

Breast weight is increased for lactation, which pulls the shoulders and scapula forward, exaggerating the thoracic kyphotic ("cuddling") posture. Prior to delivery, participants should be instructed on shoulder

external rotation and scapula retraction exercises for the postpartum period. If a participant plans to push a stroller while walking, she should make sure the handles are high or use handle extenders; handles that are too low will exacerbate thoracic kyphosis and make good spinal alignment impossible. If the handles are raised, she can focus on scapular retraction and maintenance of a neutral head and pelvis while she walks. Good breast support during postpartum exercise is essential, especially for the nursing mother. Bras that compress the breasts against the chest are preferable to those that lift, but they should be changed immediately after exercise to avoid discomfort or inhibition of milk production. Some women find layering two sports bras gives them better support during exercise.

Diastasis recti is of less concern after delivery than during pregnancy due to the fact that the internal mechanical stress on the abdominals (the baby) is no longer exerting force against them. However, participants should still be advised to evaluate their abdominal wall for the extent of separation that exists. All participants will have some separation; one to two fingers is considered normal. Although research has not shown abdominal hernias to result from postpartum crunches (Clapp, 1998), if the gap is three fingers or wider, special care and attention to strengthening is warranted. An intelligent progression from early isometric abdominal exercises to pelvic tilts and pelvic stabilization exercises to head raises and partial crunches will rapidly improve abdominal tone and facilitate closure of this gap. For participants with wide separations, it is prudent to avoid abdominal exercises that involve spinal rotation. The other abdominal muscles that are indirectly attached to the rectus abdominis can exert a pull that may widen the gap as they shorten. Noble's splinting abdominal exercises are a cautious first choice for early abdominal curl-up exercises (Noble, 1995). Remind participants that they should focus on using their abdominals throughout the day. Abdominal compression (i.e., pulling the navel toward the spine while slowly and forcibly exhaling) can be done whenever they think of it to help strengthen the transverse abdominals and improves kinesthetic awareness. To balance the abdominal workout, complete it with back extension and scapula retraction exercises.

Resuming Exercise After Caesarean Delivery

Caesarean section, also called C-section, is a major abdominal surgery and, as such, results in pain and tenderness in the abdomen for some time, as well as considerable fatigue. Most Caesarean incisions do not actually cut the abdominal muscles; the incision is made through the skin and the doctor pushes aside the muscles to open the uterus and deliver the baby. Due to the advances in surgical procedures, many women who have undergone C-section are ready to resume intermittent walking or other gentle forms of exercise by two weeks postpartum. During this time, the degree of discomfort, fatigue, and motivation will determine activity levels. Vigorous exercise is to be avoided; the goal is to encourage the healing process by performing rehabilitative exercises and getting adequate rest for the recovery process. Postpone re-entry into a structured exercise program until a doctor's clearance has been obtained after the six-week check-up. Women who have had C-sections may then participate in the

same postpartum exercise programs as women who have had vaginal births, with similar guidelines. Any activity causing pain should be avoided. While most incisions from C-section heal without complications, some may develop scar tissue or adhesions that cause discomfort months after the surgery. Massage can sometimes be of help in these cases.

Breastfeeding and Exercise

New mothers are often concerned that exercise may affect the quality or quantity of breast milk. Research has shown that regular, sustained, moderate- to high-intensity exercise does not impair the quality or quantity of breast milk (Dewey, 1998). However, in a minority of women, exercise that is anaerobic in nature (e.g., high-intensity interval training) may increase lactic acid levels in breast milk enough to cause a sour taste and decrease infant suckling (Wallace, Inbar, & Ernsthausen,1992). Only minor changes in the lactic acid content of breast milk appear after more typical workouts, and these small amounts do not affect infant suckling behavior (Wallace, Inbar, & Ernsthausen, 1994). If you encounter a participant whose baby rejects post-exercise breast milk, offer the participant several solutions: decrease exercise intensity to prevent accumulation of lactic acid, nurse the baby before exercising, collect pre-exercise breast milk for later consumption (lactic acid will clear the breast milk 30 minutes to one hour after exercise), or pump and discard the breast milk produced during the first 30 minutes after exercise (Wallace, 1993). In sum, this is an infrequent problem that should not prevent any lactating woman who wishes to exercise from doing so.

305

Summary

Exercise and Pregnancy

Summary

Attitudes about exercise during pregnancy have changed dramatically over the past 10 to 20 years. The stereotype of pregnancy being a time of "fragility" and "weakness" that necessitates near inactivity has long been discarded. This is largely due to the increasing body of scientific information regarding the safety and numerous benefits of maternal exercise, as well as anecdotal reports by thousands of active women.

Armed with the knowledge regarding the efficacy and safety of prenatal exercise, group fitness instructors have a unique opportunity to help pregnant women acquire an exercise "habit," and to realize the benefits this provides. However, ACOG has established that there are some women for whom exercise during pregnancy is absolutely contraindicated, and others for whom the potential benefits associated with exercising may outweigh the risks (American College of Obstetricians and Gynecologists, 2002). It is outside the scope of practice of a group fitness instructor to attempt to diagnose any of these contraindications (see Tables 10.1 and 10.2). It is, therefore, essential that all pregnant or postpartum women obtain a physician's clearance before beginning an exercise program.

For more detailed information on exercise and pregnancy, refer to *Pre- and Post-Natal Fitness: A Guide for Fitness Professionals* from the American Council on Exercise, available at www.acefitness.org.

References

American College of Obstetricians and Gynecologists (2002). *ACOG Committee Opinion #267: Exercise During Pregnancy and the Postpartum Period.* Washington, D.C.: American College of Obstetricians and Gynecologists.

American College of Obstetricians and Gynecologists (1994). *ACOG Technical Bulletin #194,* Washington, D.C.: American College of Obstetricians and Gynecologists.

American College of Sports Medicine (2006). *ACSM's Guidelines for Exercise Testing and Prescription,* 7th ed. Philadelphia: Lippincott, Williams & Wilkins.

American College of Sports Medicine (2000). *Current Comment: Exercise During Pregnancy.* Indianapolis: American College of Sports Medicine.

Artal, R. (1992). Exercise and pregnancy. *Clinics in Sports Medicine,* 11, 2.

Artal, R. et al. (1990). Orthopedic problems in pregnancy. *The Physician and Sportsmedicine,* 18, 9.

Boissonnault, J.S. & Blaschak, M.J. (1988). Incidence of diastasis recti abdominis during the childbearing year. *Physical Therapy,* 68, 7.

Bungum, T.J. et al. (2000). Exercise during pregnancy and type of delivery in nulliparae. *Journal of Obstetrics, Gynecology and Neonatal Nursing,* 29, 3, 258–264.

Clapp, J.F., III. (1998). *Exercising Through Your Pregnancy.* Champaign, Ill.: Human Kinetics.

Clapp, J.F., III. (1991). The changing thermal response to endurance exercise during pregnancy. *American Journal of Obstetrics & Gynecology,* 178, 3, 594–599.

Clapp, J.F., III et al. (1992). Exercise in pregnancy. (S294-S300). *Medicine & Science in Sports & Exercise,* 24, 6.

Clapp, J.F., III & Capeless, E.L. (1990). Neonatal morphometrics after endurance exercise during pregnancy. *American Journal of Obstetrics & Gynecology,* 163 (6): 1805–1811.

Clapp, J.F., III & Little, K.D. (1995). Effect of recreational exercise on pregnancy weight gain and subcutaneous fat deposition. *Medicine & Science in Sport & Exercise,* 27, 2, 170–177.

Clapp, J.F., III, Lopez, B., & Harcar-Sevcik, R. (1999). Neonatal behavioral profile of the offspring of women who continued to exercise regularly throughout pregnancy. *American Journal of Obstetrics & Gynecology,* 180, 91–94.

Clapp, J.F., III, & Rizk, K.H. (1992). Effect of recreational exercise on midtrimester placental growth. *American Journal of Obstetrics & Gynecology,* 167, 1518–1521.

Clark, N. (1992). Shower your baby with good nutrition. *The Physician & Sportsmedicine,* 20, 5.

Daly, J.M. et al. (1991). Sacroiliac subluxation: A common, treatable cause of low-back pain in pregnancy. *Family Practice Research Journal,* 11, 2.

Devine, C.M., Bov, C.F., & Olson, C.M. (2000). Continuity and change in women's weight orientations and lifestyle through pregnancy and the postpartum period: The influence of life trajectories and transitional events. *Social Science and Medicine,* 50, 4, 567–582.

Dewey, K.G. (1998). Effects of maternal caloric restriction and exercise during lactation. *Journal of Nutrition,* 128, 2 Suppl, 3865–3895.

Dunbar, A. (1992). Why Jane stopped running. *The Journal of Obstetric and Gynecologic Physical Therapy,* 16, 3.

Goodwin, A., Astbury, J., & McKeeken, J. (2000). Body image and psychological well being in pregnancy: A comparison of exercisers and non-exercisers. *Australia and New Zealand Journal of Obstetrics and Gynecology,* 40, 4, 442–447.

Hall, C. & Brody, L. (1999). *Therapeutic Exercise: Moving Toward Function.* Philadelphia: Lippincott, Williams & Wilkins.

Hummel-Berry, K. (1990). Obstetric low back pain: Part I and Part II. *The Journal of Obstetric & Gynecologic Physical Therapy,* 14, 1, 10–13 & 14, 2, 9–11.

Jacobson, H. (1991). Protecting the back during pregnancy. *American Association of Occupational Health Nurses Journal,* 39, 6.

Karsenec, J. & Grimes, D. (1984). *Hydrorobics.* Leisure Press.

Karzel, R.P. & Friedman, M.C. (1991). Orthopedic injuries in pregnancy. In *Exercise in Pregnancy,* Artal, R., Wiswell, R.A., & Drinkwater, B.L. (Eds.). Baltimore: Williams & Wilkins.

Lile, A. & Hagar, T. (1991). Survey of current physical therapy treatment for the pregnant client with lumbopelvic dysfunction. *Journal of Obstetric and Gynecologic Physical Therapy,* 15, 4.

McMurray, R.G. & Katz, V.L. (1990). Thermoregulation in pregnancy, implications for exercise. *Sports Medicine,* 10, 3.

Noble, E. (1995). *Essential Exercises for the Childbearing Year,* 4th ed. Boston: Houghton Mifflin Company.

Pivarnik, J.M. et al. (1991). Physiological and perceptual responses to cycle and treadmill exercise during pregnancy. *Medicine & Science in Sports & Exercise,* 23, 4.

Sampselle, C.M. & Seng, J. (1999). Physical activity and postpartum well-being. *Journal of Obstetrics, Gynecology, and Neonatal Nursing,* 28, 1, 41–49.

Exercise and Pregnancy

Schauberger, C.W. et al. (1996). Peripheral joint laxity increases in pregnancy but does not correlate with serum relaxin levels. *American Journal of Obstetrics & Gynecology, 174,* 667–671.

Sinclair, M. (1992). In training for motherhood? Effects of exercise for pregnant women. *Professional Nurse.* May.

Sternfeld, B. (1997). Physical activity and pregnancy outcome: Review and recommendations. *Sports Medicine, 23,* 33–47.

Sternfeld, B., Sidney, S., & Eskenazi, B. (1992). Patterns of exercise during pregnancy and effects on pregnancy outcome. *Medicine & Science in Sports & Exercise, 24,* S170.

Uzendoski, A.M. et al. (1989). Short review: Maternal and fetal responses to prenatal exercise. *Journal of Applied Sport Science Research, 3,* 4.

Wallace, J.P. (1993). Breast milk and exercise studies, *ACE Insider, 3,* 6–8.

Wallace, J.P., Inbar, G., & Ernsthausen, K. (1992). Infant acceptance of post-exercise breast milk. *Pediatrics, 89,* 1245–1247.

Wallace J.P., Inbar, G., & Ernsthausen, K. (1994). Lactate concentrations in breast milk following maximal exercise and a typical workout. *Journal of Women's Health, 3,* 91–96.

Watson, W.J. et al. (1991). Fetal responses to maximal swimming and cycling exercise during pregnancy. *Obstetrics & Gynecology, 77,* 3.

Wilder, E. (1988). *Obstetric and Gynecologic Physical Therapy.* Edinburgh: Churchill Livingstone.

Wolfe, L.A., Brenner, I., & Mottola, M. (1994). Maternal exercise, fetal well-being, and pregnancy outcome in exercise and sports science reviews. *American College of Sports Medicine, 22,* 145–194.

Wolfe, L.A. et al. (1989). Physiological interactions between pregnancy and aerobic exercise. *Medicine & Science in Sports & Exercise.* Supplement.

Work, J.A. (1989). Is weight training safe during pregnancy? *The Physician & Sportsmedicine, 17,* 3.

Yeo, S. et al. (2000). Effect of exercise on blood pressure in pregnant women with a history of gestational hypertensive disorders. *Journal of Reproductive Medicine, 45,* 4, 293–298.

Zhang, J., & Savitz, DA. (1996). Exercise during pregnancy among US women. *Annals of Epidemiology, 6,* 1, 53–59.

Suggested Reading

Anthony, L. (2006). *Pre- and Post-natal Fitness.* Monterey Calif.: Healthy Learning.

Artal, R. et al. (1991). *Exercise in Pregnancy.* Baltimore: Williams and Wilkins.

Bursch, G.S. (1987). Interrater reliability of diastasis recti abdominis measurement. *Polyform Products Inc., 67,* 7.

Clapp, J.F. et al. (1998). The one-year morphometric and neurodevelopment outcome of the offspring of women who continued to exercise regularly throughout pregnancy. *American Journal of Obstetrics and Gynecology, 178,* 3, 594–599.

Huch, R. & Erkkola, R. (1990). Pregnancy and exercise—exercise and pregnancy. A short review. *British Journal of Obstetrics and Gynecology, 97.*

Jones, R. et al. (1985). Thermoregulation during aerobic exercise in pregnancy. *Obstetrics & Gynecology, 65,* 340.

McMurray, R.G. et al. (1991). The thermoregulation of pregnant women during aerobic exercise in the water: A longitudinal approach. *European Journal of Applied Physiology, 61.*

Prentice, A. (1994) Should lactating women exercise? *Nutrition Reviews. 52,* 10, 358–360.

Schelkun, P.H. (1991). Exercise and breast-feeding mothers. *The Physician & Sportsmedicine, 19,* 4.

References and Suggested Reading

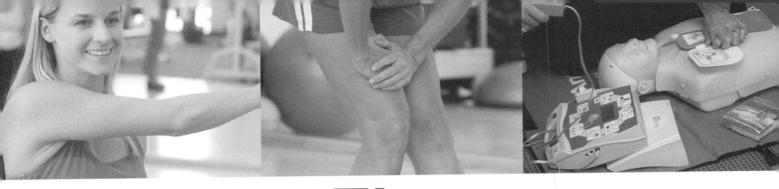

Chapter Eleven

Christine "CC" Cunningham, M.S., A.T.C., L.A.T., C.S.C.S., is a NATABOC-certified athletic trainer and a personal trainer. She is a private consultant specializing in fitness-program development and education. Cunningham is a frequent writer and industry lecturer on the issues of exercise and injury. She is a NIKE athlete and the education manager for Life Fitness.

IN THIS CHAPTER:

Injury Prevention and Emergency Procedures

By Christine "CC" Cunningham

Musculoskeletal injuries present complicated challenges for group fitness instructors. They are experienced by participants as well as instructors and can interfere with an individual's ability to participate. It is a difficult task to create an environment in which participants can achieve their varied fitness goals, while also addressing all of the individual needs to ensure everyone's safety. Doing so requires knowledge of the factors associated with injuries, methods for prevention, and appropriate modifications for specific injuries. This chapter addresses all of these areas and provides guidelines for developing a facility emergency policy.

Injury Prevention and Emergency Procedures

The injury-related responsibilities of group fitness instructors are to (1) prevent injury by careful preparation and carrying-out of every exercise session, (2) provide modifications for participants with injury limitations, and (3) properly handle injuries that may occur during a class (refer to Emergency Procedures, later in this chapter). Execution of these responsibilities is challenging because participants attending a group exercise class have a wide variety of exercise goals, backgrounds, and physical strengths or limitations. It is the job of a group fitness instructor to encourage participants to work within their own individual limits and to inform them that they ultimately have control over their workout intensity. The instructor is there for the participants' workout, not his or her own, and should appropriately set the intensity of the class by example. It is important to remember that the risk of a musculoskeletal injury occurring or being aggravated is always present. Therefore, a primary objective for a group fitness instructor is to provide a safe environment for all participants. Finally, it is beyond the scope of a group fitness instructor to diagnose an injury or prescribe rehabilitative exercise.

New class formats are constantly being introduced into group exercise schedules. They range from yoga and martial arts to group strength training and indoor cycling. Classes are even leaving the aerobics studio and moving outdoors. Equipmen ranges from traditional steps to microhurdles and treadmills. Unfortunately, there are many new risks and potential injuries emerging with each new format. Group fitness instructors must be able to manage the risks and provide modifications for participants with injury limitations. Success is dependent on understanding musculoskele-

tal injuries, their causes, and **contraindications** for participation.

Symptoms and Types of Musculoskeletal Injuries

Symptoms of Injury

Musculoskeletal injuries have several symptoms that define and determine their severity. These characteristics are:

- Pain
- Swelling and discoloration
- Loss of range of motion
- Loss of strength
- Loss of **functional capacity** or use

These symptoms indicate the presence of an injury that should be investigated and treated. Participants should always be instructed to consult their healthcare provider if symptoms are present. At no time should an instructor attempt to diagnose or treat the injury or symptoms. Instead, focus on providing the appropriate modifications for the participant so he or she can continue to participate safely.

Types of Injuries

There are two main classifications of injuries: acute and chronic. In most situations, acute refers to a rapidly occurring, new injury such as an ankle **sprain,** muscle **strain,** or broken bone. Acute injuries can be linked to a specific event that caused the injury and the symptoms are sharply defined. It is helpful to note that the term acute is also used to describe a phase of injury healing. The acute phase is when symptoms are severe, tissue damage is new, and healing has just begun.

In contrast, chronic, or overuse, injuries are usually of gradual onset, occurring as a result of repeated stress over time without allowing adequate recovery time. Exercise starts a normal cycle of tissue stress and repair. In most situations, this cycle occurs within a day or two, but its length depends on the amount of damage caused by the stress. More stress or more intense activity causes more damage. The healing process is essential for the tissue to accommodate the stress and be able to tolerate it the next time it is introduced. Healing requires recovery time. Inadequate amounts of recovery between exercise sessions can cause the tissue damage from the stress to accumulate and result in tissue breakdown. A lack of appropriate recovery time is the main cause of overuse injuries. The symptoms of a chronic injury may be less distinct, and direct diagnosis may be more difficult. Examples of chronic injuries are lateral epicondylitis, **plantar fasciitis,** and **stress fractures.** Chronic injuries may linger for months and vary in their severity. It should be noted that an **acute injury** may evolve into a chronic condition if the mechanism for injury is repeated or the injury is not properly healed. It is not uncommon for group exercise participants and instructors to continue to exercise "through" injuries, causing more damage and prolonging the healing process. This is not recommended. Proper care, treatment, and rehabilitation are essential for a successful recovery from a musculoskeletal injury.

Factors Associated With Injury

There are many factors that can lead to an injury, including flooring, footwear, equipment, movement execution, and class intensity. Other factors such as teaching technique, warm-up, and cool-down are discussed in other chapters. Be aware of all of these factors and assess each new class format for additional factors that may lead to participant or instructor injury.

Flooring/Exercise Surface

Flooring needs to absorb shock to reduce the negative effects on the bones and joints.

Repeated jarring can result in stress fractures and **tendinitis.** Hardwood flooring should be suspended to provide additional shock absorption and reduce injury risk. In addition, hardwood flooring offers good traction for dynamic movements and allows for lateral movement and pivoting. Concrete is not recommended as a surface for group exercise. It absorbs little shock and can be quite dangerous in the event of a fall. Carpeting reduces the stress on the bones and joints, but can catch the edge of shoes during dynamic lateral movements or pivoting, resulting in ankle sprains or knee injuries. Carpeting is appropriate for floorwork-based classes such as yoga or stretching.

Outdoor classes take exercise onto grass, sand, and hiking trails. Each surface offers concerns for participant safety. In general, natural surfaces offer good shock absorption, but may vary in terrain predictability and traction. Be aware of potential risks and choose the appropriate surface for the class format.

Footwear

Proper footwear will provide good cushioning, support, and flexibility. Many group exercise formats, including step training, kickboxing, and sport-conditioning classes, require that the ball of the foot absorb repetitive impact during the landing and pushing-off of dynamic movements. Footwear must provide cushion under the forefoot in addition to heel cushioning to reduce the possibility of injury to the foot from the repeated impact. Lateral movement demands support on the lateral aspect of the shoe to keep the foot from rolling over the base of support and causing an ankle sprain. Running shoes are designed for forward-movement efficiency and are not appropriate for classes with lateral or pivoting movements or repeated impact on the forefoot. Various sole designs allow for good forefoot

Injury Prevention and Emergency Procedures

flexibility without sacrificing traction. They provide freedom of movement without slipping during cutting, stopping, or rapid changes of direction. Forefoot flexibility is also necessary for many flexibility-based classes in which full range of motion is desired.

Surface, equipment, intensity, and quality of movement determine the requirements of appropriate footwear. Be sure to evaluate the class content and adhere to any footwear guidelines indicated for different formats.

Equipment

Improper equipment set-up, fit, or use can cause injury. Class formats have adopted the use of a wide variety of equipment, from steps and tubing to bikes, hurdles, and treadmills. Each piece of equipment has specific set-up and fit requirements. Adhere to these requirements at all times to minimize the risk of injury. Check equipment regularly for wear and tear and replace items when necessary. If equipment is manufactured in various sizes, have all sizes available to accommodate all participants.

Misuse of equipment can also cause injury. Use caution when incorporating new equipment and/or movements into a group situation for the first time. Be sure to learn the intended use, limitations, and safety precautions for all equipment. Apply these to the development of the class format and specific movements. Instructor creativity without adequate consideration for safety may lead to unintentionally dangerous situations for participants.

Movement Execution

Improper execution creates the greatest risk for injury in a group exercise class. Large instructor-to-student ratios make individual attention difficult and students can often repeat movements incorrectly numerous times without correction, leading to injury. The best defense against movement error is to use teaching progressions, provide modifications, and explain methods for self-evaluation.

Progressions should gradually build complicated movements in a step-by-step fashion. Along the way, participants should be instructed on modifications for range of motion, strength, and impact. Include methods for participants to use to determine if they are ready to safely go on with the next step.

When incorporating movements from other disciplines, such as elite sport training or the martial arts, be sure to learn what progressions and evaluations are used in the traditional settings to safely teach the movements. Incorporate these techniques into the class format to reduce the risk of poor execution and the resulting injury.

Class Intensity and Frequency of Participation

Class intensity needs vary from participant to participant. Training effects are achieved at individually relative exercise intensities, not absolute exercise intensities. In other words, maximum intensity for each participant occurs at a different rate of work, so one intensity may be too easy for one participant and too hard for another. Intensity applies to heart rate, loading, speed of movement, and impact. A common teaching error is to assume that the intensity needed for a good workout for the instructor is the same intensity needed for all participants. A fit and experienced instructor may direct the class at exercise intensities that are too high for the less fit or inexperienced participants. This practice can result in participant fatigue and overexertion, increasing the risk of injury. Avoid this problem by assessing the participants prior to each class. Remember, gear the intensity of the class to the participants.

Frequency of participation is a factor because individuals sometimes attend class too often without allowing for adequate recovery in between sessions. Inform participants of the appropriate frequency of participation before each class session. Promote cross-training by suggesting alternative classes that use different muscle groups or are nonimpact for days when participants should be recovering.

Overtraining is also a concern. Group fitness instructors are especially at risk for overtraining. Teaching numerous classes a day without enough recovery can lead to sleep loss, elevations in resting heart rate, and injury. Apply the alternative class approach to teaching as well.

Pre-class Evaluation

The group exercise environment makes individual participant evaluation difficult. Because instructors usually do not know who will attend class on any given day, using a health and exercise history to screen participants is not always realistic. With experience, an instructor can become very proficient at using on-the-spot indicators to assess the class prior to each session. Whenever possible, however, utilize a preparticipation screening to assess individual needs and limitations.

There are three on-the-spot indicators that can be used to gauge potential participants' limitations and alert the instructor to the type of exercise modifications he or she may need to provide during the class. These indicators are:

1. *Age*—Participants may have age-associated limitations that require the group fitness instructor to offer appropriate modification of the class content. Be sure to monitor these participants and evaluate if they are in need of modifications throughout the class.

2. *Posture*—Poor posture is associated with some muscles being short and tight and others being long and weak. This results in range of motion being limited by the short muscles and strength or endurance being affected by the weak muscles. This imbalance makes proper movement execution increasingly difficult and increases the importance of providing modifications.

3. *New participation*—New participants always make teaching more difficult. The more frequently an individual attends class, the less instruction he or she needs to change moves and perform them safely. New students require increased attention and should be watched during the class.

If possible, use the warm-up to incorporate movements that could indicate which participants need modifications or increased attention. Watch for range-of-motion or strength limitations and coordination or balance problems. As the class progresses, incorporate modifications for these individuals to ensure safety and participation success.

General Musculoskeletal Injuries

The following descriptions explain a few general types of musculoskeletal injuries. These injuries can occur at numerous sites in the body. More specific injuries are discussed later in the chapter. As a group fitness instructor, it is important to be familiar with these injuries and know enough about them to prevent their onset and provide appropriate modifications during an exercise session. The suggestions given in this chapter should only be used as guidelines for exercise modification. Diagnosis and treatment of musculoskeletal injuries is the domain of the healthcare professional. Refer all participants with complaints of injury symptoms to their healthcare providers.

Sprain

A sprain refers to an acute injury to a **ligament** caused by sudden trauma to the joint. Sprains can occur at any joint but are most common at the ankle and knee. Damage can vary from stretched ligaments to complete tears. Sprains are rated in degrees: 1st degree (mild), 2nd degree (moderate), and 3rd degree (severe). Symptoms of sprains include pain, localized swelling, discoloration, loss of motion, loss of use, and joint instability. A medical evaluation is recommended for sprains to rule out tears or associated **fractures.**

Treatment for sprains by a healthcare professional ranges from conservative, using ice and rest, to surgery. Ligaments can heal, but the healing is dependent on the degree of injury and the blood supply to the damaged ligaments. It is these factors that determine the chosen course of treatment.

Considerations for Group Exercise
- Choose exercise that does not involve the injured joint until the symptoms of sprain are minimal or no longer present.
- Gradually reintroduce activity involving the joint, since exercise introduced too early or too aggressively can increase the amount of damage.
- Avoid movement in the end ranges of motion. The instability of the joint caused by the damage to the ligament makes it more susceptible to further and recurrent injury.
- Monitor the participant for an increase or return of symptoms resulting from the activity.

Strain

A strain, often called a muscle "pull," is an injury to a muscle, usually caused by overexertion. Strains can be acute, occurring suddenly during activity, or can gradually develop from repeated overuse. Symptoms of a muscle strain are pain, loss of motion, and reduced strength. Swelling and discoloration are often difficult to see, depending on the location of the injury or how deep within the muscle the injury occurred. Bruising may be found below the actual injury site, where fluids can pool close to the surface of the skin. A healthcare professional may treat a muscle strain using ice, gentle stretching, and exercise. Gentle muscle activity promotes healing by assisting with circulation and reducing deep swelling.

Considerations for Group Exercise
- Avoid introducing strenuous or ballistic exercise after a participant experiences a muscle strain until the symptoms are minimal or no longer present.
- Gradually increase the intensity of activity.
- Incorporate additional gentle stretching of the muscle before and after exercise.
- Confine movement to the pain-free range of motion.
- Monitor the participant for an increase or return of symptoms resulting from the activity.

Tendinitis

The term tendinitis refers to the inflammation of the **tendon** or muscle–tendon junction. Tendinitis is a classic overuse injury caused by repeated stress without adequate recovery time. Symptoms of tendinitis include pain, swelling, and loss of function. There are many common locations of tendinitis, such as the patellar tendon (jumper's knee), the Achilles tendon, and the lateral epicondyle (tennis elbow). High-repetition lifting or jumping, poor lifting technique, and repeated movement throughout the same range of motion can cause this condition.

Tendinitis is very difficult to treat because the symptoms often return when activity is reintroduced. A healthcare professional may use ice, stretching, and very slow, progressive loading of the tendon to allow the tissue to heal and become able to accommodate increasing stress levels. If not treated, tendinitis can lead to failure of the tendon and rupture. Surgical intervention for tendinitis is rare. Anti-inflammatory medication and injections are used most commonly. Due to the complexity of the condition, treatment for tendinitis is best directed by a healthcare professional.

Considerations for Group Exercise

- Avoid high-repetition activity or heavy loading of the tendon.
- Assess the appropriateness of jumping, especially box jumps and other **plyometric**-type techniques with high loads.
- Use caution when incorporating ballistic movements, such as kicking and punching, that place high eccentric loads on the muscles and place the tendons at risk.
- Check equipment for proper fit. Repetitive movements, like cycling, can cause tendinitis if the equipment fit is wrong.
- Allow adequate recovery between sessions.
- Avoid very high repetitions in strength training and always focus on proper technique.
- Monitor the participant for an increase or return of symptoms resulting from the activity.

Specific Musculoskeletal Injuries

The following descriptions cover some of the most frequently seen musculoskeletal injures. There are many other injuries you will encounter as a group fitness instructor. Use these guidelines to understand prevention and modifications for activity. Do not attempt to diagnose an injury based on the symptoms given. Many injuries have similar symptoms but very different treatments and modifications for exercise. Always refer participants to their healthcare provider. In the event that the guidelines provided here are different than those provided by a physician or therapist, follow the guidelines provided by the healthcare professional. The description of each specific musculoskeletal injury presents the anatomy involved, the common treatment used by healthcare professionals during rehabilitation, and the **prognosis** for recovery. Considerations for the group fitness instructor include suggestions for modifying class content for participants who have had previous injuries and methods for preventing injury when designing a class session. It is beyond the scope of the group fitness instructor to diagnose an injury or prescribe rehabilitative exercise.

Lateral Ankle Sprain

A lateral ankle sprain occurs when the foot is inverted forcefully during weightbearing activity (Figure 11.1). Damage to the anterior talofibular ligament is most common; however, the calcaneofibular ligament can

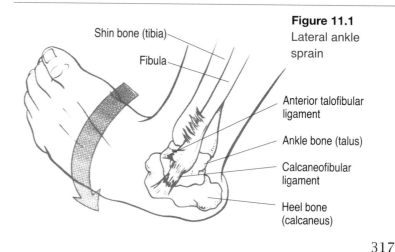

Figure 11.1
Lateral ankle sprain

Shin bone (tibia)

Fibula

Anterior talofibular ligament

Ankle bone (talus)

Calcaneofibular ligament

Heel bone (calcaneus)

317

also be involved. Sprains range in severity from slight tears or stretching of the ligament to complete ruptures of one or more of the lateral ligaments (Malone & Hardaker, 1990). Lateral ankle sprains are commonly treated with **RICE** (rest, ice, compression, and elevation) and progressive exercise to regain normal function. Surgical intervention is less common but may be used to correct chronic instability. The prognosis for a lateral ankle sprain is very positive and most individuals recover full range of motion, strength, and function to preinjury levels.

Considerations for Group Exercise

- Limit motion to a pain-free range and intensity.
- Remind participants to resume activity only when released by a physician or when all symptoms of the injury are gone.
- Avoid incorporating cutting, jumping, and lateral movements until full strength and **proprioception** of the ankle have returned.
- Encourage workouts that are predominantly nonimpact to minimize ankle discomfort until the ankle has fully healed.
- Load **closed-chain** strengthening of the lower extremity, such as squats and lunges, according to the tolerance of the ankle joint.
- Double-check that participants are wearing footwear appropriate for the class. Ankle sprains frequently occur when participants wear running shoes in classes that involve dynamic lateral movement.
- Use lateral movement cautiously on carpet or uneven surfaces.
- Monitor the participant for an increase or return of symptoms resulting from the activity.

Plantar Fasciitis

Plantar fasciitis is microtearing of the fascia at or near its attachment to the calcaneus bone (heel) and is thought to be caused by repetitive overloading of the tissue at its calcaneal attachment (Kibler, Goldberg, & Chandler, 1991). Common treatment for plantar fasciitis is rest, ice massage, stretching, modifications in training intensity, and strengthening of the muscles of the foot and ankle. Orthotics to correct abnormal foot mechanics and surgery are used in some cases of plantar fasciitis. Evaluation of exercise footwear to ensure proper fit and support is also recommended. Full return to preinjury range of motion, strength, and function, including athletic participation, is expected in most cases of plantar fasciitis. However, the condition may recur in some individuals.

Considerations for Group Exercise

- Encourage an extended warm-up prior to class.
- Incorporate additional stretching of the gastrocnemius, soleus, and plantar fascia.
- Avoid sudden increases in training intensity or frequency.
- Do not introduce plyometric exercises such as jumping or high-force loading of the foot until full strength and range of motion have returned.
- Monitor the progression in the increase of the impact of the given activity.
- Suggest strengthening the muscles of the lower leg and foot to reduce the chance of recurrence of plantar fasciitis.
- Double-check that participants are wearing footwear appropriate for the class.
- Watch for an increase or return of symptoms resulting from the activity.

Rotator Cuff Strain

A rotator cuff strain is the overstretching, overexertion, or overuse of the musculotendinous unit of one or more of the rotator cuff muscles (Kisner & Colby, 1990). Symptoms of a rotator cuff strain include pain, loss of motion, loss of strength, and loss of function. Rotator cuff strains can be acute or chronic. Rest, stretching, and gradually progressive strengthening exercises are used to return the shoulder to preinjury function. The prognosis for return to full range of motion, full strength, and full functional capacity is good following a rotator cuff strain.

Considerations for Group Exercise

- To aid shoulder stabilization, avoid loading of the shoulder joint in excess of the tolerance of the rotator cuff. Overloading might occur in the dumbbell press or pec flyes, where the rotator cuff is too weak to stabilize the shoulder against the load needed to effectively stimulate the chest muscles.
- Watch for complaints of pain and altered mechanics that indicate that the load is too much for the shoulder.
- Do not fatigue the rotator cuff muscles with isolated exercise prior to executing movements that require their activity for stabilization. These movements include punches, medicine ball throws, some stretching positions, and strength exercises. Doing so is likely to exacerbate the rotator cuff strain and prolong healing.
- Monitor the participant for an increase or return of symptoms resulting from the activity.

Rotator Cuff Impingement

Rotator cuff impingement is a common overuse syndrome of the shoulder in athletes who participate in overhead sports (swimming, baseball, volleyball) or individuals who perform repetitive overhead work (carpenters, painters). It is characterized as a pinching of the rotator cuff tendon under the coracoacromial arch when the arm is abducted (Roy & Irvin, 1983) (Figure 11.2). Rotator cuff impingement is treated conservatively with rest, stretching, and gradual strengthening exercises. Other treatments for impingement include various surgical techniques and anti-inflammatory injections. Each treatment is different in its approach to relieving the disorder and in the exercise guidelines. Impingement syndrome treated early, before anatomical damage has occurred, will likely return to full functional capacity, including participation in athletic competition (Jobe & Pink, 1993).

Considerations for Group Exercise

- Encourage additional stretching of the posterior cuff.

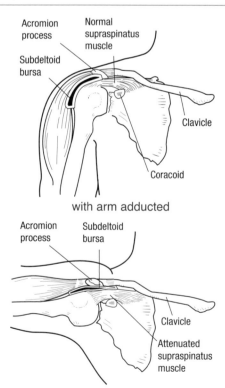

Figure 11.2
Impingement of bursa and supraspinatus under the coracoacromial arch with abduction movement

with arm adducted

with arm abducted

- Discourage stretching of the anterior shoulder.
- Avoid active abduction and overhead arm movements unless pain-free.
- Minimize the repetition of abduction or overhead motion, including lifts and arm swings.
- Do not have participants perform military presses, triceps pull-overs, lat pull-downs behind the neck, and pull-ups behind the neck, as they are likely to exacerbate shoulder impingement (Litchfield et al., 1993).
- Monitor the participant for an increase or return of symptoms resulting from the activity.

Anterior Shoulder Instability

Anterior shoulder instability is a weakness in the anterior wall musculature (subscapularis, pectoralis major, latissimus dorsi, and teres major) and/or stretching of the anterior capsule and ligaments that allows the humeral head to sublux or dislocate anteriorly (Jobe & Pink, 1993). This condition can be caused acutely from a fall or blow to the shoulder. Chronic instability is a gradual onset of muscle weakness and progressive damage of the anterior structures.

Anterior shoulder instability is treated conservatively with rest, stretching, and gradual strengthening of weak muscles. Significant anatomical damage to the anterior structures is repaired surgically. If conservative treatment is appropriate and started early, there is a high rate of return to full activity. Postsurgical prognosis is dependent upon the surgical procedure used and the adherence to rehabilitation guidelines (Jobe & Pink, 1993). Different surgical procedures result in varying losses in range of motion and function and, therefore, an exercise that is allowed after one type of repair may not be allowed after another. Always follow the guidelines for exercise provided by the healthcare provider.

Considerations for Group Exercise

- Limit motion to avoid humeral abduction with external rotation or horizontal extension. An unstable shoulder can dislocate or sublux if put in these positions.
- Be very cautious during all movements that place the shoulder in an externally rotated position, even with stretching.
- Avoid pec flyes, lat pull-downs behind the neck, and full-range or wide-grip chest presses because of the stress they place on the anterior shoulder (Litchfield et al., 1993).
- Encourage stretching of the posterior cuff.
- Discourage stretching of the anterior shoulder.
- Monitor the participant for an increase or return of symptoms resulting from the activity.

Lateral Epicondylitis (Tennis Elbow) and Medial Epicondylitis (Golfer's Elbow)

Lateral epicondylitis, **tennis elbow,** is an overuse injury affecting the musculotendonus junction of the wrist extensor muscles at the lateral epicondyle of the humerus (Figure 11.3). Repetitive activities involving the wrist, such as playing tennis, carpentry, or pruning shrubs, result in microdamage to the tissue. Medial epicondylitis, golfer's elbow, is an overuse injury affecting the musculotendonus junction of the wrist flexor muscle at the medial epicondyle of the humerus. Repetitive activities involving the wrist, such as throwing, striking a golf ball, or carrying a heavy suitcase, result in microdamage to the tissue. These elbow injuries

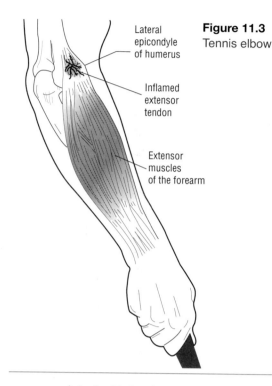

Figure 11.3
Tennis elbow

Lateral epicondyle of humerus

Inflamed extensor tendon

Extensor muscles of the forearm

are associated with inadequate strength, power, endurance, and flexibility in the wrist extensors or flexors. The onset for both conditions is usually gradual. Conservative treatment consists of rest, ice, gradual stretching, and strengthening of the wrist extensors or flexors. Cortisone injections and surgery are used when conservative management is not successful. Return to full activity is expected.

Considerations for Group Exercise

• Encourage stretching for all motions of the wrist, including flexion, extension, radial/ulnar deviation, and pronation/ supination.

• Perform wrist flexion and/or extension stretching before all activities that involve the wrist (e.g., punching, push-ups, jumping rope).

• Use lighter loads for the wrist during repetitive motion to avoid overloading the tissue and causing pain during or after the exercise.

• Do not include high repetitions of wrist exercises.

• Avoid having participants hold hand positions for a prolonged period of time during cycling. Encourage frequent changes of position to avoid irritation.

• Monitor the participant for an increase or return of symptoms from the activity.

Anterior Cruciate Ligament Tear and Reconstruction

The anterior cruciate ligament (ACL) lies within the joint capsule of the knee (Figure 11.4). It attaches superiorly on the femur and inferiorly on the tibia. The ACL is instrumental in preventing the tibia from shifting forward on the femur, especially during forceful quadriceps contraction. Injuries to the ACL are commonly caused by rapid deceleration, such as a basketball player stopping suddenly, or by a direct blow to the knee that causes the knee to hyperextend (Roy & Irvin, 1983).

Instability of the knee, or the tendency for the tibia to shift during quadriceps contraction or weightbearing, is a concern when the integrity of the ACL is disrupted. This shifting can cause additional damage to the structures

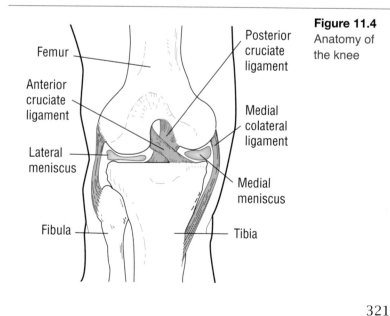

Figure 11.4
Anatomy of the knee

Femur

Anterior cruciate ligament

Lateral meniscus

Fibula

Posterior cruciate ligament

Medial colateral ligament

Medial meniscus

Tibia

of the knee, such as the meniscus. The amount of instability is related to the extent of the damage to the ACL. ACL injuries range from a partial tear to a complete rupture of the ligament. Partial tears are frequently treated with RICE and an extensive rehabilitation program to return the knee to full range of motion and strength. Throughout rehabilitation, and all activity thereafter, the ACL is protected to prevent additional damage to the ligament, which may result in increased instability. Reconstructive surgery is often encouraged after large tears and complete ruptures to restore the stability of the knee and avoid further damage.

The most common procedure for ACL reconstruction involves taking a portion of the patellar tendon out and using it as a graft to replace the torn ligament. The lengthy rehabilitation after an ACL reconstruction is a careful progression to return full range of motion, strength, proprioception, and function to the knee without damaging the graft. Range-of-motion limitations are used to avoid premature stress on the graft. A person's ability to contract the quadriceps reflects the state of tissue healing and the integrity of the

graft during each phase of rehabilitation (Wilk & Andrews, 1992). All exercise involving the knee should be directed by a physician or therapist to avoid complications. Successful ACL reconstruction and rehabilitation results in the return to full activity, including participation in athletic competition.

Considerations for Group Exercise

- Do not allow participation in group exercise until the participant is released by a physician or therapist.
- Adhere closely to all limitations in range of motion and loading provided by the physician or physical therapist.
- Avoid cutting, jumping, sprinting, kicking, and pivoting unless specifically approved by a physician or therapist.
- Watch for difficulty with balance and movement execution caused by the loss of strength and proprioception after the injury. Provide safe modifications for these activities.
- Encourage participation in cycling or aquatic exercise classes after an ACL injury if directed by a physician or therapist.
- Incorporate additional stretching of the lower-extremity muscles before and after class.
- Monitor the participant for an increase or return of symptoms resulting from the activity.

Patellofemoral Pain Disorders

The patellofemoral pain disorders (PFPD) may involve the patella, the femoral condyles, the quadriceps muscle, and/or patellar tendon (Figure 11.5). Together, these components are referred to as the extensor mechanism. Numerous conditions affect the extensor mechanism, including

Figure 11.5
Components typically involved in some knee injuries

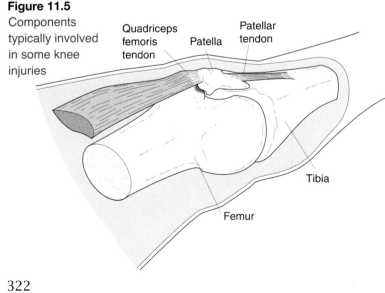

Quadriceps femoris tendon Patella Patellar tendon

Tibia

Femur

chondromalacia, patellar tendinitis, anterior knee pain, and patellofemoral malalignment (Shelton & Thigpen, 1991).

The majority of PFPD are considered overuse syndromes and, thus, are associated with overload or repetitive microtrauma to the knee. Training errors, improper footwear, anatomical abnormalities, and postsurgical complications all contribute to PFPD (Rintala, 1990). There are many similarities among the conditions, which allow the exercise guidelines to be generalized. It should be noted, however, that each specific condition requires modifications that should be determined by a healthcare professional to ensure appropriateness.

Conservative treatment of PFPD is highly effective and generally used prior to surgical treatment. If nonoperative treatment fails, surgical management may be used. Rest, ice, lower-extremity strengthening emphasizing the quadriceps, lower-extremity stretching, and gradual functional progressions are all used in conservative management of PFPD. Nonsteroidal anti-inflammatory medication and bracing or taping may also be included. Prognosis for recovery depends on the specific cause of PFPD.

Considerations for Group Exercise
- Avoid full squats or excessive knee flexion.
- Use strengthening within a mid-range of eight to 20 repetitions, since most PFPD disorders are sensitive to overuse.
- Encourage additional stretching of the lower extremity, as full range of motion is essential for extensor-mechanism function and the reduction of PFPD (Hertling & Kessler, 1996; Shelton & Thigpen, 1991; Woodall & Welsh, 1990).
- With indoor cycling, elevate the seat as high as possible without causing the pelvis

to rock. This reduces the amount of knee flexion at the top of the pedal stroke.
- Avoid repeated jumping or plyometrics.
- Monitor the participant for an increase or return of symptoms from the activity.

Shin Splints

Shin splints are also known as **tibial stress syndrome.** The exact pathology involved in shin splints is not known. It is theorized that shin splints are a microtearing of the attachment of the muscles of the lower leg on the tibia (Figure 11.6). Pain is the major symptom associated with shin splints. The anterior tibialis is frequently involved, but all of the muscles that attach below the knee on the anterior tibia may be affected. Shin splints are an overuse injury caused by repetitive loading of the lower leg with weak musculature. Runners frequently experience shin splints from the repetitive impact. An inability of the foot to absorb shock due to weak

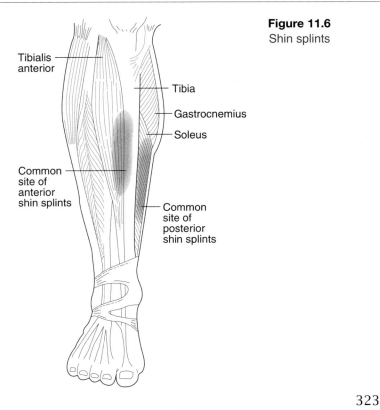

Figure 11.6
Shin splints

Tibialis anterior

Tibia

Gastrocnemius

Soleus

Common site of anterior shin splints

Common site of posterior shin splints

arches can contribute to the onset of the condition. Lack of flexibility of the posterior muscles can also overload the anterior musculature, causing the microtearing. Footwear and exercise surface are major factors in the onset of shin splints. Treatment for shin splints includes ice, rest, stretching, and strengthening of the muscles of the foot and lower leg. Footwear should be evaluated and orthotics may be prescribed. With treatment and rehabilitation, shin splints can be managed to allow full return to activity.

Considerations for Group Exercise

- Avoid repetitive impact on hard surfaces.
- Do not drastically change the amount of impact in a class format, as this can lead to shin splints.
- Use shock-absorbing surfaces for all class formats involving impact.
- Encourage additional stretching of the anterior and posterior muscles of the lower leg.
- Incorporate additional warm-up before class.
- Double-check that participants are wearing footwear with adequate support and cushioning in both the forefoot and heel.
- Watch indoor cyclists who do not regularly participate in weightbearing/impact class formats for signs of shin splints when taking a class with impact.
- Monitor participants for an increase or return of symptoms from the activity.

Low-back Pain

Low-back pain is one of the most difficult conditions to understand. Low-back pain itself is a symptom that can be caused by a number of underlying conditions, including genetic abnormalities, muscle strains, sprains, disc herniations, and bony abnormalities. In general, symptoms of low-back pain include loss of motion, loss of strength, and reduced function. Each condition has contraindications and modifications specific to the injury. It is far beyond the scope of the group fitness instructor to try to determine the cause of a participant's low-back pain. Refer all complaints of low-back pain to a healthcare provider. The following guidelines can be used to provide modifications for movement and create a safe environment for exercise.

- *Avoid motion that causes an increase in pain.* It is not always true that back extension is bad. In some cases, trunk extension is preferred over flexion. In other cases, this is reversed. For example, spinal stenosis, a narrowing of the spinal canal due to aging, is a contraindication for lumbar extension. It is therefore always a good rule to offer a modification for activity that requires the trunk to move into extremes of flexion or extension. This is necessary for loaded and unloaded (stretching) movements. Rotation of the lumbar spine may also be contraindicated, especially with herniated discs. Disc compression is greatest in the seated position, so seated rotation can be a risk. Modify the movement by using a standing or **supine** position.

- *Always engage the abdominal muscles for protection of the lumbar spine during motion.* The abdominal and back muscles work in concert to support and move the trunk without overloading the spine. Abdominal strength and endurance is essential and should be trained in the supine and standing positions. When standing, training involves the functional incorporation of abdominal contraction into movement, so the pelvis is stabilized throughout the movement. Always cue participants to remember to actively contract the abdominals for lumbar support. Modify movements that place high demand on abdominal support to accommodate participants who do not have the strength or coordination. Loaded squats, ballistic kicks, and end-range trunk motion are examples of high-demand activity. Failure to provide modifications can result in injury to the low back.

• *Emphasize the maintenance of good posture.* Poor posture can cause low-back strains and sprains, as well as potentially damage the discs and bony structures. Good postural alignment has the head aligned so that the ears are over the shoulders. The shoulders should be pulled back to align with the hips. The back is slightly curved forward at the lumbar region, with the top of the pelvis parallel to the ground. Excessive lumbar or thoracic curvature indicates poor posture and high risk of low-back problems. Cueing for posture is essential and participants with poor posture may require movement modifications to reduce the risk of injury. Avoid loading of the spine with increased curvatures (e.g., **lordosis** or **kyphosis**) or poor posture.

• *Encourage stretching of the trunk and lower extremities to maintain full range of motion.* Limited range of motion, especially in the hamstrings, has been associated with the onset of low-back pain. It is theorized that the hamstring tension reduces the ability of the pelvis to move properly, placing more mobility demands on the intervertebral joints. This can cause sprains and strains of the low back, especially with ballistic movements. Tight hip flexors can also alter pelvic mobility and cause lordosis (i.e., an increase in the lumbar curve). Flexibility is essential for proper execution of many group exercise movements. Participants without the necessary flexibility may stress their backs when trying to execute certain movements. Offer modifications for movements such as kicks, leg lifts, and advanced stretching.

Emergency Policy

Despite the most vigilant attention to careful preparation of class content and in-class modifications, emergency situations will arise. Being prepared to handle the emergency appropriately is one of the responsibilities of a group fitness instructor. Since emergencies do not occur frequently, the procedures for dealing with them can be unfamiliar or forgotten if they are not attended to on a regular basis. Unfortunately, in an emergency situation, lack of familiarity with the emergency plan can result in the loss of valuable time, and possibly a life. An instructor must review emergency policies and procedures frequently, rehearse the handling of different events, and always be prepared to act quickly to assist in any situation. Every club or exercise facility must have a written emergency plan with detailed procedures for contacting the local emergency services. If a group fitness instructor teaches at numerous locations, a copy of the existing plan for each site should be obtained and reviewed on a regular basis.

The Emergency Plan

The following information provides an outline of the necessary content for a group exercise emergency plan. Use these guidelines to develop or assess the plan at any facility at which you teach.

A group exercise emergency plan will include five main areas of information:
1. How to contact emergency services
2. Where to locate the closest AED (automated external defibrillator)
3. Necessary emergency medical supplies
4. Who to alert within the facility in the event of an emergency
5. Documentation of procedures

A written version of the plan is essential to ensure that all staff members are equally

Injury Prevention and Emergency Procedures

> Be ready for an emergency by making the following responsibilities as much a part of the job as teaching each class.
>
> - Review emergency policies and procedures frequently.
> - Rehearse dealing with different events.
> - Always be prepared to assist in any situation.

informed about the plan and to allow easy review and updating of the plan as necessary.

How to Contact Emergency Services

When an emergency occurs, stay with the victim to provide first aid and send another staff member or class participant to make the necessary phone call. The following details are needed for this to occur efficiently.

- *Phone numbers:* In most areas, the emergency services can easily be accessed through the use of 911. However, this is not always the case and the emergency number must be provided. If an additional digit is needed to reach an outside line, this must be stated in the plan. Post all emergency phone numbers on or near each phone in the facility.
- *Phone locations:* Indicate the phone location nearest the group exercise room. If the closest phone is a pay phone, and change is needed to access the emergency services, carry the necessary change at all times. If there is a locked door between the group exercise area and the phone, this door must be unlocked during classes or the instructor must be provided with a key.
- *Building access information:* Once the phone call is made, the emergency services will need to know the facility address and the exact location of the group exercise area within the facility. Include this

information in the written plan. Also, provide a written description of how to verbally direct the emergency personnel to the nearest accessible facility entrance.

Remember to let the emergency services individual end the phone call by allowing him or her to hang up first to ensure that all the information needed has been given.

Where to Locate the Nearest AED

An AED should be located in the facility near all workout areas. An instructor must be sure to know where the AED is located and be able to direct someone to the location for quick access. If possible, have two different people contact emergency services and retrieve the AED. Remember, for cardiac arrest, early use of an AED can save a life.

Emergency Medical Supplies

All facilities should have a first-aid kit and blood clean-up supplies available for possible group exercise emergencies. Their location and contents should be indicated in the emergency plan so that all staff members are aware of where to find needed supplies.

First-aid kit: A stocked first-aid kit should be kept near the group exercise area. The following supplies are recommended:
- Assorted bandage materials
- Sterile gauze pads
- Elastic wraps
- Liquid soap
- Topical antibiotic cream
- Triangular bandages
- Splinting material
- Blood pressure cuff and stethoscope
- Penlight
- Scissors
- Paper bag
- Chemical cold packs or small plastic bags if ice is available

Emergency
Policy

- Latex gloves (multiple sizes)
- Resuscitation masks

Blood clean-up supplies: For all incidents where blood or body fluids are involved, the following supplies must be provided. (For more information on dealing with blood, refer to OSHA's Blood-Borne Pathogen Rule.)

- Latex gloves (multiple sizes)
- Liquid soap
- Mixture of water and household bleach in accordance with the Centers for Disease Control and Prevention guidelines

Who to Alert Within the Facility

In the event of an emergency, contacting emergency services and providing the necessary first aid have priority over contacting additional staff and management. However, it is critical to make sure that the front desk and other area staff members (fitness floor, child care, etc.) are aware of the situation and can direct emergency services if they should happen to arrive in the wrong location. Staff members should also be prepared to address other members' questions about the situation. Facility management should also be notified. Additionally, in the event that assistance is needed in handling the emergency while awaiting emergency services, the method for reaching other staff members in the facility should be included in the emergency plan.

Documentation

The emergency plan should indicate which facility forms need to be completed following an emergency situation. Include the location of these forms in the emergency plan. Separate forms should be available for incidents involving class participants or other members and for incidents involving staff.

Emergency Procedure

In the event of an emergency, quick and efficient response by the instructor can be critical to minimizing the injury or preventing death. Every situation has to be handled differently, whether it is a sprained ankle or cardiac arrest. The details of how to cope with each situation are covered in first-aid and CPR/AED courses; hence, every instructor should be up to date with these certifications at all times. In general, however, the following procedure can be used to organize an efficient response.

1. EVALUATE
   - Evaluate the victim/situation by assessing consciousness, bleeding, and immediate danger.
   - Follow first-aid or CPR/AED procedures.
2. GET HELP*
   - Direct someone to alert the necessary emergency service and meet them at the facility entrance.
   - Provide this person with a condition description (**vital signs,** bleeding, obvious injury, etc.) and indicate if a medical alert tag is found on the victim. (Do not assume that the condition on the medical alert tag is the cause of the situation; allow a medical professional to make that determination.)
3. GET THE AED
   - If the situation appears to be cardiac arrest, send someone for the AED as quickly as possible while initiating CPR. Follow the instructions on the unit to apply and activate the AED.
4. ALERT THE FACILITY
   - Assign someone to control the crowd and alert the other facility locations of the situation.

---

*In the event that there is not someone available to contact the emergency services, follow the guidelines established by CPR or first aid for caring for the victim before leaving to phone for help.

5. CONTINUE VICTIM SUPPORT
   - Continue to provide necessary victim support until emergency personnel arrive.
6. CLEAN UP
   - Clean area appropriately. Restock the first-aid kit.
7. DOCUMENT
   - Complete the necessary documentation. Review the situation with management to determine what steps, if any, could be taken to reduce the chance of the emergency occurring again.

Summary

Group fitness instructors have several responsibilities regarding musculoskeletal injuries. They must (1) prevent injury by carefully preparing and executing every exercise session, (2) provide modifications for participants with injury limitations, and (3) properly handle injuries that may occur during a class. Success is dependent on knowing the factors associated with injuries, methods for prevention, and contraindications and appropriate modifications for specific injuries.

Symptoms of many musculoskeletal injuries include pain, swelling, loss of motion and strength, and reduced functional capacity. These symptoms are present in various degrees and combinations in most injuries. Acute injuries are the result of an immediate trauma. Chronic injuries are developed gradually from repeated stress over time. Both types of injuries can be caused by any number of factors, including footwear, flooring or exercise surface, equipment, movement execution, class intensity, and frequency of participation. Other factors such as teaching technique, warm-up, and cool-down are discussed in other chapters.

Three general descriptions of injuries encompass many of those seen in a group exercise setting: sprains, strains, and tendinitis. Sprains are acute injuries of the ligaments surrounding a joint. Strains involve the muscles and can be caused by exercise-intensity overloads. Tendinitis is an overuse injury frequently seen in participants and instructors who do not incorporate appropriate recovery into their exercise schedule.

Specific musculoskeletal injuries can be described based on the structures involved and their symptoms. Every injury has different recommendations for modifying movements or class formats to avoid exacerbating the condition. Diagnosis and treatment of musculoskeletal injuries is the responsibility of a physician or other healthcare professional and is not within the scope of practice for a group fitness instructor.

Continuously changing class formats introduces new potential for injuries in every class. Group fitness instructors cannot forget their responsibility for preventing injury through proper design and execution of the class. Providing modifications for all participants based on their needs is difficult but essential to ensure an outstanding group exercise experience for everyone.

Emergency situations can occur at any time and, therefore, a group fitness instructor has to be prepared to handle the situation appropriately. It is essential to have a written emergency plan that includes all necessary information for contacting local emergency services. Frequently review the plan for each facility and practice the procedures for coping with a variety of different emergencies. Prepare and manage each class to minimize the chance of an emergency and always be prepared to respond if one does occur.

References

Hertling, D. & Kessler, R.M. (1996). *Management of Common Musculoskeletal Disorders* (3rd ed.). Philadelphia: Lippincott Williams & Wilkins.

Jobe, F.W. & Pink, M. (1993). Classification and treatment of shoulder dysfunction in the overhead athlete. *Journal of Orthopaedic and Sports Physical Therapy,* 18, 2, 427–432.

Kibler, W.B., Goldberg, C., & Chandler, T.J. (1991). Functional biomechanical deficits in running athletes with plantar fasciitis. *American Journal of Sports Medicine,* 19, 1, 66–71.

Kisner, C. & Colby, L.A. (1990). *Therapeutic Exercise: Foundations and Techniques* (2nd ed.). Philadelphia: F.A. Davis.

Litchfield, R. et al. (1993). Rehabilitation for the overhead athlete. *Journal of Orthopedic and Sports Physical Therapy,* 18, 2, 433–441.

Malone, T.R. & Hardaker, W.T. (1990). Rehabilitation of foot and ankle injuries in ballet dancers. *Journal of Orthopaedic and Sports Physical Therapy,* 11, 8, 355–361.

Rintala, P. (1990). Patellofemoral pain syndrome and its treatment in runners. *Journal of Athletic Training,* 25, 2, 107–110.

Roy, S. & Irvin, R. (1983). *Sports Medicine: Prevention, Evaluation, Management, and Rehabilitation.* Englewood Cliffs, N.J.: Prentice-Hall.

Shelton, G.L. & Thigpen, L.K. (1991). Rehabilitation of patellofemoral dysfunction: A review of literature. *Journal of Orthopedic and Sports Physical Therapy,* 14, 6, 243–249.

Wilk, K.E. & Andrews, J.R. (1992). Current concepts in the rehabilitation of the athletic shoulder. *Journal of Orthopedic and Sports Physical Therapy,* 15, 6, 279–289.

Woodall, W. & Welsh, J. (1990). A biomechanical basis for rehabilitation programs involving the patellofemoral joint. *Journal of Orthopaedic and Sports Physical Therapy,* 11, 11, 535–542.

Suggested Reading

American College of Sports Medicine (2007). *ACSM's Health/Fitness Facility Standards and Guidelines* (3rd ed.). Champaign, Ill: Human Kinetics.

Alter, M.J. (2004). *Science of Flexibility* (3rd ed.). Champaign, Ill.: Human Kinetics.

Balady, G.J. et al. (1998). Recommendations for cardiovascular screening, staffing, and emergency policies at health/fitness facilities. *Circulation,* 97, 2283–2293.

Baumgartner, T.A., & Jackson A.S. (1999). *Measurement for Evaluation in Physical Education and Exercise Science* (6th ed.). Madison, Wisc.: WCG/McGraw-Hill.

Brukner, P. & Khan, K. (2003). *Clinical Sports Medicine* (2nd ed.). Sydney: McGraw-Hill.

Garrick, J.G. & Webb, D.R. (1999). *Sports Injuries: Diagnosis and Management* (2nd ed.). Philadelphia: W.B. Saunders Co.

McHugh, M.P. et al. (1998). Preoperative indicators of motion loss and weakness following anterior cruciate ligament reconstruction. *Journal of Orthopaedic and Sports Physical Therapy,* 27, 6, 407–411.

Oestmann, R.E. (2004). *Proven Therapeutic Exercise Techniques: Best Practices for Therapists and Trainers.* Springfield, Ill.: Charles Thomas.

Radcliffe, J.C. & Farentinos, T.C. (1999). *High Powered Plyometrics.* Champaign, Ill.: Human Kinetics.

Starkey, C. & Johnson, G. (Eds.) (2006). *Athletic Training and Sports Medicine* (4th ed.). Sudbury, Mass.: Jones and Bartlett.

References and Suggested Reading

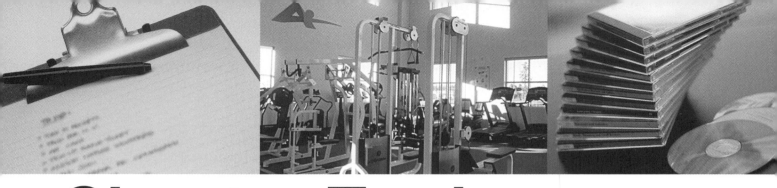

Chapter Twelve

David K. Stotlar, Ed.D., is a professor in the School of Kinesiology and Physical Education at the University of Northern Colorado, where he teaches sport law, sport administration, and finance. He has served as a consultant to school districts, sports professionals, attorneys, and international sports administrators, and has been published extensively on sports law issues.

IN THIS CHAPTER:

Legal and Professional Responsibilities

By David K. Stotlar

Most people who teach or administer group fitness programs have received some form of training in exercise instruction and supervision. Often their experience with the law, if any, has been limited to cases involving common sports injuries. However, the rapid expansion of the fitness industry has created new forms of legal liability. The purpose of this chapter is to explain basic legal concepts that concern group fitness instructors and to show how these concepts can be applied to reduce injuries to program participants, thus reducing the likelihood that an instructor or studio owner will be involved in a lawsuit.

Legal and Professional Responsibilities

Liability and Negligence

The term **liability** refers to responsibility. Legal liability concerns the responsibilities recognized by a court of law. Every instructor or exercise leader who stands in front of a class faces the responsibilities of knowing the capacities of, and setting limitations on, participants before they begin an exercise program.

Studio owners and managers have the added responsibility of ensuring that the facilities and equipment are appropriate and safe. Fitness professionals cannot avoid liability any more than they can avoid assuming the responsibilities inherent in their positions. However, those liabilities may be reduced through adherence to the appropriate standard of care and the implementation of certain risk-management principles.

The responsibilities arising from the relationship between the group fitness instructor and the participant produce a legal expectation, commonly referred to as the standard of care. **Standard of care** means that the quality of services provided in a fitness setting is commensurate with current professional standards. In the case of a lawsuit alleging negligence, the court would ask the question, "What would a reasonable, competent, and prudent group fitness instructor do in a similar situation?" An instructor or studio owner who failed to meet that standard could be found negligent by a court of law.

Negligence is usually defined as "failure to act as a reasonable and prudent person would act under a similar circumstance." For the group fitness instructor, this definition has two important components. The first deals specifically with actions: "Failure to act" refers to acts of omission as well as acts of commission. In other words, an instructor can be sued for not doing something that should have been done,

as well as for doing something that should not have been done. The second part of the definition of negligence pertains to the appropriateness of the action in light of the standard of care, or a "reasonable and prudent" professional standard. If other qualified instructors would have acted similarly under the same circumstances, a court would probably not find an instructor's action negligent.

To legally substantiate a charge of negligence, four elements must be shown to exist. As stated by Wong (2002), they are: (1) that the **defendant** (person being sued) had a duty to protect the **plaintiff** (person filing the suit) from injury; (2) that the defendant failed to exercise that standard of care necessary to perform that duty; (3) that such failure was the proximate cause of the injury; and (4) that the damage or injury to the plaintiff did occur.

Consider this situation: A participant in an aerobics class badly sprains her ankle while following instructions for an aerobic-dance routine. The movement that led to the injury consisted of prolonged and excessive hopping on one foot, something not recommended by reasonable and prudent group fitness instructors. If the participant sues the instructor for negligence, the following questions and answers might surface in court: Was it the instructor's duty to provide proper instruction? Yes. Was that duty satisfactorily performed? Probably not. Was the instructor's failure to provide safe instruction the direct cause of the injury? It probably was. Did actual damages occur? The plaintiff's doctor concluded that they did.

Areas of Responsibility

The duties assigned to fitness professionals vary from one position to another and from organization to organization. Overall, there are seven major areas of responsibility: **health screening,** testing and programming, instruction, supervision, facilities, equipment, and risk management. Each area poses unique questions for the professional that are important even to the beginning instructor. The American Council on Exercise (ACE) has developed a statement on ethics that is quite helpful in guiding the actions of fitness professionals (see Appendix A).

Health Screening

A fitness professional's responsibility begins when a new participant walks in the door. Most prospective participants will be generally healthy people with the goal of improving their personal health and fitness level. Others, however, may come as part of their recovery from heart attacks or other serious health conditions. Therefore, it is imperative that instructors compile a medical history for each participant to document any existing conditions that might affect performance in an exercise program (see Chapter 5). For a complete review, consult the *AHA/ACSM Scientific Statement: Recommendations for Cardiovascular Screening, Staffing, and Emergency Policies at Health/Fitness Facilities* (American Heart Association/American College of Sports Medicine, 1998).

An instructor's responsibility does not end with collecting information. The health history and other data must be examined closely for information that affects programming decisions. Instructors have been charged with negligence for not accurately assessing available information that could have prevented an injury. Every club or studio needs to establish policies and procedures to ensure that each participant's personal history and medical information are taken into account in designing an exercise program.

Fitness Testing and Exercise Programming

Many states require "medical prescriptions" to be developed by licensed medical doctors. Once the medical prescription is developed, a physical therapist is legally allowed to administer and supervise its implementation. The purpose of an exercise "prescription" is to induce a physiological response that will result in a clinical change in a given condition. As a result, fitness professionals are usually limited to providing exercise programs, not exercise prescriptions, which may be construed as medical prescriptions under these circumstances. Although the difference between the terms "program" and "prescription" may seem like a technicality, it may be important in a court of law.

Fitness testing presents similar issues. The health and fitness level of the participant, the purpose of the test, and the testing methods should all be calculated before test administration. The use of relatively simple tests, such as a skinfold caliper to measure body-fat percentage, would not normally pose significant legal problems. On the other hand, the use of a **graded exercise test** on a treadmill with a multiple-lead **electrocardiogram** could expose an unqualified instructor to a charge of practicing medicine without a license. Therefore, it is important that the test be recognized by a professional organization as appropriate for the intended use, be within the qualifications and training of the instructor, and that an accepted protocol (testing procedure) be followed exactly.

Instruction

To conduct a safe and effective exercise program, fitness professionals are expected to provide instruction that is both adequate and proper. Adequate instruction refers to the amount of direction given to participants before and during their exercise activity. For example, an instructor who asks a class to perform an exercise without first demonstrating how to do it properly could be found negligent if a participant performs the exercise incorrectly and is injured as a result. Proper instruction is factually correct. In other words, an instructor may be liable for a participant's injury resulting from an exercise that was not demonstrated or was demonstrated improperly or from an unsafe exercise that should not have been included in a group fitness routine.

In the courtroom, the correctness of instruction is usually assessed by an expert witness who describes the proper procedures for conducting the activity in question. Therefore, the instructional techniques used by a group fitness instructor should be consistent with professionally recognized standards. Proper certification from a nationally recognized professional organization, as well as appropriate documentation of training (degrees, continuing education, etc.) can enhance an instructor's competence in the eyes of a court, should he or she ever be charged with negligence.

In addition to providing adequate and proper instruction, fitness professionals should also be careful not to diagnose or suggest treatment for injuries. This includes not only injuries received in the instructor's exercise class, but also those injuries acquired through other means. When participants ask for advice, it may be best to suggest they call their doctor. In general, only physicians and certain other healthcare providers are allowed to diagnose, prescribe treatment, and treat injuries. An instructor can provide first aid, but only if he or she is qualified to do so.

Simple advice for a sprained ankle once resulted in a nasty lawsuit. When a partici-

pant sprained her ankle during a fitness routine, the instructor told her to go home and ice the ankle to reduce the swelling. Because the ice made the injury feel much better, the participant kept her foot in ice water for two to three hours. As a consequence, several of her toes had to be amputated because of frostbite.

This example may be extreme, but it serves as a valuable warning. There are several ways the instructor could have avoided this unfortunate situation. First, the instructor could have advised the participant to see a physician. While this approach protects the instructor, it would be costly if every participant who suffered a sprained ankle had to see a doctor. Second, the instructor could have provided a more precise description of the first-aid ice treatment. The third and best approach would be a combination of the first two; the instructor would provide specific instructions (both written and verbal) on the first-aid procedures recommended by the American Red Cross and suggest that if the injury did not respond well, then the participant should seek the advice of a physician.

Supervision

The instructor is responsible for supervising all aspects of a class. The standards that apply to supervision are the same as those for instruction: adequate and proper. A prerequisite to determining adequate supervision is the ratio of participants to instructors and supervisors. A prudent instructor should allow a class to be only as large as can be competently monitored. The participant/instructor ratio will, of course, vary with activity, facility, and type of participant. An exercise class of 30 may be appropriate in a large gymnasium, but too big for an aquatic exercise class. Adequate and proper supervision may be different for a class of fit 20-year-olds than for a class of 55-year-old beginning exercisers.

General, or nonindividualized, supervision can be used when the activity can be monitored from a position in general proximity to the participants. For example, in an aerobics class a conscientious instructor can give enough attention to all participants to keep them relatively safe through general but systematic observation. On the other hand, a series of fitness tests administered to a participant before an exercise program calls for specific, or individualized, supervision. The person qualified to administer the testing must provide continuous attention in immediate proximity to the participant to ensure safety. Whether general or specific, required supervision should be based on one's own judgment of the nature of the activity and the participants involved, compared with what other prudent professionals would do under the same circumstances.

Facilities

Safety is the basic issue for a fitness facility. Is the environment free from unreasonable hazards? Are all areas of the facility appropriate for the specific type of activity to be conducted in that area? For example, martial arts require a floor surface that will cushion the feet, knees, and legs from inordinate amounts of stress. Similarly, workout areas or stations of a circuit-training class should have adequate free space surrounding them to ensure that observers will not be struck by an exercising participant.

Some facilities provide locker room and shower facilities. These areas must be sanitary, the floors must be textured to reduce accidental slipping, and areas near water must be protected from electrical shock. Although group fitness instructors may not be responsible for designing and maintaining the exercise facility,

any potential problem should be detected, reported, and corrected as soon as possible. Until then, appropriate warning signs should be clearly posted to warn participants of the unsafe conditions and access to the area should be restricted.

In some cases, an instructor may be assigned to teach in an area that is unsafe or inappropriate for the activity. Under these circumstances, a prudent instructor would refuse to teach and would document that decision in writing to the club or studio management so that constructive action may be taken.

Equipment

For a program that uses exercise equipment, the legal concerns center primarily on selection, installation, maintenance, and repair. Equipment should meet all appropriate safety and design standards in the industry. If the equipment has been purchased from a competent manufacturer, these standards will probably be met. However, some organizations may try to save money by using homemade or inexpensive equipment. If an injury is caused by a piece of equipment that fails to perform as expected, and the injured party can show that the equipment failed to meet basic safety and design standards, the club or studio would be exposed to increased liability.

It is also important that trained technicians assemble and install all equipment. Having untrained people assemble some types of machinery may void the manufacturer's warranty and expose the program to additional risks. A schedule of regular service and repair should also be established and documented to show that the management has acted responsibly. Defective or worn parts should be replaced immediately, and equipment that is in need of repair should be removed for service.

Legal and Professional Responsibilities

Instructors and supervisors should instruct each participant on equipment safety. In addition, each instructor and participant should be required to examine the equipment before each use and report any problems to the person in charge.

Several states have begun to require that automated external defibrillators (AEDs) be available in spas and health and fitness clubs. This move means that group fitness instructors should be competent in using AEDs should a critical incident arise.

Another equipment-related situation arises when participants ask their instructor about which shoes to wear or what exercise equipment to purchase for home use. An exercise professional should be extremely cautious when giving such recommendations. Before an instructor is qualified to give advice, he or she must have a thorough knowledge of the product lines available and the particular characteristics of each product. If this condition cannot be met, an instructor should refer the participant to a retail sporting-goods outlet. Otherwise, the instructor could be held liable for a negligent recommendation. An instructor who makes a recommendation based solely on personal experience should clearly state that it is a personal, and not a professional, recommendation. Instructors who are receiving money for endorsing a particular product must be particularly careful not to portray themselves as experts giving professional advice.

Risk Management

One of the duties of professionals in the fitness industry is to effectively manage risk. The process of **risk management** is more than just avoiding accidents; it encompasses a total examination of risk areas for the fitness professional. Each of the responsibilities identified above presents various levels of risk that should be assessed. The steps involved in a comprehensive risk-management review include the following:
- Identification of risk areas
- Evaluation of specific risks in each area
- Selection of appropriate treatment for each risk
- Implementation of a risk-management system
- Evaluation of success

Risk management is an important professional duty. Too often, it is considered merely a process by which to avoid lawsuits. Professionals in the fitness industry should approach risk management as a way to provide better service to their participants. With this philosophy, risk management can become a method of conducting activities, not just a way to avoid legal trouble. The end goal is to create a safe, enjoyable experience for participants.

Guidelines

The following guidelines reflect the general areas described in preceding sections of this chapter and are intended to provide group fitness instructors with criteria necessary for reducing injuries to participants and the accompanying legal complications.

Health Screening

Each participant beginning a fitness program should receive a thorough evaluation. Specific risk-management criteria may include the following:
- Evaluation is conducted prior to participating in exercise.
- Screening methods concur with national guidelines (ACE, ACSM, AHA, etc.).

Programming

Primary responsibilities of all fitness instructors include program design and exercise selection. Specific risk-management criteria may include the following:

- Health history data is used appropriately in program design.
- Programs and tests selected are recognized by a professional organization as appropriate for the intended use.
- Programs and tests are within the qualifications and training of the group fitness instructor.
- Accepted protocols are followed exactly in all programs and procedures.

Instruction

A fitness professional must provide instruction that is both "adequate and proper." To fulfill this standard, the following criteria would apply to instruction:

- Instructions or directions given to participants prior to, and during, activity are sufficient and understandable.
- The instructor conforms to a "standard of care" (what a reasonable and prudent instructor would provide in the same situation).

Supervision

Group fitness instructors must perform their supervisory duties in accordance with the following professionally devised and established guidelines:

- Continuous supervision is provided in immediate proximity to the participant to ensure safety.
- Larger groups are supervised from the perimeter of the exercise area to ensure all participants are in full view of the instructor.
- Specific supervision is employed when the activity merits close attention to an individual participant.

Facilities

The basic issue regarding facilities centers on the safety of the premises (Table 12.1). The central focus is whether the environment is free from unreasonable hazards. Examples of risk-management criteria include the following:

- The floor surface is appropriate for each activity.
- The free area around equipment is sufficient for the exercise.
- Lighting is adequate for performance of the skill and for supervision.
- Entrances and exits are well marked.

Equipment

In the equipment area, the legal concerns center primarily on selection, maintenance, and repair of the equipment. A risk-management plan should examine the following points:

- Equipment selected meets all safety and design standards within the industry.
- Assembly of equipment follows manufacturers' guidelines.
- A schedule of regular service and repair is established and documented.
- Caution is exercised in relation to recommending equipment.
- Homemade equipment is avoided if at all possible.

Accident Reporting

Regardless of the safety measures provided, some injuries are going to occur in the conduct of fitness activities. When someone is injured, it is necessary for the instructor to file an accident report, which should include the following information:

- Name, address, and phone number of the injured person
- Time, date, and place of the accident

Legal and Professional Responsibilities

Table 12.1
Standards for Health/Fitness Facilities

1. All facilities offering exercise equipment or services must offer a general pre-activity cardiovascular risk screening (e.g., PAR-Q) and/or a specific pre-activity screening tool (e.g., HRA, MHQ) to all new members and prospective users. (Chapter 2)

2. All specific pre-activity screening tools (e.g., HRA, MHQ) must be interpreted by qualified staff and the results of the screening must be documented. (Chapter 2)

3. If a facility becomes aware that a member/user has a known cardiovascular, metabolic, or pulmonary disease, or two or more major cardiovascular risk factors, or any other major self-disclosed medical concern, that person must be advised to consult with a qualified healthcare provider before beginning a moderate-to-vigorous physical-activity program. (Chapter 2)

4. All facilities with qualified staff must offer each new member a general orientation to the facility, including identification of resources available for personal assistance with developing a suitable physical-activity program and the proper use of any exercise equipment to used in that program. (Chapter 3)

5. Facilities must have in place a written system for sharing information with users and employees/independent contractors regarding the handling of potentially hazardous materials, including the handling of bodily fluids by the facility staff in accordance with the Occupational Safety and Health Administration (OSHA). (Chapter 4)

6. Facilities must have written emergency-response system policies and procedures that must be reviewed and rehearsed regularly. These policies must be capable of handling basic first-aid situations and emergency cardiac events. (Chapter 4)

7. Facilities must have as part of their written emergency response system a public access defibrillation (PAD) program. (Chapter 4)

8. The fitness and healthcare professionals who have supervisory responsibility for the physical-activity programs (supervise and oversee members, users, staff and/or independent contractors) of the facility must demonstrate the appropriate professional education, certification, and/or experience. (Chapter 5)

9. The fitness and healthcare professionals who serve in counseling, instructional, and physical-activity supervision roles for the facility must demonstrate the appropriate professional education, certification, and/or experience. (Chapter 5)

10. Fitness and healthcare professionals engaged in pre-activity screening, instructing, monitoring, or supervising physical-activity programs for facility members/users must have current AED/CPR (automated external defibrillator and cardiopulmonary resuscitation) certification from an organization qualified to provide such certification. (Chapter 5)

11. Facilities, to the extent required by law, must adhere to the building design standards that relate to the designing, building, expanding, or renovating of space as presented by the Americans with Disabilities Act (ADA). (Chapter 6)

12. Facilities must be in compliance with all federal, state, and local building codes. (Chapter 6)

13. The aquatic and pool facilities must provide the proper safety equipment and signage, per state and local codes and regulations. (Chapter 7)

14. Facilities must have a system in operation that monitors the entry to, and usage of, the facility by all individuals, including members and users. (Chapter 8)

15. Facilities that offer a sauna, steam room, or whirlpool must make sure that these areas are maintained at the proper temperature and that the appropriate warning systems are in place to notify members/users of any unwarranted changes in temperature. (Chapter 8)

16. Facilities that offer members/users access to a pool or whirlpool must make sure that the pool-water chemistry is maintained in accordance with state and local codes. (Chapter 8)

17. A facility that offers youth services or programs must provide appropriate supervision. (Chapter 8)

18. Facilities must post the appropriate caution, danger, and warning signage in conspicuous locations where existing conditions and situations warrant such signage. (Chapter 9)

19. Facilities must post the appropriate emergency and safety signage pertaining to fire and related emergency situations, as required by federal, state, and local codes. (Chapter 9)

20. Facilities must post all required ADA and OSHA signage. (Chapter 9)

21. All cautionary, danger, and warning signage must have the required signal icon, signal word, signal color, and layout, as specified by the American National Standards Institute (ANSI) and reflected in the American Society of Testing and Materials (ASTM) standards for fitness equipment and fitness facility safety signage and labels. (Chapter 9)

Note: Chapters in parentheses refer to *ACSM's Health/Fitness Facility Standards and Guidelines*.

- A brief description of the part of the body affected and nature of the injury (e.g., "cut on the right hand")
- A description and model number of any equipment involved
- A reference to any instruction given and the type of supervision in force at the time of the injury
- A brief, factual description of how the injury occurred (no opinions as to cause or fault)
- Names, addresses, and phone numbers of any witnesses
- A brief statement of actions taken at the time of the injury (e.g., first aid given, physician referral, or ambulance called)
- Signatures of the supervisor and the injured person

Accident reports should be kept for three to five years, depending on each state's **statute of limitations.** If the person was injured in a formal class setting, it may also be helpful to file a class outline or lesson plan with the accident report. In addition, a yearly review of injuries can be helpful in reducing accidents causing injuries to participants.

Common Approaches for Managing Risks

The most common approaches for the management of potential risks are: avoidance, retention, reduction, and transfer.

Avoidance—This simply means that the activity is judged to be too hazardous to justify its use. Some examples of this include high-risk exercises such as full squats and straight-leg sit-ups.

Retention—In some instances, instructors will simply want to budget for the situation. This might include paying for the cost of an emergency room visit for an injured participant. It's much cheaper than litigation!

Reduction—Instructors should continue to compare their instruction, facilities, equipment, and procedures to national standards. Implementing changes constitutes reduction.

Transfer—This usually is accomplished through insurance. Fitness personnel and clubs should have viable programs of insurance that will cover the cost of legal defense and any claims awarded. Read the coverage carefully, because company policies vary considerably. The general types of coverage that should be obtained include the following:

- **General liability insurance** covers basic trip-and-fall-type injuries.
- **Professional liability insurance** covers claims of negligence based on professional duties.
- **Disability insurance** provides income protection in the event of an injury to the instructor.
- **Individual medical insurance** provides hospitalization and major medical coverage.

Group fitness instructors who are independent contractors should pay special attention to their coverage. They should make sure that if they work for clubs, all aspects of coverage are understood and included in the written agreements for services.

Duties also include enforcing conduct and ensuring adherence to safety guidelines. Clearly written safety guidelines for each type of activity should be posted in appropriate areas of the facility and rigidly enforced by the supervisor.

Of particular importance are the policies and procedures for emergencies. All employees should be thoroughly familiar with the policies and should have actual practice in carrying out an emergency plan. For example, every club or studio should conduct a "heart attack drill," requiring all

Legal and Professional Responsibilities

staff to carry out emergency plans and procedures such as those recommended by the American Heart Association. The program manager should maintain records of these simulations.

Many group fitness instructors and supervisors are needlessly exposed to liability because they permit indiscriminate use of the facility. Supervisory personnel should restrict the facility to people who have a legitimate entitlement. Each staff member should have a list of the people scheduled to use the equipment and facilities during specific time periods, and the supervisor should allow access only to those people. This policy should be enforced with the same vigor as the safety procedures.

Implementation of a Risk-management System

Implementation is a management function. For a complete review of considerations regarding the creation and implementation of policy and staffing concerns, consult the *AHA/ACSM Scientific Statement: Recommendations for Cardiovascular Screening, Staffing, and Emergency Policies at Health/Fitness Facilities*. Attention must be given to all subject areas identified in this chapter. This process is normally called a safety audit and should be conducted regularly. Many professionals in the field develop safety checklists, while clubs often have professional consultants conduct safety audits. Regardless, a systematic evaluation of the risks in group fitness activities is essential for safe program operation.

Waivers and Informed Consent

The staff members of many facilities attempt to absolve themselves of liability by having all participants sign a liability **waiver** to release the instructor and fitness center from all liability associated with the conduct of an exercise program and any resulting injuries. In some cases, these documents have been of little value because the courts have enforced the specific wording of the waiver and not its intent. In other words, if negligence was found to be the cause of injury, and negligence of the instructor or fitness center was not specifically waived, then the waiver would not be effective. Therefore, waivers must be clearly written and include statements to the effect that the participant waives all claims to damages, even those caused by the negligence of the instructor or fitness center.

Some fitness centers use an **informed consent** form. While this document may look similar to a waiver, its purpose is different. The informed consent form is used to make the dangers of a program or test procedure known to the participant and thereby provide an additional measure of defense against lawsuits.

Obtaining informed consent is very important. It should be an automatic procedure for every person who enters the program, and it should be done before every fitness test. The American Council on Exercise suggests the following procedures:

- Inform the participant of the exercise program or testing procedure, and explain the purpose of each. This explanation should be thorough and unbiased.
- Inform the participant of the risks involved in the testing procedure or program, along with the possible discomforts.
- Inform the participant of the benefits expected from the testing procedure or program.
- Inform the participant of any alternative programs or tests that may be more advantageous to him or her.

- Solicit questions regarding the testing procedure or exercise program, and give unbiased answers to these inquiries.
- Inform the participant that he or she is free, at any time, to withdraw consent and discontinue participation.
- Obtain the written consent of each participant.

For extensive guidance on many of these issues, you may want to consult *IHRSA's Guide to Club Membership and Conduct,* which provides specific standards, sample forms, and suggested policies and procedures that could be used in risk-management implementation.

Basic Defenses Against Negligence Claims

It is important for instructors to know and understand that they are not without protection under the law. Several defenses are available for use by fitness professionals as defendants in litigation in fitness-related personal-injury cases.

Assumption of Risk

This defense is used to show that the participant voluntarily accepted dangers known to exist with participation in the activity. The two most important aspects of this definition are "voluntary" and "known danger." If the participant does not voluntarily engage in a program or test, this defense cannot normally be used. Also, if the participant was not informed of the specific risks associated with the program or test, then he or she cannot be held to have assumed them. The best way to prove that a participant was knowledgeable of the risks involved is to utilize the assumption-of-risk documents (e.g., informed consent and waivers) described earlier.

Contributory Negligence

This defense means that the plaintiff played some role in his or her own injury. Although this legal doctrine is viable in only a few states (check applicable state law), it provides a total bar to recovery for any damages. An example might consist of a participant exceeding the designated maximum heart rate in a prescribed exercise program. A salient factor would also be whether an instructor was there to monitor the participant, or if the participant was exercising alone and following program guidelines.

Comparative Negligence

In this defense, the relative fault of both the plaintiff and the defendant are measured to see who was most at fault for the injury. The result is an apportionment of guilt and any subsequent award for damages. The court (or jury) determines the percentage of responsibility of each party and then prorates the award. This can be useful if a participant is somewhat to blame for his or her own injury.

Act of God

Although this defense is not often used in fitness and sport law cases, it may be of interest. It involves injury caused by unforeseeable acts of nature. The foreseeability aspect is the most crucial. If, during an exercise session, an earthquake opened the floor and a participant was engulfed, it may be applicable.

Other Legal Considerations

Group fitness instructors are providers of a special service. As a result, professionals in this field must be familiar with the special aspects of

Legal and Professional Responsibilities

the law that are most frequently encountered in the conduct of their business.

Contracts

Fitness personnel must have an adequate knowledge of legal **contracts** to perform their tasks, get paid, and avoid costly legal battles with participants and/or clubs. Some instructors will want to work as individuals not affiliated with one particular club, while others may want to be employed by a club or fitness center, yet specialize in one-on-one instruction.

Whatever the nature of the work arrangement, an instructor must be aware of the essentials of contract law. Basic contract law indicates that the following elements are necessary to form a binding contract:

- An offer and acceptance—mutual agreement to terms
- Consideration—an exchange of items of value
- Legality—acceptable form and subject under the law
- Capacity—such as majority age and mental competency

The general considerations that should be addressed in contracts for use with participants, as well as contracts between exercise professionals and clubs for which they intend to work, should include the following:

- Identification of the parties (trainer and participant/club)
- Description of the services to be performed (fitness training and consultation)
- Compensation ($X.00 per hour, day, month, or class, and payment method)
- Confidential relationship (agreement by each party not to divulge personal or business information gained through the relationship)

- Business status (confirmation of employment status)
- Term and termination (express definition of the length of the contract and the conditions under which termination is allowed by either party)

Employment Status

As noted above, another prominent concern for many fitness professionals deals with employment status: **independent contractor** versus **employee**. Both of these terms can apply to those who work in a fitness center. However, only the independent contractor status applies to self-employed instructors working independently from a club. However, most clubs still require independent contractors hired by the club to follow club rules.

Clients who hire a fitness professional do not intend, for the most part, to hire that person as an employee, but prefer to lease their services for a brief period of time. Hence, most self-employed fitness instructors are independent contractors and not employees of their clients.

In some instances, owners of fitness centers or clubs have used the term independent contractor for employees. Club owners are often motivated to hire independent contractors in place of regular employees because the company does not have to train, provide medical or other benefits, arrange for social security withholding, or pay into worker's compensation or unemployment funds for independent contractors. Club owners also find an advantage in having independent contractors because it is more complicated, from a legal standpoint, to fire existing employees than it is to simply not renew contracts with independent contractors.

A legal dichotomy exists between regular employees and independent contractors. Most commonly, the courts have considered 10 "tests" to determine if the business relationship in question between a club and a fitness professional is that of a regular employee or an independent contractor. These tests are:

1. *The extent of control that, by agreement, the employer can exercise over the details of the work.* The existence of a right to control is indicative of an employer–employee relationship.

2. *The method of payment, whether by time or by the job.* Generally, those persons scheduled to be paid on a regular basis at an hourly or weekly rate have been considered employees. Conversely, those paid in a single payment for services rendered have more easily qualified as independent contractors.

3. *The length of time for which the person is employed.* Individuals hired for short periods of time (a few days or weeks) have more often been seen as independent contractors, whereas employment periods that extended upward of a full year have been ruled as establishing an employer–employee relationship.

4. *The skill required for the provision of services.* When the worker needs no training because of the specialized or technical skills that the employer intends to utilize, the independent contractor status has prevailed. On the other hand, if an employer provides training to a recently hired individual, that person will more than likely be judged to be an employee.

5. *Whether the person employed is in a distinct business or occupation.* If a worker offers services to other employers or clients, a status of independent contractor would probably be found. If, however, the worker only intended to provide

services for one employer, and failed to offer the services to others as an independent business, the employee status could be found.

6. *Whether the employer of the worker provides the equipment.* If independent contractor status is desired, group fitness instructors will have a better chance getting it if they provide their own equipment.

7. *Whether the work is a part of the normal business of the employer.* Court rulings have favored classifying individuals as regular employees when services rendered are integral to the business of the employer. Supplemental, special, or one-time services are more likely to be provided by independent contractors.

8. *Whether the work is traditionally performed by a specialist in similar businesses.* Employers and employees must examine their field of business to gain an understanding of current practices and align themselves with the prevailing trends.

9. *The intent of the parties involved in the arrangement.* The courts will attempt to enforce intent of the parties at the time the agreement was executed. If a professional thought that he or she was hired as an independent contractor, as did the club, it would influence the court's determination. Therefore, a clear understanding of the arrangement is a must.

10. *Whether the employer is engaged in a business.* The intent here is to protect clients from being construed as employers when a fitness professional is hired to perform work of a "private" nature. This is most common when fitness professionals sell their services to

Legal and Professional Responsibilities

private citizens rather than to clubs or corporations.

The process of determining employment status is marked by careful analysis of the facts and the weighing of interpretations on both sides of the issue. All of the issues addressed above have been used in court cases dealing with this matter, each with varying degrees of authority. It is, therefore, imperative that all fitness professionals and club owners understand and examine these factors when initiating agreements.

For more specific information on the legal aspects surrounding the independent contractor versus employee issue, you may want to consult the guidelines published by the Internal Revenue Service (www.irs.gov).

Copyright Law

One of a group fitness instructor's major legal responsibilities is compliance with copyright law. All forms of commercially produced creative expression are protected by **copyright** law, but music is the area most pertinent to exercise instructors. This has become an extremely important issue with the availability of downloadable music. Simply stated, almost all musical compositions that one can hear on the radio or television or buy from music outlets are owned by artists and studios and are protected by federal copyright law. Whether an instructor makes a tape or burns a CD from various songs on the radio or from media he or she has purchased does not matter; the instructor who uses that music in a for-profit exercise class—legally speaking, a **public performance**—is in violation of copyright law.

Performance Licenses

To be able to use copyrighted music in an exercise class, one must obtain a performance license from one of the two major **performing rights societies**, the **American Society of Composers, Authors and Publishers (ASCAP)** or **Broadcast Music, Inc. (BMI)**. These organizations vigorously enforce copyright law for their memberships and will not hesitate to sue a health club, studio, or freelance instructor who plays copyrighted music without a license.

Accordingly, most clubs and studios obtain a **blanket license** for their instructors. The license fees for the clubs are determined either by the number of students who attend classes each week, by the number of speakers used in the club, or by whether the club has a single- or multifloor layout.

Instructors who teach as independent contractors at several locations may have to obtain their own licenses. They should check with the clubs where they teach to see if each club's blanket license covers their classes. If freelance instructors teach at several different locations with their own music, they will have to obtain their own performance licenses.

Given that the fees for either getting licenses or paying damages for copyright infringement may be prohibitive, independent instructors in particular may want to consider other options. One is to create rhythm CDs of their own using a drum machine, an electronic instrument that can range in sophistication from toy to professional recording device. A professional model is not needed, however, to make an appealing rhythm CD. A local music store owner or salesperson could probably steer the instructor to someone who could help create such a disk.

Other options include buying licensed music expressly made for fitness and aerobic exercise classes, where the copyright holder expressly permits the original music to be used in a class, or asking exercise class students to bring their own recordings for the workouts, in effect using them for the participants' own noncommercial use. Another trend is for clubs to buy "packaged" group fitness programs where all of the advertising, music, and instructor training are provided and the fitness center is allowed to use the name brand of the program in its advertising.

Obtaining Copyright Protection

Some group fitness instructors may want to obtain copyright protection for certain aspects of their work, including the following:

- *Pantomimes and choreographic work*—If an instructor creates more than a simple routine, and publicly distributes (through a dance notation system), performs, or displays the choreography, it can be copyrighted.
- *Books, videos, and films*—If a choreographed work by an instructor is sold to a **publisher,** video distributor, or movie studio, that business entity will own the copyright for the material and the instructor will be compensated with either an advance or a certain portion of the proceeds (royalties), or both. Through negotiation with the producing or distributing company, the instructor may be able to retain certain rights to the material.
- ***Compilations*** *of exercise routines*—If an instructor makes an original sequence of routines, it may be protected by copyright and licensed to others for a book, video, film, or other presentation form.
- *Graphic materials*—If an instructor creates pictures, charts, diagrams, informational handouts, or other graphic materials for instructional aids or promotional material, these too may be copyrighted.

For copyright information or applications, write to:

Register of Copyrights
United States Copyright Office
Library of Congress
Washington, D.C. 20559
www.copyright.gov

Liability Insurance

Every group fitness instructor will want to assess his or her liability insurance needs. An instructor employed at a club should inquire about the general liability policy and any other liability insurance the owner might have.

Independent contractors may not be covered by a club's general policy and, if not, should ask the club if they can be added by special endorsement.

Many nonprofit groups, such as churches and recreation centers, may not have coverage that includes their contract instructors. The instructors at these venues should have their own general liability coverage.

General liability coverage will cover an accident where a student trips over a loose floorboard or falls and breaks an arm. What about a student hurting herself in a routine that she says was improperly demonstrated? For this kind of claim, instructors would be wise to have professional liability insurance.

Since professional standards in the exercise field are becoming the norm, the expectations of students (and courts, as well) are rising to include all facets of exercise-class management, from screening participants correctly to adequately supervising them.

Professional liability insurance will not cover an instructor for copyright infringement claims or offer protection in suits involving libel, slander, invasion of privacy, or defamation of character. These sorts of

Legal and Professional Responsibilities

actions may be considered intentional torts and are not typically covered.

Instructors seeking affordable liability policies should check with their certifying agency or discuss their needs with insurance agents who may suggest liability coverage be added onto the instructor's residence insurance as a "business pursuits rider."

Liability insurance is a must for exercise instructors. They should not begin a class anywhere without knowing what the insurance coverage is and what is excluded. The key thing for instructors to do if they are not given adequate insurance information by a club supervisor is to ask specific questions related to a club's liability insurance policy.

Americans With Disabilities Act

Fitness professionals can be affected by legislative mandates beyond insurance regulations. One of the laws that affects the profession is the **Americans with Disabilities Act,** which became law in 1992. Modeled after the Civil Rights Act, it prohibits discrimination on the basis of disability. The law provides for equal treatment and equal access to programs for disabled Americans. The act extends provisions to all areas of public accommodation, including businesses such that all participants, regardless of disability, are guaranteed access to all programs and spaces within the facility. Therefore, it is essential that fitness professionals make sure that their buildings, equipment, and programs are available to persons with disabilities. Employers must also provide reasonable accommodations for employees with disabilities, including adjusted work stations and equipment as necessary. Therefore, whether a person with a disability is an employee or a participant, steps must be taken to ensure that the professional and business environment is one that respects the dignity, skills, and contributions of those individuals.

Scope of Practice in the Profession

Group fitness instructors are generally in the business of providing exercise leadership and exercise-related advice. They are not normally physicians, physical therapists, or dietitians (although some may be certified or licensed in these areas).

The primary area in which the **scope of practice** comes into question is generally the health-history or wellness-history form. As described earlier, this form is used as a general screening document prior to the participant's entry into a fitness program. Fitness law expert David Herbert says that "wellness-assessment documents should be utilized for…determination of an individual's level of fitness…*never* for the purpose of providing or recommending *treatment* of any condition." Use of such a form in recommending treatment could constitute the practice of medicine without a license.

Another area of interaction between fitness professionals and participants that can cause issues related to the scope of certain professional practices is in dietary and nutritional counseling. With the tremendous growth in the nutritional supplements market, this is an issue that affects many professionals in the industry. According to the American Dietetic Association, most states have statutes that regulate or license nutritionists. In the other states, anyone is able to claim to be a nutritionist. Laws in each state should be examined to ensure that healthcare-practice statutes are not violated by fitness professionals who may be surpassing their training and expertise. If a participant has complex dietary questions, referral should be made to a registered dietitian (R.D.) or other qualified healthcare professional.

Similarly, group fitness instructors are not psychologists or marriage counselors and therefore should not provide advice or counseling on issues related to a participant's emotional and/or psychological status. Participants should always be referred to licensed practitioners in these and other related areas.

Summary

No program, regardless of how well it is run, can completely avoid all injuries. In an attempt to reduce injuries to participants and the accompanying legal complications, a group fitness instructor would be wise to adhere to the following guidelines:

- Obtain professional education, guided practical training under a qualified exercise professional, and current certification from an established professional organization.
- Design and conduct programs that reflect current professional standards.
- Formulate and enforce policies and guidelines for the conduct of the program in accordance with professional recommendations.

- Establish and implement adequate and proper procedures for supervision in all phases of the program.
- Establish and implement adequate and proper methods of instruction in all phases of the program.
- Post safety regulations in the facility and ensure that they are rigidly enforced by supervisory personnel.
- Keep the facility free from hazards and maintain adequate free space for each activity.
- Establish and document inspection and repair schedules for all equipment and facilities.
- Formulate policies and guidelines for emergency situations, rehearse the procedures, and require all instructors to have current first-aid training and CPR/AED certification.

By applying these recommendations, fitness professionals can help reduce the probability of injury to participants. Should legal action result from an injury, the facts of the case would be examined to determine whether negligence was the cause. A properly trained, competent, and certified instructor conducting a program that was in accordance with current professional standards would probably prevail.

References

American College of Sports Medicine (2007). *ACSM's Health/Fitness Facility Standards and Guidelines* (3rd ed.). Champaign, Ill.: Human Kinetics.

American Heart Association/American College of Sports Medicine (1998). *AHA/ACSM Scientific Statement: Recommendations for Cardiovascular Screening, Staffing, and Emergency Policies at Health/Fitness Facilities.* Philadelphia: Lippincott Williams & Wilkins.

Wong, G. (2002). *Essentials of Sports Law.* Westport, Conn.: Praeger.

Suggested Reading

Carpenter, L.J. (2000). *Legal Concepts in Sport: A Primer.* Champaign, Ill.: Sagamore Publishing.

Cotten, D. (1997). *Legal Aspects of Waivers in Sport, Recreation & Fitness Activities.* Canton, Ohio: PRC Pub.

Dougherty, N.J. (2002). *Sport, Physical Activity, and the Law.* Champaign, Ill.: Sagamore Publishing.

Herbert, D.L. & Herbert, W.G. (1989). *Legal Aspects of Preventative and Rehabilitative Exercise Programs* (2nd ed.). Canton, Ohio: Professional and Executive Reports and Publications.

International Health & Racquetball & Sportsclub Association. *IHRSA's Guide to Club Membership and Conduct* (3rd ed.). http://download.ihrsa.org/pubs/club_membership_conduct.pdf

Koeberle, B.E. (1990). *Legal Aspects of Personal Training.* Canton, Ohio: Professional and Executive Reports and Publications.

Appendix A

Code of Ethics

ACE-certified Professionals are guided by the following principles of conduct as they interact with participants, the public, and other health and fitness professionals.

ACE-certified Professionals will endeavor to:

✔ Provide safe and effective instruction

✔ Provide equal and fair treatment to all participants

✔ Stay up-to-date on the latest health and fitness research and understand its practical application

✔ Maintain current CPR/AED certification and knowledge of first-aid services

✔ Comply with all applicable business, employment, and intellectual property laws

✔ Maintain the confidentiality of all client information

✔ Refer participants to more qualified health or medical professionals when appropriate

✔ Uphold and enhance public appreciation and trust for the health and fitness industry

✔ Establish and maintain clear professional boundaries

Code of Ethics

Provide Safe and Effective Instruction

Providing safe and effective instruction involves a variety of responsibilities for ACE-certified Professionals. Safe means that the instruction will not result in physical, mental, or financial harm to the participant. Effective means that the instruction has a purposeful, intended, and desired effect toward the participant's goal. Great effort and care must be taken in carrying out the responsibilities that are essential in creating a positive exercise experience for all participants.

Screening

ACE-certified Professionals should have all potential participants complete an industry-recognized health-screening tool to ensure safe exercise participation. If significant risk factors or signs and symptoms suggestive of chronic disease are identified, refer the participant to a physician or primary healthcare practitioner for medical clearance and guidance regarding which types of assessments, activities, or exercises are indicated, contraindicated, or deemed high-risk. If an individual does not want to obtain medical clearance, have the participant sign a legally prepared document that releases you and the facility in which you work from any liability related to any injury that may result from exercise participation or assessment. Once the participant has been cleared for exercise and you have a full understanding of the participant's health status and medical history, including their current use of medications, a formal risk-management plan for potential emergencies must be prepared and reviewed periodically.

Assessment

The main objective of a health assessment is to establish the participant's baseline fitness level to design an appropriate exercise program. Explain the risks and benefits of each assessment and provide the participant with any pertinent instructions. Prior to conducting any type of assessment, the participant must be given an opportunity to ask questions and read and sign an informed consent. The types and order of assessments are dictated by the participant's health status, fitness level, symptoms, and/or use of medications. Remember that each assessment has specific protocols and only those within your scope of practice should be administered. Once the assessments are completed, evaluate and discuss the results objectively as they relate to the participant's health condition and goals. Educate the participant and emphasize how an exercise program will benefit the participant.

Program Design

You must not prescribe exercise, diet, or treatment, as this is outside your scope of practice and implies ordering or advising a medicine or treatment. Instead, it is appropriate for you to design exercise programs that improve components of physical fitness and wellness while adhering to the limitations of a previous injury or condition as determined by a certified, registered, or licensed allied health professional. Because nutritional laws and the practice of dietetics vary in each state, province, and country, understand what type of basic nutritional information is appropriate and legal for you to disseminate to your participant. The participant's preferences and short- and long-term goals, as well as current industry standards and guidelines must be taken into consideration as you develop a formal yet realistic exercise program. Provide as much detail for all exercise parameters such as intensity, type of exercise, frequency, duration, progression, and termination points.

Program Implementation

Do not underestimate your ability to influence a participant on becoming active for a lifetime. Be sure that each class or session is well-planned, sequential, and documented. Instruct the participant on how to safely and properly perform the appropriate exercises and communicate this in a manner that the participant will understand and retain. Each participant has a different learning curve that will require different levels of attention, learning aids, and repetition. Supervise the participant closely, especially when spotting or cueing is needed. If supervising a group of two or more, ensure that you can supervise and provide the appropriate amount of attention to each individual at all times. Ideally, the group will have similar goals and will be performing similar exercises or activities. Position yourself so that you do not have to turn your back to any participant performing an exercise.

Facilities

Although the condition of a facility may not always be within your control, you are still obligated to ensure a hazard-free environment to maximize safety. If you notice potential hazards in the health club, communicate these hazards to the participant and the facility management. For example, if you notice that the clamps that keep the weights on the barbells are getting rusty and loose, it would be prudent of you to remove them from the training area and alert the facility that immediate repair is required.

Equipment

Obtain equipment that meets or exceeds industry standards and utilize the equipment only for its intended use. Arrange exercise equipment and stations so that adequate space exists between equipment, participants, and foot traffic. Schedule regular maintenance and inspect equipment prior to use to ensure it is in proper working condition. Avoid the use of homemade equipment, as your liability is greater if it causes injury to a class participant.

Provide Equal and Fair Treatment to All Participants

ACE-certified Professionals are obligated to provide fair and equal treatment for each participant without bias, preference, or discrimination against gender, ethnic background, age, national origin, basis of religion, or physical disability.

The Americans with Disabilities Act protects individuals with disabilities against any type of unlawful discrimination. A disability can be either physical or mental, such as epilepsy, paralysis, HIV infection, AIDS, a significant hearing or visual impairment, mental retardation, or a specific learning disability. ACE-certified Professionals should, at a minimum, provide reasonable accommodations to each individual with a disability. Reasonable simply means that you are able to provide accommodations that do not cause you any undue hardship that requires additional or significant expense or difficulty. Making an existing facility accessible by modifying equipment or devices, assessments, or training materials are a few examples of providing reasonable accommodations. However, providing the use of personal items or providing items at your own expense may not be considered reasonable.

Code of Ethics

This ethical consideration of providing fair and equal treatment is not limited to behavioral interactions with participants, but also extends to exercise programming and other business-related services such as communication, scheduling, billing, cancellation policies, and dispute resolution.

Stay Up-to-Date on the Latest Health and Fitness Research and Understand its Practical Application

Obtaining ACE certification required you to have broad-based knowledge of many disciplines; however, this credential should not be viewed as the end of your professional development and education. Instead, it should be viewed as the beginning or foundation. The dynamic nature of the health and fitness industry requires you to maintain an understanding of the latest research and professional standards and guidelines, and their impact on the design and implementation of exercise programming. To stay informed, make time to review a variety of industry resources such as professional journals, position statements, trade and lay periodicals, and correspondence courses, as well as to attend professional meetings, conferences, and educational workshops.

An additional benefit of staying up-to-date is that it also fulfills your certification-renewal requirements for continuing education credit (CEC). To maintain your ACE certification status, you must obtain an established amount of CECs every two years. CECs are granted for structured learning that takes place within the educational portion of a course related to the profession and presented by a qualified health and fitness professional.

Maintain Current CPR/AED Certification and Knowledge of First-aid Services

ACE-certified Professionals must be prepared to recognize and respond to heart attacks and other life-threatening emergencies. Emergency response is enhanced by training and maintaining skills in CPR, first aid, and using automated external defibrillators (AEDs), which have become more widely available. An AED is a portable electronic device used to restore normal heart rhythm in a person experiencing a cardiac arrest and can reduce the time to defibrillation before EMS personnel arrive. For each minute that defibrillation is delayed, the victim's chance of survival is reduced by 7 to 10%. Thus, survival from cardiac arrest is improved dramatically when CPR and defibrillation are started early.

Comply With All Applicable Business, Employment, and Intellectual Property Laws

As an ACE-certified Professional, you are expected to maintain a high level of integrity by complying with all applicable business, employment, and copyright laws. Be truthful and forthcoming with communication to participants, co-workers, and other health and fitness professionals in advertising, marketing, and business practices. Do not create false or misleading impressions of credentials, claims, or sponsorships, or perform services outside of your scope of practice that are illegal, deceptive, or fraudulent.

All information regarding your business must be clear, accurate, and easy to understand for all potential participants. Provide disclosure about the name of your business, physical address, and contact information, and maintain a working phone number and email address. Provide detailed information regarding schedules, prices, payment terms, time limits, and conditions so participants can make an informed choice about paying for your services. Cancellation, refund, and rescheduling information must also be clearly stated and easy to understand. Allow the participant an opportunity to ask questions and review this information before formally agreeing to your services and terms.

Because employment laws vary between each city, state, province, and country, familiarize yourself with the applicable employment regulations and standards to which your business must conform. Examples of this may include conforming to specific building codes and zoning ordinances or making sure that your place of business is accessible to individuals with a disability.

The understanding of intellectual property law and the proper use of copyrighted materials is an important legal issue for all ACE-certified Professionals. Intellectual property laws protect the creations of authors, artists, software programmers, and others with copyrighted materials. The most common infringement of intellectual property law in the fitness industry is the use of music in an exercise class. When commercial music is played in a for-profit exercise class without a performance or blanket license, it is considered a public performance and a violation of intellectual property law. Therefore, make sure that any music, handouts, or educational materials are either exempt from intellectual property law or permissible under laws by reason of fair use. You may also obtain express written consent from the copyright holder for distri-

bution, adaptation, or use. When in doubt, obtain permission first or consult with a qualified legal professional who has intellectual property law expertise.

Maintain the Confidentiality of All Participant Information

Every participant has the right to expect that all personal data and discussions with an ACE-certified Professional will be safeguarded and not disclosed without the participant's express written consent or acknowledgement. Therefore, protect the confidentiality of all participant information such as contact data, medical records, health history, progress notes, and meeting details. Even when confidentiality is not required by law, continue to preserve the confidentiality of such information.

Any breach of confidentiality, intentional or unintentional, potentially harms the productivity and trust of your participant and undermines your effectiveness as a fitness professional. This also puts you at risk for potential litigation and puts your participant at risk for public embarrassment and fraudulent activity such as identity theft.

Most breaches of confidentiality are unintentional and occur because of carelessness and lack of awareness. The most common breach of confidentiality is exposing or storing a participant's personal data in a location that is not secure. This occurs when a participant's file or information is left on a desk, or filed in a cabinet that has no lock or is accessible to others. Breaches of confidentiality may also occur when you have conversations regarding a participant's performance or medical/health history with staff or others and the participant's first name or other identifying details are used.

Post and adhere to a privacy policy that communicates how participant information will

Code of Ethics

be used and secured and how a participant's preference regarding unsolicited mail and email will be respected. When a participant provides you with any personal data, new or updated, make it a habit to immediately secure this information and ensure that only you and/or the appropriate individuals have access to it. Also, the participant's files must only be accessed and used for purposes related to health and fitness services. If participant information is stored on a personal computer, restrict access by using a protected password. Should you receive any inquiries from family members or other individuals regarding the progress of a participant or other personal information, state that you cannot provide any information without the participant's permission. If and when a participant permits you to release participant information to an authorized individual or party, utilize secure methods of communication such as certified mail, sending and receiving information on a dedicated private fax line, or email with encryption.

Refer Participants to More Qualified Health or Medical Professionals When Appropriate

A fitness certification is not a professional license. Therefore, it is vitally important that ACE-certified Professionals who do not also have a professional license (i.e., physician, physical therapist, dietitian, psychologist, and attorney) refer their participants to a more qualified professional when warranted. Doing so not only benefits your participants by making sure that they receive the appropriate attention and care, but also enhances your credibility and reduces liability by defining your scope of practice and clarifying what services you can and cannot reasonably provide.

Knowing when to refer a participant is, however, as important as choosing a professional for referral. For instance, just because a participant complains of symptoms of muscle soreness or discomfort or exhibits signs of fatigue or lack of energy is not an absolute indication to refer that individual to a physician. Because continual referrals are not practical, familiarize and educate yourself on expected signs and symptoms, taking into consideration the participant's fitness level, health status, chronic disease, disability, and/or background as they are screened and as they begin and progress with an exercise program. This helps you better discern between emergent and non-emergent situations and know when to refuse to offer your services, continue to monitor, and/or make an immediate referral.

It is important that you know the scope of practice for various health professionals and which types of referrals are appropriate. For example, some states require that a referring physician first approve visits to a physical therapist, while other states allow people to see a physical therapist directly. Only registered or licensed dietitians or physicians may provide specific dietary recommendations or diet plans; however, a participant who is suspected of an eating disorder should be referred to an eating disorders specialist. Refer participants to a clinical psychologist if they wish to discuss family or marital problems or exhibit addictive behaviors such as substance abuse.

Network and develop rapport with potential allied health professionals in your area before you refer participants to them. This demonstrates good will and respect for their expertise and will most likely result in reciprocal referrals for your services and fitness expertise.

Uphold and Enhance Public Appreciation and Trust for the Health and Fitness Industry

The best way for ACE-certified Professionals to uphold and enhance public appreciation and trust for the health and fitness industry is to represent themselves in a dignified and professional manner. As the public is inundated with misinformation and false claims about fitness products and services, your expertise must be utilized to dispel myths and half-truths about current trends and fads that are potentially harmful to the public.

When appropriate, mentor and dispense knowledge and training to less experienced fitness professionals. Novice fitness professionals can benefit from your experience and skill as you assist them in establishing a foundation based on exercise science, from both theoretical and practical standpoints. Therefore, it is a disservice if you fail to provide helpful or corrective information—especially when an individual, the public, or other fitness professionals are at risk for injury or increased liability. For example, if you observe an individual using momentum to perform a strength-training exercise, the prudent course of action would be to suggest a modification. Likewise, if you observe a fitness professional in your workplace consistently failing to obtain informed consents before participants undergo fitness testing or begin an exercise program, recommend that he or she consider implementing these forms to minimize liability.

Finally, do not represent yourself in an overly commercial or misleading manner. Consider the fitness professional who places an advertisement in a local newspaper stating: Lose 10 pounds in 10 days or your money back! It is inappropriate to lend credibility to or endorse a product, service, or program founded upon unsubstantiated or misleading claims; thus a solicitation such as this must be avoided as it undermines the public's trust of health and fitness professionals.

Establish and Maintain Clear Professional Boundaries

Working in the health and fitness industry requires fitness professionals to come in contact with many different people. It is imperative that a professional distance be maintained in relationships between instructor and participant. Instructors are responsible for setting and monitoring the boundaries between a working relationship and friendship with their participants. To that end, ACE-certified Professionals should:

- Never initiate or encourage conversation of a sexual nature
- Avoid touching participants unless it is essential to instruction
- Inform participants about the purpose of touching and find an alternative if the participant objects
- Discontinue all touching if it appears to make the participant uncomfortable
- Take all reasonable steps to ensure that any personal and social contacts between themselves and their participants do not have an adverse impact on the instructor-participant relationship

If you find yourself unable to maintain appropriate professional boundaries with a participant (whether due to your attitudes and actions or those of the participant), the prudent course of action is to terminate the relationship and, perhaps, refer the participant to another professional. Keep in mind that charges of sexual harassment or assault, even if groundless, can have disastrous effects on your fitness career.

Appendix B

For the most up-to-date version of the
Exam Content Outline please go to
www.acefitness.org/GFIexamcontent
and download a free PDF.

Group Fitness Instructor Certification Exam Content Outline

The Examination Content Outline is essentially a blueprint for the exam. As you prepare for the exam, it is important to remember that all exam questions are based on this outline.

Target Audience Statement

The certified Group Fitness Instructor is responsible for planning and leading group exercise sessions to enhance the general well-being (e.g., fitness, health) and exercise skills of participants. The certified Group Fitness Instructor is at least 18 years of age and possesses a valid certificate in cardiopulmonary resuscitation (CPR).

Domains, Tasks, and Knowledge and Skill Statements

A Role Delineation Study completed for the Group Fitness Instructor certification first identified the major categories of responsibility for the professional. These categories are defined as "Domains" and it was determined that the profession could be divided into four Performance Domains, or major areas of responsibility. These Performance Domains are:

- Domain I: Exercise Programming and Class Design
- Domain II: Group Instructional Methods
- Domain III: Group Leadership Methods
- Domain IV: Professional Responsibilities

The Group Fitness Instructor draws upon knowledge from four foundational sciences, which are included within a Content Domain called Applied Exercise Science.

These sciences are:

- Kinesiology (anatomy, kinesiology, biomechanics)
- Physiology
- Nutrition and weight control
- Exercise psychology

This Content Domain includes all topics important to the competence of Group Fitness Instructors and applies primarily to the following Performance Domains: Exercise Programming and Class Design, Group Instructional Methods, and Group Leadership Methods.

Within each Performance Domain, there is additional Domain-specific information referring to tests, procedures, and techniques.

Each Domain is composed of Task Statements, which detail the job-related functions under each Domain. Each Task Statement is further divided into Knowledge and Skill Statements that detail the scope of information required and how that

Group Fitness Instructor Certification Exam Content Outline

Table 1: Exam Content Outline: Group Fitness Instructor Certification

Applied Exercise Science

| Performance Domain | Total Items | KINESIOLOGY | | | Physiology | Nutrition & Weight Control | Exercise Psychology |
		Anatomy (17)	Kinesiology (17)	Biomechanics (21)			
Exercise Programming and Class Design	61	9	9	11	19	5	8
Group Instructional Methods	39	6	6	7	12	3	5
Group Leadership Methods	17	2	2	3	6	2	2
Professional Responsibilities	8	0	0	0	0	0	0
Total:	**125**	**17**	**17**	**21**	**37**	**10**	**15**

information is applied in a practical setting.

The Domains are presented in Table 1 in two ways to demonstrate how the Content and Performance Domains are interconnected:

• Performance Domains are listed vertically: Exercise Programming and Class Design, Group Instructional Methods, Group Leadership Methods, and Professional Responsibilities

• Content Domains are listed horizontally: Kinesiology (Anatomy, Kinesiology, Biomechanics), Physiology, Nutrition and Weight Control, and Exercise Psychology

DOMAIN I: EXERCISE PROGRAMMING AND CLASS DESIGN   49%

Task 1

Construct a group fitness class of basic exercise components using appropriate movements, music, and/or equipment to promote the health and wellness of class participants.
(Chapters 6, 7, Appendix E & DVD)

Knowledge of:

1. Basic components of a class (e.g., warm-up, conditioning, cool-down, flexibility)
2. Music styles and tempos appropriate for

each class format or class component

3. Use and application of various group fitness–related equipment (e.g., steps, indoor cycles, free weights, elastic resistance, medicine balls, stability balls, balance-related tools)
4. Varied class formats (e.g., traditional high-impact/low-impact, step, kickboxing, indoor cycling, aquatic exercise, interval, circuit, muscular conditioning, sports conditioning, flexibility, mind-body activities)
5. Functional-training principles to improve the quality of life

Skill in:

1. Lesson planning to determine the content and sequence of various types of general group exercise classes
2. Demonstrating proper use of group fitness–related equipment
3. Integrating functional-training principles into a group fitness class setting

Task 2

Accommodate varied fitness levels of participants by applying general fitness principles (e.g., varying frequency, intensity, duration, mode, sets, reps) to provide safe and effective classes.
(Chapters 1, 6, 7 & Glossary)

Group Fitness Instructor Certification Exam Content Outline

Knowledge of:

1. Major health-related components of fitness including cardiovascular endurance, muscular strength, muscular endurance, flexibility, and body composition
2. The current and established guidelines for improving and maintaining cardiorespiratory endurance, muscular fitness, and flexibility with reference to mode of activity, intensity, duration, and frequency
3. Skill-related fitness components including balance, agility, speed, power, coordination, and reaction time

Skill in:

1. Adapting the health-related fitness components to accommodate various fitness levels within the class
2. Incorporating the skill-related fitness components, where appropriate
3. Manipulating various exercises, equipment, music, and approaches within any class format

Task 3

Incorporate progression in class design consistent with established standards and guidelines with variation in exercise selection, equipment, music, and approach to achieve fitness goals, reduce potential injury and attrition, and alleviate boredom.
(Chapters 7 & 8)

Knowledge of:

1. Methods to vary the exercises, equipment, music, and approach selected within a class format
2. The concepts of variety and progression as they relate to the prevention of injury and boredom

Skill in:

1. Varying the class in accordance with fitness principles

2. Varying music, exercise selection, equipment, and approach
3. Recognizing the need for progression
4. Implementing appropriate progression rates

Task 4

Accommodate the needs of special populations by recognizing their limitations and making appropriate exercise adaptations to provide safe and effective classes.
(Chapters 5, 6, 9 & 10)

Knowledge of:
General

1. General medical conditions such as diabetes, hypertension, heart disease, arthritis, osteoporosis, musculoskeletal disorders, respiratory disorders, obesity
2. How exercise impacts each of these medical conditions
3. Common physical disabilities

Older Adults:

1. Aging process and its impact on the cardiorespiratory, muscular, skeletal, metabolic, neurologic, thermoregulatory, and psychological systems
2. Health and medical concerns of mature adults and appropriate exercise selection and modifications for each
3. Appropriate music for older-adult classes

Youth:

1. Thermoregulation, anaerobic capacity, intensity monitoring, muscular conditioning, safety, and adult supervision
2. Importance of program design (e.g., programming, equipment, mechanics, adaptations, progression):
   (a) Gradual increase in exercise intensity
   (b) Improvement in adequate muscular strength and flexibility
   (c) Improvement in adequate cardiorespiratory function

(d) Proper body mechanics

(e) Appropriate equipment

(f) Short-term intermittent activity

Pregnant and Postpartum Participants:

1. American College of Obstetricians and Gynecologists (ACOG) recommendations for exercise during pregnancy and the postpartum period, as well as contraindications and warning signs requiring cessation of exercise

2. Risks associated with exercise during pregnancy that are related to musculoskeletal, cardiorespiratory, metabolic, and thermoregulatory processes

3. Appropriate method for monitoring intensity

Obesity:

1. Medical and physical problems specific to obesity, including cardiorespiratory, musculoskeletal, and thermoregulatory problems

2. Appropriate class modifications for obesity-related problems, including cardiorespiratory, musculoskeletal, and thermoregulatory changes

Skill in:

General:

1. Recognizing and understanding medical conditions that affect a participant's ability to exercise safely in class, such as diabetes, hypertension, heart disease, arthritis, osteoporosis, musculoskeletal disorders, asthma, chronic obstructive pulmonary disease, obesity

2. Integrating appropriate exercise for participants with medical conditions who have been cleared by a physician

3. Recognizing health problems that interfere with a participant's ability to exercise safely within a specific class format

Older Adults:

1. Recognizing changes associated with the aging process and the implications on exercise

2. Modifying class design based on American College of Sports Medicine (ACSM) guidelines (e.g., frequency, intensity, duration, mode, sets, reps)

3. Designing safe and effective classes that address the specific health and medical concerns of the older adult

Youth:

1. Recognizing special concerns related to teaching youth

2. Modifying the class based on established guidelines (e.g., frequency, intensity, duration, mode, sets, reps)

3. Using appropriate body mechanics and equipment

Pregnant and Postpartum Participants:

1. Modifying the class based on established ACOG guidelines (e.g., frequency, intensity, duration, mode, sets, reps).

2. Adapting class exercises and transitions to accommodate postural, weight, cardiorespiratory, and musculoskeletal changes

Obesity:

1. Recognizing special concerns related to teaching obese or overweight participants

2. Modifying class design based on American College of Sports Medicine (ACSM) guidelines (e.g., frequency, intensity, duration, mode, sets, reps)

3. Designing safe and effective classes that address the specific health and medical concerns of the obese or overweight client

Task 5

Adjust class design for various environmental conditions (e.g., cold, heat, humidity, altitude, acoustics, pollution) to ensure a safe and comfortable exercise

setting for all participants.
(Chapters 1 & 7)

Knowledge of:

1. Specific environmental factors as they relate to the safety of the class participants (e.g., cold, heat, humidity, altitude, acoustics, exercise surface, exercise area)
2. Physiological responses and adaptations that result from variations in environmental conditions
3. Recommendations and precautions for exercising in heat, cold, humidity, altitude, and pollution

Skill in:

1. Adapting class content and/or programming based on specific environmental conditions to maximize participants' safety
2. Adapting class formats relative to environmental conditions

DOMAIN II: GROUP INSTRUCTIONAL METHODS 31%

Task 1

Choose an appropriate and effective teaching method to accommodate various learning styles and cultural differences by analyzing the skills, interests, lifestyles, and preferences of the class participants.
(Chapter 7)

Knowledge of:

1. Teaching styles (e.g., command, practice, reciprocal, self-check, inclusion) appropriate for a group fitness class
2. Teaching strategies (e.g., slow-to-fast, repetition reduction, spatial, part-to-whole, simple-to-complex) used to facilitate participant

learning
3. Choreographic methods (e.g., freestyle vs. structured)
4. Domains and stages of learning
5. Various learning styles (e.g., visual, auditory, kinesthetic)

Skill in:

1. Using teaching styles (e.g., command, practice, reciprocal, self-check, inclusion) appropriate for a group fitness class
2. Selecting appropriate teaching strategies (e.g., slow-to-fast, repetition reduction, spatial, part-to-whole, simple-to-complex) to accommodate participant fitness and skill levels and class modality
3. Accommodating participants in the various stages of learning

Task 2

Monitor intensity using a variety of methods so that participants can exercise at the most appropriate levels for improving health and fitness.
(Chapters 1, 6, 7, 9, 10, & Appendix D)

Knowledge of:

1. Reasons for monitoring exercise intensity
2. Significance of resting, exercise, and recovery heart rates
3. Methods for monitoring exercise intensity: heart rate, talk test, Borg's rating of perceived exertion (RPE), dyspnea scale, and metabolic equivalents (METs)
4. Heart-rate response to various class components (warm-up, cardiovascular phase, muscular conditioning, and cool-down)
5. Applications and limitations in the calculations of target heart rate: percent of heart-rate reserve, age-predicted maximum heart rate, and measured maximum heart rate
6. Techniques, precautions, and limitations for monitoring heart rate

7. Precautions and limitations to monitoring heart-rate intensity (abnormal heart-rate responses, effects of medications, pregnancy and other special populations)

Skill in:

1. Implementing and explaining the procedures for monitoring heart-rate intensity (e.g., carotid and radial sites)
2. Using and explaining the talk test, RPE, and dyspnea scales as methods for monitoring exercise intensity
3. Modifying exercise intensity
4. Identifying signs and symptoms of over-exercising and making appropriate modifications
5. Selecting an appropriate intensity-monitoring method to accommodate special populations (e.g., pregnancy) and/or the effects of medications on heart-rate response

Task 3

Instruct participants using succinct and timely cues to prepare participants for the next movement and facilitate safe and effective exercise performance.
(Chapters 6 & 7)

Knowledge of:

1. Various types of verbal, visual, and kinesthetic cueing methods
2. When to cue an exercise
3. Appropriate use of music
4. Voice projection, vocal control, and how to avoid vocal stress
5. Appropriate volume levels needed for effective cueing and prevention of vocal stress

Skill in:

1. Using the various types of verbal and visual cueing methods effectively
2. Cueing exercises at the appropriate time
3. Stating cues in as few words as possible

4. Projecting the voice effectively
5. Using visual cues to accommodate special needs (language barriers, hearing impaired)
6. Cueing and teaching movement of exercise (e.g., 32-count phrase when applicable)

Task 4

Correct improper technique using appropriate strategies to prevent injury and/or improve performance of participants.
(Chapters 6 & 7)

Knowledge of:

1. Appropriate body alignment and posture for various exercises
2. How to apply effective instructional techniques for correcting technique and movements
3. Precautions when using touch to correct improper form

Skill in:

1. Executing exercises with proper form and technique
2. Identifying improper exercise form and technique
3. Providing cues to encourage participants to correct their form and exercise execution
4. Applying effective instructional techniques for error correction
5. Correcting improper exercise form and technique in a friendly manner
6. Reminding participants to use proper form and technique
7. Walking around the room to make appropriate corrections while maintaining class control

Task 5

Provide educational and motivational feedback using specific statements and demonstrations to maintain and improve

exercise performance.
(Chapters 2, 6, 7 & 8)

Knowledge of:

1. The types of feedback (e.g., corrective, value, and neutral statements)
2. Appropriate use of feedback (e.g., corrective, value, and neutral statements)
3. Components of effective feedback (e.g., informational rather than controlling, based on performance standards, specific and immediate)
4. Benefits of various exercises and how they improve the health- and skill-related components of fitness
5. Factors that affect participants' self-esteem and body image

Skill in:

1. Applying appropriate feedback based on participant skill, fitness level, and/or cultural background
2. Providing information regarding the benefits of various exercises and how they improve the health- and skill-related components of fitness
3. Using feedback to motivate participants and encourage adherence
4. Maintaining class control while providing individualized feedback
5. Using positive reinforcement to enhance participants' self-esteem and body image

Task 6

Provide exercise modifications to accommodate multiple fitness levels and special populations by demonstrating variations and options.
(Chapters 9 & 10)

Knowledge of:

1. The contraindications and musculoskeletal, cardiorespiratory, and metabolic

adaptations to exercise affecting participants who have been cleared by a physician or appropriate medical professional
2. Methods used to accommodate various fitness levels and populations within a class

Skill in:

1. Teaching multiple options for most exercises to accommodate various fitness levels and populations in the same class
2. Incorporating adaptations for various special populations (e.g., musculoskeletal, cardiovascular, respiratory, and metabolic conditions)
3. Modifying exercises for older adults, youth, pregnant and postpartum women, and obese participants

DOMAIN III: GROUP LEADERSHIP METHODS 14%

Task 1

Apply interpersonal skills by interacting with participants to build individual rapport, relationships, and adherence.
(Chapters 6, 7 & 8)

Knowledge of:

1. Communication techniques that enhance participant/instructor relationships (e.g., active listening, open-ended questioning, acknowledgement)
2. Participant-centered teaching approaches
3. Strategies to facilitate conflict resolution

Skill in:

1. Mirroring and matching
2. Establishing an atmosphere of trust
3. Establishing rapport (e.g., learning participant names, being accessible and approachable)
4. Identifying individual and group needs
5. Building group camaraderie

Group Fitness Instructor Certification Exam Content Outline

6. Recognizing and interpreting nonverbal communication
7. Addressing and alleviating class conflicts

Task 2

Facilitate a sense of belonging by building a comfortable exercise environment for class participants to encourage success.
(Chapters 6, 7 & 8)

Knowledge of:

1. Effective verbal and nonverbal communication methods
2. Verbal articulation and inflection to enhance the quality of the message (e.g., word emphasis, volume, speed of delivery)
3. Empathy and compassion
4. Various personality types
5. Various communication and learning styles

Skill in:

1. Observing and interpreting nonverbal communication
2. Listening effectively (e.g., use of minimal encouragement, reflecting, summarizing)
3. Using and maintaining eye contact to build relationships
4. Recognizing the special needs of participants

Task 3

Motivate participants to set realistic exercise goals and take ownership of their exercise experience to achieve optimal results and develop a lifelong exercise habit.
(Chapter 8)

Knowledge of:

1. Effective goal-setting techniques

2. Motivational strategies that engage participants with various skills, limitations, preferences, and expectations
3. Techniques to develop self-confidence and self-efficacy
4. Support systems to foster accountability and improve adherence
5. Potential barriers to exercise adherence

Skill in:

1. Selecting appropriate motivational techniques for desired outcomes
2. Selecting appropriate communication styles
3. Recognizing opportunities to create support systems within the class setting
4. Recognizing the special needs of participants
5. Providing tools to establish support systems outside of the class setting

Task 4

Educate participants about lifestyle, fitness, and health using credible resources for participants to achieve optimal results.
(Chapters 7, 8 & Glossary)

Knowledge of:

1. Current and relevant research material and information
2. Effective delivery systems for communicating
3. Basic behavior theory (e.g., health-belief model, stages of change)
4. Strategies for behavior modification

Skill in:

1. Recognizing appropriateness and timeliness of delivering educational material
2. Obtaining credible material and information for class participants

3. Identifying stages of learning (e.g., cognitive, associative, autonomous)

DOMAIN IV: PROFESSIONAL RESPONSIBILITIES   6%

Task 1

Adhere to applicable law and industry guidelines by maintaining a working knowledge of current principles and accepted professional practices to protect the interests of participants and minimize the risk of litigation.
(Chapters 6 & 12)

Knowledge of:

1. Assumption of risk, including risk assessment, waiver, and informed consent
2. Liability, including health screening, exercise recommendations, supervision, instruction, facilities, and equipment
3. Negligence, both contributory and comparative
4. Copyright law as it applies to music, print media, and film
5. Scope of practice
6. Standard of care
7. Employment status (e.g., independent contractor, employee)
8. Americans with Disabilities Act
9. Standards governing confidentiality
10. Important practices and behaviors when seeking employment (e.g., attire, audition procedures), subbing, and interacting with peers and participants

Skill in:

1. Completing an accident/injury report
2. Safeguarding confidential information
3. Following industry guidelines to minimize risk of injury and litigation (e.g., adequate warm-up and cool-down, recognizing potential hazards, providing proper instruction)

4. Behaving in a professional manner when auditioning, subbing, and interacting with peers and participants

Task 2

Adhere to the ACE Code of Ethics by upholding its principles consistently to protect the interests of participants, enhance consumer confidence in the industry, and maintain professional responsibilities.
(Appendices A & C)

Knowledge of:

1. American Council on Exercise Code of Ethics
2. Standards governing confidentiality
3. Establishing and maintaining clear professional boundaries
4. Upholding and enhancing public appreciation and trust for the health and fitness industry
5. Scope of practice
6. Current CPR, AED, and first-aid services
7. Fair and equal treatment for all clients
8. American Council on Exercise Professional Practices and Disciplinary Procedure

Skill in:

1. Providing safe and effective exercise instruction
2. Safeguarding confidential information
3. Mentoring and dispensing knowledge and training
4. Referring clients to more qualified fitness, medical, or health professionals when appropriate
5. Administering CPR and AED if accessible
6. Administering basic injury-management procedures

Task 3

Respond to acute medical conditions and injuries as they arise by implementing CPR, AED, and first aid, obtaining necessary assistance, and following documentation procedures to provide appropriate care and risk-management.
(Chapters 11, 12 & Appendix C)

Knowledge of:

1. CPR, AED, and basic first-aid procedures
2. Symptoms and types of musculoskeletal injuries
3. Factors associated with injury
4. Contraindications to exercise
5. Basic injury-management procedures (e.g., RICE: rest, ice, compression, elevation)
6. Facility risk-management and emergency protocols

Skill in:

1. Administering CPR and AED if accessible
2. Administering basic injury-management procedures

Task 4

Respond to emergencies as they arise by following established procedures and incident-reporting requirements to maximize participants' safety and manage risk.
(Chapters 11 & 12)

Knowledge of:

1. EMS activation
2. Risk-management implementation protocols
3. Facility-evacuation procedures

Skill in:

1. Completing an incident report
2. Leading the evacuation process of class participants in accordance with facility-evacuation procedures

Task 5

Protect clients and other interested parties by assessing insurance needs as they relate to group exercise instruction to minimize financial risk.
(Chapter 12)

Knowledge of:

1. Professional liability insurance
2. General liability insurance
3. Worker's compensation insurance
4. Health and disability insurance
5. Property insurance
6. Business interruption insurance

Task 6

Enhance professional competence through ongoing education in current research and exercise modalities to optimize group fitness instruction.
(Chapter 12)

Knowledge of:

1. Appropriate sources for acquiring continuing education offered by individuals, conferences, colleges, universities, seminars, workshops, etc.
2. Credible and current health and physical-activity information and research

Skill in:

1. Staying current with updated information and recommendations and applying them to teaching a class

CONTENT DOMAIN: APPLIED EXERCISE SCIENCE

The Group Fitness Instructor draws upon knowledge from four foundational sciences, which are included within a Content Domain called Applied Exercise Science.

Group Fitness Instructor Certification Exam Content Outline

These sciences are:

- Kinesiology (anatomy, kinesiology, biomechanics)
- Physiology
- Nutrition and weight control
- Exercise psychology

This Content Domain includes all topics important to the competence of Group Fitness Instructors and applies primarily to the following Performance Domains: Exercise Programming and Class Design, Group Instructional Methods, and Group Leadership Methods.

Kinesiology (Anatomy, Kinesiology, Biomechanics)
(Chapters 1, 2 & 3)
Knowledge of:
Anatomy

1. General anatomy and function of the following systems: cardiovascular, musculoskeletal, cardiorespiratory, and neuromuscular
2. Function of the different types of joints of the body
3. Anatomical terminology (e.g., landmarks, directional, planes of movement, position, muscle roles)
4. Major functions of the muscles (e.g., agonist, antagonist, stabilizer, assister)
5. Flow of blood through the heart

Knowledge of:
Kinesiology

1. Human movement as it relates to making decisions concerning the safety of participants
2. Strategies for identifying areas of weakness and designing exercise and providing feedback to encourage improvement
3. Range of motion of the hip, knee, and ankle; hip flexion; hip extension; and hyperextension for improved strength and flexibility
4. Proper postural alignment, including lordo-

sis, kyphosis, scoliosis, and hyperextension of the spine
5. Strategies for identifying abnormalities and neutral spine position
6. Prime movers in any given movement
7. Types of muscle contractions: isokinetic, isometric, isotonic (eccentric and concentric)
8. Principles of balance
9. Actions and application of major muscle groups of the upper extremity, lower extremity, and trunk
10. Factors affecting movement: neurological, proprioceptive, biomechanical, kinesthetic awareness
11. Difference between dorsiflexion and plantarflexion
12. Shoulder joint complex: scapulothoracic articulation, scapulohumeral rhythm
13. Concentric and eccentric movement
14. The term "winging" as it applies to the scapula
15. Scapular movements: elevation, depression, adduction, abduction, upward rotation, downward rotation
16. Relationship between joint mobility and muscular flexibility
17. Strategies for identifying participants with kinesthetic-awareness dysfunction

Knowledge of:
Biomechanics

1. Joint mobility (e.g., torque, force)
2. Appropriate exercises based on biomechanics
3. Risks associated with muscular-strength training, improper body mechanics, and lifting techniques that may result in acute and chronic overuse
4. Newton's Law as it relates to the analysis of human movement
5. Use of the laws of inertia, acceleration, and reaction as they apply to exercise

Physiology

(Chapter 1)

Knowledge of:

Basic and Applied Exercise Physiology

1. Components of physical fitness (e.g., muscular strength, muscular endurance, cardiorespiratory endurance, flexibility, body composition)

2. Cardiorespiratory terms as they apply to endurance training (e.g., cardiac output, stroke volume, heart rate, oxygen consumption, ventilation, respiration, aerobic capacity)

3. Principles of training as they apply to cardiorespiratory endurance (e.g., overload, specificity, reversibility, progression, training effect, adaptation)

4. Metabolic physiology, including anaerobic metabolism (e.g., phosphagen system, anaerobic glycolysis) and aerobic metabolism (e.g., aerobic glycolysis, fatty-acid oxidation)

5. Anaerobic and aerobic energy systems in terms of rate and amount of ATP produced, limitations, and major use during physical activity

6. Roles of carbohydrates, fats, and proteins used as fuel for energy production

7. Acute responses to aerobic exercise

8. Cardiovascular and cardiorespiratory systems with respect to oxygen-carrying capacity, delivery, and extraction

9. Benefits of aerobic exercise for healthy participants and those with chronic disease (e.g., type 2 diabetes, arthritis, pulmonary disease, coronary heart disease)

10. Terminology as it applies to muscular fitness: training effect, resistance, overload, specificity, repetitions, sets, frequency, rest periods, progression, muscular atrophy, and hypertrophy

11. Benefits of muscular strength and endurance

12. Training principles to improve muscular strength and endurance training

13. Definition of, and risks associated with, performing the Valsalva maneuver during resistance training

14. Characteristics of fast- and slow-twitch muscle fibers (e.g., ability to use anaerobic and aerobic pathways)

15. Neuromuscular system, including the basic organization of the nervous and muscular systems

16. Sliding filament theory of muscle contraction

17. Types of muscle contractions (e.g., isotonic, isometric, isokinetic)

18. Roles of the Golgi tendon organ and muscle spindle in the regulation of muscle contraction

19. Static, dynamic, ballistic, and proprioceptive neuromuscular facilitation (PNF) stretches and the risks and benefits associated with each

Nutrition and Weight Control

(Chapters 1, 4 & 5)

Knowledge of:

Nutrition

1. Function and types of carbohydrate, protein, and fat

2. Recommended percentage of calories from carbohydrate, protein, and fat in a balanced diet

3. Number of calories per gram in carbohydrate, protein, and fat

4. Current recommendations contained in the MyPyramid Food Guidance System

5. Current recommendations contained in the USDA's Dietary Guidelines for Americans

6. Dietary concerns for vegetarians

7. Specific functions and food sources of major vitamins and minerals

8. Function and food sources of antioxidants and phytochemicals
9. Function and food sources of fiber
10. Role of nutrition in various diseases (e.g., cardiovascular disease, hypertension, diabetes, cancer, osteoporosis, anemia)
11. Signs and symptoms of eating disorders (e.g., anorexia, bulimia, compulsive overeating)
12. Uses and potential hazards of supplements and ergogenic aids
13. Fitness instructor's scope of practice when discussing nutrition information and when to refer to a dietitian or other qualified healthcare professional
14. Recommended hydration guidelines
15. How to read a nutrition label

Knowledge of:
Weight Control
1. Energy balance and how to modify diet and exercise to affect weight
2. Number of calories in a pound of fat
3. How to calculate desired body weight based on current weight and lean-body-mass percentage
4. Safe and effective weight-loss methods
5. Recommended amount of weight loss per week for unsupervised, safe, and effective weight loss (lean-muscle gain per month and body-fat loss per month)
6. Metabolic terminology (e.g., kilocalories, caloric expenditure, caloric deficit, caloric intake, energy balance)
7. Definition of body mass index, its limitations, and how it is used to classify weight status
8. Extreme approaches to weight loss

Exercise Psychology
(Chapters 7 & 8)
Knowledge of:
1. Attributes of an ideal fitness instructor
2. Motivational techniques used to optimize exercise adherence and other healthy lifestyle behaviors
3. Factors that influence adherence (e.g., social factors, personal factors, program factors, environmental factors)
4. Principles of learning theory with respect to effective teaching in a group exercise setting
5. Theories of behavioral change (e.g., health belief model, stages of change)
6. Issues related to body image
7. Use of relaxation/visualization to enhance the exercise experience
8. Importance of delivery in communicating feedback to a participant

Appendix C

Effects of Medications on Heart-rate (HR) Response and Exercise Performance

Medications	Resting HR	Exercise HR	Exercise Performance	Comments
Beta-adrenergic blocking agents	↓*	↓	↑ in individuals with angina ↓ or ↔ in individuals without angina	Dose-related response
Diuretics	↔	↔	usually ↔	Can cause postexercise hypotension
Antihypertensives	↑, ↔, or ↓	↑, ↔, or ↓	usually ↔	Many antihypertensive medications are used. Some may decrease, a few may increase, and others do not affect heart rates. Some exhibit a dose-related response.
Calcium channel blockers	↑, ↔, or ↓	↑, ↔, or ↓	↑ in individuals with angina ↓ or ↔ in individuals without angina	Variable and dose-related responses
Antiarrythmic agents	↔	↔	↔	
Antilipemic agents (cholesterol medication)	↔	↔	↔	
Hypoglycemic agents (diabetes medication)	↔	↔	↔	Can cause postexercise hypoglycemia
Thyroid medications	↑	↑	↔	
Bronchodilators	↔	↔	usually ↔	An improvement in exercise capacity in individuals limited by bronchospasm
Cold medications: without sympathomimetic activity (SA)	↔	↔	↔	
with SA	↔ or ↑	↔ or ↑	↔	Magnitude of effects is usually mild or moderate

* Beta-blockers with intrinsic sympathomimetic activity only slightly lower resting heart rate.

Effects of Medications on Heart-rate (HR) Response and Exercise Performance

Medications	Resting HR	Exercise HR	Exercise Performance	Comments
Tranquilizers	◀▶ , or if anxiety-reducing may ▼	◀▶	◀▶	
Antidepressants and some antipsychotic medication	◀▶ or ▲	◀▶ or ▼	◀▶	
Alcohol	◀▶	◀▶	◀▶	Exercise prohibited while under the influence; effects of alcohol on coordination increase possibility of injuries
Antihystamines	◀▶	◀▶	◀▶	
Diet pills:				Discourage as a poor approach to weight loss; acceptable only with physician's written approval
with SA	▲ or ◀▶	▲ or ◀▶	◀▶	
containing amphetamines	▲	▲	◀▶	
without SA or amphetamines	◀▶	◀▶	◀▶	
Caffeine	◀▶ or ▲	◀▶ or ▲	◀▶ or ▲	Variable effects depending on history of use
Nicotine	◀▶ or ▼	◀▶ or ▼	▲ in individuals with angina ▼ or ◀▶ in individuals without angina	Discourage smoking; suggest lower target heart rate and exercise intensity for smokers

▲ = increase   ◀▶ = no significant change   ▼ = decrease

Note: Many medications are prescribed for conditions that do not require clearance. Do not forget other indicators of exercise intensity (e.g., participant's appearance, rating of perceived exertion). Also, consult the most current edition of the *Physician's Desk Reference* to obtain detailed information regarding a specific medication's actions and side effects.

Appendix D

Group Fitness Specialties

Traditional Aerobics

Following the publication of Dr. Kenneth Cooper's book *Aerobics* in 1968, movement forms reflecting a shared cultural value of health and fitness proliferated. Traditional aerobics was among these, tracing its early lineage to such pioneers as Jacki Sorensen, founder of Aerobic Dancing, Inc., and Judi Sheppard Missett, president of Jazzercise, Inc. These women and others adapted Dr. Cooper's concept of aerobic exercise to exercise classes with music, creating what became known as aerobic dance-exercise or, simply, aerobics. With the release of "Jane Fonda's Workout" video in 1982, the dissemination of traditional aerobics to a mass market via electronic media forever changed fitness culture worldwide.

Traditional aerobics continues to provide the form, methodology, and objectives upon which subsequent group fitness forms have been modeled. While the three primary types of traditional aerobics—high-impact, combination high-low impact, and low-impact—continue to appear on group fitness class schedules, many of these classes have taken on new forms to appeal to a wide range of participants. Hip hop and African dance classes, for example, are variations on a traditional aerobics class. Creative fitness professionals continue to come up with new ways to keep participants engaged in group exercise classes.

Benefits

The main benefits of traditional aerobics are improved cardiorespiratory endurance and body composition. In addition, the social interaction and sense of community that develops from frequent participation in a group exercise program promotes adherence and motivation.

The potential for freedom of movement is greater in traditional aerobics than many other modes of aerobic training. Only the anatomical limits of the body and the boundaries of the room dictate the form of the movement. Because traditional aerobics is a weightbearing activity, it has important implications for postural balance and bone mineral density. Individuals who participate in a high- or low-impact aerobics class are required to move quickly in many directions while keeping their balance intact. This promotes dynamic stability as the muscles work to stabilize the joints during movement in various planes, and has a high carryover to the activities of daily living. Bone mass is also positively affected by weightbearing exercise. Several research studies have reported that performing land-based, standing exercise increases participants' bone mineral density in the lumbar and hip regions. This benefit is increased significantly when exercisers add impact (e.g., hopping, jumping) to their programs. Furthermore, older adults who regularly participate in aerobic weightbearing exercise programs are less likely to fall due to loss of balance, thereby potentially reducing their risk of fractures.

Participant Suitability

Traditional aerobics classes are well-suited for individuals who enjoy choreography-based exercise and are fond of pacing their movements to rhythms in music. Historically, more women than men have participated in aerobics classes, possibly due to the classes' dance-like characteristics. However, both men and women can benefit from the cardiorespiratory-endurance and balance-training opportunities provided by this type of weightbearing, land-based exercise.

Individuals who are new to exercise, are overweight or obese, or who have certain joint injuries or chronic diseases may find an entire traditional aerobics class too difficult. Furthermore, individuals who are at risk for falling (e.g., seniors with osteoporosis, late-term pregnant women) should consult with their physicians prior to engaging in this type of activity. Individuals with health risks may find that modifying the choreography to include only low-impact moves allows them to safely enjoy a traditional aerobics class.

For more information on Traditional Aerobics:

Traditional Aerobics: ACE's Group Fitness Specialty Series

ACE's Traditional Aerobics and Step Training Online Learning Course

Step Training

Introduced in the late 1980s, step aerobics has become a staple in group exercise programming. Also called bench aerobics, step/bench training, and aerobic stepping, step training is a relatively low-impact exercise program that utilizes a platform ranging from 4 to 12 inches in height. Participants step up and down while performing a variety of movement skills and sequences to music and utilizing large muscle groups to tax the cardiovascular, respiratory, and muscular systems.

The physiological response to stepping up and down off a bench has been known for decades. Exercise physiologists in the early 20th century developed fitness tests based on the heart-rate response to repetitive stepping, such as the Harvard Step Test. Further step-

test protocols have been developed and validated in major universities for estimating physical work capacity and aerobic fitness. For example, Fred Kasch, Ph.D., of San Diego State University developed the Three-Minute Step Test, which is currently used by YMCAs for mass testing of participants. Stepping is also used in sports medicine rehabilitation, most specifically as a standard form of knee rehabilitation exercise. Stepping emphasizes conditioning the quadriceps muscles, which are important for knee stability, provides low injury potential to the recovering knee due to its low-impact nature, and is an ideal progressive exercise for knee rehabilitation because of its adjustability and control. It was the use of stepping in knee rehabilitation that ultimately led to its application in the fitness industry.

Step exercise evolved primarily out of a need for another type of challenging, interesting, and effective cardiovascular activity. Despite the advent of complex choreography and power step training, which utilizes hops and jumps to increase intensity, it is the relatively low-impact nature of the exercise that has largely contributed to the popularity of step training.

Benefits

Step training is a moderate- to high-intensity aerobic activity that effectively challenges the cardiorespiratory system. In a study at San Diego State University, testing on an 8-inch platform revealed that a class utilizing non-propulsive step patterns and arm movements averaged 7.7 METs, a value comparable to traditional hi/lo aerobic dance (Francis et al. 1992). Woodby-Brown, Berg, and Latin (1993) studied the oxygen cost of aerobic dance bench stepping and found that step has oxygen requirements similar to other forms of aerobic dance, providing appropriate intensity challenges for improving aerobic fitness. Stanforth, Stanforth, and Velasquez (1993) and Williford et al. (1998) also found step training to significantly improve aerobic capacity.

Several studies have evaluated the energy expenditure of step training to determine its usefulness in weight control. Scharff-Olson et al. (1991) studied step exercise and energy expenditure. It was determined that for participants desiring weight or fat loss, step exercise must be performed for longer than 20 minutes to expend the minimum 200 calories per session recommended by the American College of Sports Medicine (ACSM). Combining all factors, including step height, step rate, body weight, and step patterns, makes it difficult to determine the actual number of calories expended in a step-training session (Scharff-Olson & Williford, 1998).

Participant Suitability

Similar to traditional aerobics, step aerobics provides a choreography-based workout to music where the music sets the pace or stepping cadence for the class. Therefore, step training typically appeals to participants who enjoy following combinations and routines set to musical rhythms.

One of the greatest appeals of step training is its appropriateness for a variety of fitness levels. Many studies have demonstrated that step is easily modified according to fitness needs by adjusting step height (Scharff-Olson et al., 1991; Stanforth, Stanforth, & Velasquez, 1993). Participants at a beginning level can use the 4-inch step height. As they become familiar with stepping techniques and their fitness level improves, the height of the platform can be increased, demanding greater intensity. If step height adjustments are not appropriate, you can also increase step cadence to achieve greater intensity (Goss et al.,

1989; Darby, Browder, & Reeves, 1995). According to Reebok Step Training Guidelines, beginners are easily and appropriately challenged at music speeds of 118 to 122 bpm. Safe cadences of 122 to 128 bpm are acceptable for participants at intermediate to advanced fitness levels seeking greater aerobic challenges.

Although step training may be performed safely with low levels of impact, individuals with health risks, such as obesity, low-back pain, or arthritis of the hips and knees, may find a step training class too difficult. Similar to traditional aerobics classes, individuals who are at risk for falling should consult with their physicians prior to engaging in this type of activity. Modifications to the choreography that allow all of the step movements to be performed on the floor without using the step may be an option for participants with health risks to be able to safely enjoy a step training class.

References

Darby, L., Browder, K., & Reeves, B. (1995). The effects of cadence, impact, and step on physiological responses to aerobic dance exercise. *Research Quarterly for Exercise and Sport, 66,* 231–238.

Francis, P. et al. (1992). Effects of choreography, step height, fatigue and gender on metabolic cost of step training (Abstract). *Medicine & Science in Sports & Exercise, 23* (S839).

Goss, F. et al. (1989). Energy cost of bench stepping and pumping light handweights in trained subjects. *Research Quarterly for Exercise and Sport, 60,* 369–372.

Scharff-Olson, M. & Williford, H. (1998). Step aerobics fulfills its promise. *ACSM's Health and Fitness Journal, 2,* 32–37.

Scharff-Olson, M. et al. (1991). The cardiovascular and metabolic effects of bench stepping exercise in females. *Medicine & Science in Sports & Exercise, 23,* 1311–1316.

Stanforth, D., Stanforth, P., & Velasquez, K. (1993). Aerobic requirement of bench stepping. *International Journal of Sports Medicine, 14,* 129–133.

Group Fitness Specialities

Williford, H. et al. (1998). Bench stepping and running in women. *The Journal of Sports Medicine and Physical Fitness, 38,* 221–226.

Woodby-Brown, S., Berg, K., & Latin, W. (1993). Oxygen cost of aerobic dance bench stepping at three heights. *Journal of Strength and Conditioning Research, 7,* 163–167.

For more information on Step Training:

Step Training: ACE's Group Fitness Specialty Series

ACE's Traditional Aerobics and Step Training Online Learning Course

Kickboxing Fitness

Kickboxing is a cardiovascular workout that uses the hands, feet, knees, and elbows, and mimics kickboxing training to obtain health and fitness benefits. Workouts based on boxing and kickboxing entered the mainstream in the late 1990s and appeal equally to men and women. Today, most health clubs and martial arts schools offer some type of boxing or kickboxing classes.

Equipment-based Workouts

Equipment-based workouts are designed to allow participants to spend a defined amount of time performing kickboxing skills using the heavy bag, punching mitts, kicking pads, speed bags, and/or jump rope, and may be made up of several components. Following a general warm-up, for instance, you may spend 10 to 15 minutes leading participants through basic footwork, punches, kicks, and combinations before moving to performance drills using equipment. The participants may then work together performing the drills for two or three work periods and then be assigned another skill.

It is expected that participants in equipment-based workouts will naturally experience accidental contact. For example, when teaching defensive drills, you may assign participants to work in pairs, with one throwing slow-speed punches while the other practices slipping. Participants may react slowly or move in the wrong direction and occasionally be tapped with a glove on the chin or forehead. Although contact may be slow and controlled, you must still supervise these types of exercises. Participants should never be allowed to perform any sparring. It increases the liability of risk and is clearly outside the scope of practice for a fitness professional.

Workouts may also be structured as circuits, where stations are set up in a circle or row and participants rotate between pieces of equipment. Stations may include exercises for strength, flexibility, and conditioning. If equipment is limited, arrange for participants to alternate between equipment stations and non-equipment stations or work in pairs.

Non-equipment-based Workouts

Non-equipment-based workouts mirror a traditional aerobics class in that the instructor leads participants through a warm-up and specific boxing and/or kickboxing skills designed to elicit a certain intensity. Movements and combinations are typically based on 32-count phrasing. One punch is typically performed every two counts and a kick is usually performed every two or four counts. Higher-intensity combinations may be performed at a faster tempo of one count (punches) or two counts (punches and/or kicks) for brief work periods.

Benefits

Research continues to support the efficacy of martial arts and kickboxing training as means of improving fitness and health. A 1997 study (Bellinger et al.) found that a 60-minute boxing training session (without kicking) was equivalent in energy expenditure to running about 5.6 mph (9 kph) for 60 minutes on the treadmill. In 1999, the American Council on Exercise (ACE) investigated the physiological effects and benefits of kickboxing (American Council on Exercise, 1999). The researchers found that the activity provides a workout sufficient to improve and maintain cardiovascular fitness, and noted some additional benefits, such as increased strength and flexibility, improved coordination, and sharper reflexes. Jumping rope may also be an integral part of kickboxing training, and its benefits have been acknowledged in several studies. Jumping rope develops neuromuscular skills, muscular strength, and cardiovascular endurance, and thus is an excellent complement to kickboxing training. Furthermore, regular participation in weightbearing activities that provide impact, such as jumping rope and some of the movements performed in kickboxing, have been shown to improve bone mineral density.

Participant Suitability

Kickboxing fitness classes are enjoyed by various types of individuals for different reasons. Typically, kickboxing fitness classes are performed to music. However, the pacing of the movements may or may not be influenced by the beats and rhythms of the music. For example, a non-equipment-based workout may resemble a traditional aerobics class with choreography matched to the music, whereas an equipment-based workout may consist of participants moving through circuit-training stations with music being played in the background for enjoyment. This range in styles of kickboxing workouts ensures that most exercise participants can find a class that suits their needs. That is, participants who enjoy structured choreography programmed to music may enjoy the non-equipment-based workout and individuals who prefer a more athletic, non-choreographed routine may feel more comfortable in an equipment-based class.

Individuals with health risks, such as obesity, low-back pain, or arthritis, may find kickboxing fitness classes too difficult. Similar to traditional aerobics classes, individuals who are at risk for falling should consult with their physicians prior to engaging in this type of activity. Modifications to the exercises that limit the impact and speed of the movements may be appropriate for some special populations. In addition, participants who are inflexible may need to limit the range of motion of certain kickboxing moves (e.g., front kick, side kick, roundhouse kick).

References

American Council on Exercise (1999). Cardio kickboxing packs a punch. *ACE FitnessMatters,* 5, 4, 4–5.

Bellinger, B. et al. (1997). Energy expenditure of a non-contact boxing training session compared with submaximal treadmill running. *Medicine & Science in Sports & Exercise,* 29, 12, 1653–1656.

For more information on Kickboxing Fitness:

Kickboxing Fitness: A Guide for Fitness Professionals from the American Council on Exercise

ACE's Kickboxing Fitness Correspondence Course

Group Fitness Specialities

Group Indoor Cycling

Group indoor cycling has evolved into a fitness phenomenon. In the mid-1980s, Johnny Goldberg, who is better known as Johnny G, partnered with Schwinn® to create Spinning® and develop a bike specifically for the program. This program was introduced to the fitness industry in 1995 and focuses on visualizing an outdoor ride, complete with wind, hills, and butterflies. The primary goal of Johnny G's program is empowerment. One year later, both Keiser and Reebok developed their own programs.

Both outdoor and indoor cycling activity has increased dramatically in recent years. More and more participants are training indoors with a commitment to stay in shape and perfect their cycling techniques. In addition, there are individuals who prefer to train aerobically without adding stress to their joints, and indoor cycling fits this need. Indoor cycling programs can be adapted for a variety of populations and are currently being used successfully for individuals with spinal cord injuries, arthritis, and cerebral palsy, and as rehabilitation following surgery.

Benefits

Cycling is an excellent cardiorespiratory activity and a good alternative for those who do not like to jog or run, or who have orthopedic limitations to weightbearing exercise.

The many physical benefits of indoor cycling include improved cardiorespiratory endurance, an increase in muscular strength and endurance, and a decrease of body fat and increase of lean body mass. It is also a great weight-management tool when used in conjunction with a well-balanced diet. Psychological benefits include stress relief, an increase in beta-endorphins, and the enjoyment drawn from participating in a fun, social activity.

In addition to convenience, another advantage of indoor cycling is its relative safety, which can lead to a more intense workout. Distractions are minimized, allowing participants to focus on maximizing or maintaining heart rate for the session without worrying about cars, potholes, and other road hazards. The workout can also be more precise, since participants can lend more focus to the program.

There are a number of additional benefits to the indoor cycling format. Participants improve pedal stroke action by focusing on a smooth and complete pedal cycle on each leg independently. Also, participants achieve personalized workouts within a group setting by modifying resistance, cadence, and body position. Indoor cycling may also be used for recovery. By working at a lower intensity, riders enhance venous return and speed up lactic acid clearance from the muscle and diminish post-training stiffness and soreness.

Participant Suitability

Group cycling classes are generally suitable for participants of varying fitness levels and for those with health risks because this format is nonimpact, nonweightbearing, and the participants have complete control over the amount of resistance, and thus intensity, used during the workout. As with any mode of exercise, an extended warm-up and cool-down and intensity modification may be necessary for participants with special needs.

Participants who have some experience training on a cycle (indoor or outdoor) usually have an easier transition into a group indoor cycling class. Experienced cyclists are accustomed to the flexed-forward spinal posture and hand-gripping techniques used in most indoor cycling classes. Individuals who are new to cycle exercise, however, may need to incorporate several modifications to the riding technique until they become more comfortable on the bike. For example, it is recommended that novice riders adjust the handle bars so that they are slightly higher than the seat, take frequent postural breaks (i.e., sit upright in the saddle during class), and use a preferred cycling cadence instead of focusing on pedaling as fast as possible.

While not an absolute necessity, participants often choose to invest in specialized shoes that attach to the pedals to enhance their in-class cycling experience. Most cyclists use clipless pedals that allow the foot to "float" a few degrees inward or outward on the pedal as it moves through the pedal cycle. Research has shown that these pedal systems put less strain on the knees and allow a more natural pedaling motion. The floating-pedal systems allow the tibia to move in and rotate as riders push down on the pedal. In a fixed-pedal system, the knee and its ligaments absorb much of this rotation, which can potentially cause knee problems (Burke, 1995). In addition, cycling shorts and/or seat pads may be purchased to decrease the discomfort often experienced by participants new to training on a cycle. Participants who see the value in purchasing the accessories that accompany training on an indoor cycle may be more likely to adhere to the program.

Reference

Burke, E. (1995). *Serious Cycling*. Champaign, Ill.: Human Kinetics.

For more information on Group Indoor Cycling:

Group Indoor Cycling: ACE's Group Fitness Specialty Series

Aquatic Exercise

Aquatic exercise is one of the most adaptable and versatile exercise training modalities. Water's natural resistance allows for a healthy, balanced workout with little risk of injury, while its buoyancy allows for minimal impact on joints. Because of water's myriad other properties, the aquatic environment provides a unique opportunity for participants to develop both physical and motor fitness, along with a variety of skills that aid movement on land. It is not surprising, then, that aquatic exercise participation is at an all-time high for both trained and untrained exercisers.

Aquatic fitness instructors have a multitude of options when it comes to teaching methods and formats and choosing equipment for their participants. Instructors may choose to teach from the deck, in the water, or a combination of both. Several different aquatic exercise formats have been successfully established (e.g., circuit, interval, aquatic step, water tai chi). A variety of aquatic exercise equipment makes the possibility of exercise progression in the water a more realistic task. For example, instructors can choose from different pieces of equipment that provide balance, resistance, traction, safety, comfort, warmth, buoyancy, drag, cardiovascular work, sports training, and functional training.

Benefits

Aquatic exercise is unique in that it can provide training effects in all of the recommended fitness components (cardiorespiratory conditioning, muscular strength and endurance, and flexibility) with minimal risk of injury for exercisers of all ages and fitness levels. Because of water's versatility and safety, due mostly to its physical properties, water provides an ideal training medium for healthy fitness enthusiasts, competitive athletes, older adults, sedentary individuals, prenatal women, people recovering from injury or surgery, or those with chronic medical conditions such as arthritis or low-back pain.

One of the key benefits of water is injury prevention. Depending on water depth, the body is significantly less weightbearing in water than on land. Bearing less weight reduces joint stress and allows for full range of motion, while also allowing for greater overall intensity because of the water's resistance. Additionally, since buoyancy offsets the effects of gravity, participants can move unrestrained without fear of falling. Athletes can continue training in the cushioning environment of the water and maintain performance, while reducing the risk of injury from impact forces.

Another key benefit to aquatic exercise is progression. Properly using the properties of water (e.g., buoyancy, surface area, drag) allows exercisers to cater their workouts to their individual needs. Aquatic exercise involves progressive resistance by allowing for training in multiple ranges of motion and with uninterrupted overload. Because of water's properties, an exerciser can instantly alter a movement, such as increasing or decreasing movement speed, to adjust intensity.

Aquatic exercise provides a wide variety of additional benefits. It promotes postural stability and enhances balance, due to the effects of water currents on trunk musculature. Performing exercise in heart-to-neck-level water strengthens respiratory musculature, due to the effects of hydrostatic pressure on the lungs. Water also provides a somewhat private, less-intimidating exercise environment for certain special populations, as being submerged allows them to feel comfortable while exercising, rather than feeling as though they are on display.

Participant Suitability

During the past decade, numerous research studies have shown without question the value and versatility of aquatic fitness as an exercise modality. Its widespread and growing popularity among exercisers of all levels, ages, and abilities simply validates these research outcomes.

The benefits of water therapy for rehabilitation have long been known (Koury, 1996). The properties of water, such as buoyancy, help prevent injuries because of reduced impact (Sanders, 1999). Further, hydrostatic pressure reduces tissue swelling and blood pooling in the extremities during exercise, and increases metabolic waste product excretion (Becker & Cole, 1997).

Training in the water has also been shown to improve performance of activities of daily living (ADL) for a variety of populations. Sufferers of chronic back pain who undergo therapeutic aquatic exercise programs experience reduced pain and improved ADL performance (Landgridge & Phillips, 1988). Studies that looked at joint motion and ADL performance for persons with arthritis and rheumatic diseases also reported decreased pain and increased range of motion after water-therapy exercise programs.

Results have been just as positive in healthy (nondiseased or injured) older adults who gained functional postural mobility through aquatic exercise. An aquatic exercise study conducted through the Sanford Center on Aging at the University of Nevada, Reno evaluated ADL performance in older adults (Sanders, Constantino, & Rippee, 1997). The authors found that water training significantly improved functional abilities, increased muscle strength and flexibility, decreased body fat, and improved self-esteem.

References

Becker, B. & Cole, A.J. (1997). *Comprehensive Aquatic Therapy.* Boston, Mass.: Butterworth-Heinemann.

Landgridge, J. & Phillips, D. (1988). Group hydrotherapy exercises for chronic back pain sufferers. *Physiotherapy, 74,* 269–273.

Koury, J. (1996). *Aquatic Therapy Programming Guidelines for Orthopedic Rehabilitation.* Champaign, Ill.: Human Kinetics.

Sanders, M.E. (1999). Cross over to the water. *IDEA Health & Fitness Source,* March, 53–58.

Sanders, M., Constantino, N., & Rippee, N. (1997). A comparison of results of functional water training on field and laboratory measures in older women. *Medicine & Science in Sports & Exercise, 29,* ixx.

For more information on Aquatic Exercise:

Aquatic Exercise: ACE's Group Fitness Specialty Series

ACE's Aquatic Exercise Online Learning Course

Fitness Yoga

Yoga as an exercise activity has become a permanent fixture in the fitness arena. Long recognized as an effective stress-management technique and a great way to improve flexibility, yoga has more recently become known for what it can do for building strength and stamina. Yoga classes are now a standard feature of class schedules in gyms, health clubs, and spas.

Yoga, however, is much more than another form of exercise. It is part of an extensive ancient East Indian philosophical tradition. What is referred to as "yoga"—the exercise activity—is really hatha yoga, the physical aspect of this philosophy. There are many different ways in which hatha may be practiced. Guidelines govern the practice and reflect the basic principles of yoga, regardless of style. It takes education, maturity, and experience to teach yoga safely and effectively.

Hatha yoga, initially created to prepare the body for meditation, includes exercises designed to strengthen the body and nervous system, thereby creating the appropriate psychophysiological state for a higher level of consciousness. The repertoire consists of postures, movements, breathing, and relaxation techniques that affect every system of the body, bringing about an optimal state of health and well-being. You will undoubtedly encounter questions regarding yoga's religious and spiritual components. When you do, stress that yoga is not a religion. However, its philosophy has been embraced by religious traditions in India and elsewhere.

Yoga's current status reflects the growing interest in the mind-body connection. Continuing research in both the medical and fitness communities supports the important role the mind plays in promoting wellness, reducing stress, and combating disease. Yoga techniques provide both a blueprint for stress management and a system for physical fitness. There is also a therapeutic aspect to the practice of yoga. This area deals with specific breathing techniques, poses, and meditations to remedy various structural, physiological, and psychological conditions.

Whereas fitness experts once paid little attention to what yoga had to offer, leaders in the field now recognize its value as a viable fitness choice. While not all styles of hatha cover all the essential facets of a fitness regimen—aerobic, strength, and flexibility training—many do. At the very least, hatha yoga can provide a balanced strength and flexibility workout that can be supplemented with a cardiovascular routine.

Styles of Hatha Yoga

As indicated earlier, there are many different styles, or systems, of hatha practice. Some are vigorous and intense while others are gentle and more meditative. While yoga itself is a very ancient practice, most of the hatha systems practiced today have been refined and developed in the twentieth century. You should be aware of newly emerging hybrids of these systems, developed by teachers interested in creating their own variations on these traditional forms. Many yoga teachers teach in eclectic styles, having been influenced by a number of methods. Hatha has proven to be a practice that continues to change and evolve with the times, while remaining true to the essential principles of the philosophy. Physical health and fitness level and personal goals will determine which style is best for the individual. The following list describes the styles most commonly practiced today.

Ananda: This gentle and meditative approach developed by Swami Kriyananda places emphasis on deeply relaxing into the poses along with the use of affirmations, with the view that hatha's ultimate purpose is to heighten self-awareness.

Ashtanga: This is an intense and vigorous system developed by K. Pattabhi Jois that is characterized by equal emphasis on strength, flexibility, balance, and stamina. A modified version of this system is taught and often called "power yoga."

Bikram: Developed by Bikram Choudhury, this intense routine consists of 26 postures, including many standing single-leg balances, and begins and ends with a pranayama, or breath awareness, technique. The focus of this style is to detoxify the system and to warm up the muscles, allowing for maximum mastery of the poses. Therefore, teachers often use a humidifier and set the thermostat at 90° F (27° C) or higher for this practice.

Integral: This system was developed by Swami Satchidananda and reflects the teachings of Swami Sivananda. This method promotes the integration of yoga principles into lifestyle and thought, with the advice to be "easeful, peaceful, and useful."

Iyengar: A precise and detailed system developed by B.K.S. Iyengar, this style emphasizes correct postural alignment and proper body mechanics. The use of props and therapeutic applications are also characteristic of this style.

Kripalu: An internally directed approach developed by Yogi Amrit Desai, Kripalu is characterized by focusing on the breath and monitoring of the physical, mental, and emotional effects of the practice. Intensity ranges from gentle to vigorous.

Kundalini: A moderate-to-intense practice developed by Yogi Bhajan, this style focuses on the activation of the kundalini (serpent power) energy, believed to be stored at the base of the spine. Many breathing techniques are employed, along with poses and meditation, to facilitate the release of this energy.

Sivananda: This is a five-point method of practice that includes proper exercise, breathing, deep relaxation, vegetarian diet, and positive thinking through meditation. Swami Sivananda's system was popularized by Swami Vishnu-devananda and follows a standard format that includes breathing techniques, Sun Salutations, 12 yoga postures, relaxation, and chanting and prayers at the beginning and end of each class.

Viniyoga: Developed by T.K.V. Desikachar, this style employs a step-by-step approach (vinyasa krama) and emphasizes the use of the breath during asana practice. Another characteristic of this technique is the focus on tailoring the practice to the individual. Teachers of this system often design therapeutic applications.

Benefits

Yoga offers many benefits. While the ultimate goal of this age-old philosophy is to realize your divine nature, the positive effects on physical health and mental well-being are impressive. Hatha yoga's methodology dictates a balance between effort and relaxation and positively influences every system of the body. The repertoire includes poses for strength, flexibility, and balance. Some styles even include a cardiovascular component. The breathing techniques in yoga improve respiration while producing a cognitive quiescence, or "mental stillness," and an associated decrease in central nervous system activity. In fact, the breathing and meditative techniques of yoga, long known as effective stress- and pain-management tools, have been employed by Western physicians and therapists for a good portion of the 20th century. Many modern-day methods such as biofeedback and Dr. Herbert Benson's Relaxation Response (Benson, 1976) are patterned after these techniques. In addition to promoting strength and flexibility, it is believed that yoga can promote healing if practiced under supervision in a controlled fashion.

Participant Suitability

As noted previously, the health and fitness benefits of yoga are well established, making this mode of exercise appealing to individuals of various fitness levels and abilities. Background music and dim lighting may be used to create an atmosphere of peace and mind-body-connection enhancement. Specific poses and breathing techniques are thought to prevent or even remedy many physical and mental conditions. Similarly, there are poses and techniques that are contraindicated for specific health issues. The following are the most common contraindications:

Menstruation

Back bends, certain standing postures, and inverted postures, such as head, hand, and shoulder stands, are discouraged for women during menstruation. However, for women with menstrual discomfort, forward bends and relaxation techniques may be effective at thwarting symptoms.

Pregnancy

Pregnant women should avoid inverted postures and holding of the breath during yoga practice. Additionally, abdominal contractions, such as the stomach lift, are prohibited for a woman during pregnancy. After obtaining the appropriate training and experience, many yoga instructors specialize in prenatal yoga instruction.

Sciatica

Extreme flexion and intense hamstring-stretching poses should be avoided by individuals with sciatica. Back-extension poses, such as the cobra, may be more suitable for participants diagnosed with sciatica or who have with sciatica-type symptoms.

Hypertension, Glaucoma, Eye Problems, and Ear Congestion

Holding of the breath, inverted poses, or prolonged standing forward bends should be avoided by individuals with these conditions. A practice that promotes relaxation is more appropriate for participants with these health limitations.

High-risk Postures

Controversial poses, such as the shoulder stand, plow, headstand, and back bend, should be taught only by an experienced instructor who understands the precise biomechanical benefits and limitations of each posture. Generally, instructors who teach fitness-based yoga should stick to modifications of these postures to ensure the safety of their participants and reduce their risk of liability.

Reference

Benson, H. (1976). *The Relaxation Response.* New York: Avon Books.

For more information on Fitness Yoga:

Fitness Yoga: A Guide for Fitness Professionals from the American Council on Exercise

ACE's Fitness Yoga Correspondence Course

Pilates Mat Training

Joseph Hubertus Pilates created the Pilates method of exercise at the beginning of the 20th century. Born in 1880 near Düsseldorf, Germany, Pilates suffered a sickly childhood with asthma, rickets, and rheumatic fever. To improve his health as a youth, he turned to physical training and pursued diving, skiing, gymnastics, boxing, and bodybuilding. By age 14, his physique was so well developed that he worked as a model for anatomical charts. He pursued a varied career as a boxer, fitness trainer, and circus performer, among other activities.

In 1912, Pilates moved to England, where he had many jobs, including self-defense instructor to detectives at Scotland Yard. When World War I erupted, the British government labeled Pilates as an enemy alien and placed him in an internment camp. While imprisoned, he provided exercise training to other internees and worked in a hospital to help bedridden patients. He used his time to develop physical-conditioning methods to rehabilitate these patients and created training equipment from hospital beds, using springs to facilitate exercise. These inventions formed the basis for the now popular reformer, which still resembles a cot, and for the trapeze table, sometimes called the "Cadillac," which looks like a table with hanging springs and bars. In 1926, Pilates immigrated to New York and opened a training studio with his wife, Clara, whom he met on the ship as he traveled to America. The Pilates' clientele included many prominent ballet and modern dancers of the era. Today, Pilates exercises remain a staple of dance conditioning.

In 2001, the Pilates Method Alliance (PMA) was founded by Kevin A. Bowen and Colleen Glenn as a nonprofit, unbiased information resource dedicated to the teachings of Joseph H. and Clara Pilates. Unlike other organizations that offer instructor training and certification programs, the PMA is a separate body with an organizational mission to protect the public by establishing certification and continuing education standards for Pilates professionals. The PMA has created a national certification test for the Pilates method.

The many variations of Pilates are united by their common foundation and adherence to the basic principles of Pilates. Due to similarities between Pilates and yoga, fusion-styled classes that blend Pilates exercises with hatha yoga postures are becoming increasingly popular. While these two disciplines are distinct, both yoga and Pilates have much to offer consumers on both a physical and mental level, because they not only offer physical-conditioning benefits, but also require mental concentration that enhances the mind-body connection.

Benefits

The regular practice of Pilates mat exercise offers the following benefits for apparently healthy participants, in addition to improvements in overall strength, flexibility, stability, and mobility:

- Improved posture
- Stronger abdominal and back muscles
- Stronger pelvic and shoulder stabilizer muscles
- Balanced muscle development
- Improved breathing
- Better coordination and balance
- Reduced likelihood of back pain or injury
- Enhanced confidence and self-esteem
- Enhanced mind-body connection
- Enhanced athletic performance

Practicing Pilates provides these benefits because the exercises combine the use of the core musculature to stabilize the torso with rhythmic, coordinated movements accompanied by deep breathing. Precise attention to detail and form creates a stronger core and more efficient movement habits. This translates into better posture and more effective movement mechanics in both functional activities and in sports. In addition, imbalances in muscular development immediately become apparent and can be corrected by performing the exercises regularly and by progressing the level of difficulty over time.

Participant Suitability

The various difficulty levels and class formats available to consumers make Pilates mat classes an appropriate mode of exercise for any individual who is comfortable in a group fitness setting. Class size is typically limited so that participants can receive focused attention from the instructor. In addition, knowledgeable and experienced instructors can provide modifications to the exercises to accommodate participants with special needs or health limitations.

With Pilates mat exercises, as with any exercise program, there is always a risk of injury. For this reason, it is important that fitness professionals ensure that adequate prescreening has been conducted in accordance with industry standards and guidelines and that medical clearances are obtained as necessary. In particular, because Pilates mat exercises involve spinal flexion, rotation, and extension, there is a higher risk of injury for individuals with orthopedic problems. In addition, certain Pilates exercises include high-risk hatha yoga poses such as the plow and the shoulder stand that should not be taught unless the instructor is highly experienced and trained and the participants are ready and individually supervised.

Although Pilates is widely accepted in rehabilitation, trainers should not provide any training services beyond the appropriate scope of practice as defined by their specific training, certification, or licensure. As with all forms of exercise, fitness professionals should always consider the safety of the participant first, and only offer instructional services that are based on solid and in-depth training. Fitness professionals should not teach any movements without a complete understanding of the benefits and risks and of the necessary modifications for people with different body types and needs.

For more information on Pilates:

Pilates Mat Training: A Guide for Fitness Professionals from the American Council on Exercise

ACE's Pilates Mat Training Correspondence Course

Stability Ball Training

Known by many names, from Swiss Ball to Gymnastic Ball to Physioball, the "stability ball" is a large, inflated vinyl rubber ball that comes in a variety of sizes, colors, and even shapes. Its most common use is, not surprisingly, in the area of balance training, with advocates continually promoting core musculature stabilization. In addition, the stability ball is a valuable exercise tool that offers cardiovascular, muscle strength, muscle endurance, and flexibility training for the entire body. Most importantly, this is an exercise prop that is both challenging and fun, offering options to exercisers of virtually all skill and ability levels.

Contrary to what many fitness professionals might think, the stability ball is not a new invention. In fact, use of the ball began in the physical therapy arena more than 90 years ago. The stability ball was first used by Dr. Susanne Klein-Vogelbach in Switzerland in 1909, where it came to be known as the Swiss Ball. Dr. Klein-Vogelbach introduced the Swiss Ball in her physical therapy work with children with cerebral palsy, helping them to maintain reflex response as well as improve their balance. Recognizing the value of the ball, the physical therapy community used it in the treatment of neurological and orthopedic disorders as well as spinal injuries. The ball made

its appearance in the United States in the late 1970s and early 1980s, where it continued to be used as an exercise, balance, and therapy aid in the medical rehab arena, primarily by physical therapists. It is only in the past 10 to 15 years that the stability ball made the transition to the fitness industry.

In 1992, Mike and Stephanie Morris developed a total-body fitness-training program around the ball and are credited by many as having led the way for use of the stability ball in both the group exercise and personal training fields. Their Resist-A-Ball® program introduced this unique piece of exercise equipment, along with an extensive educational program, to the mainstream health and fitness market. Since then, the stability ball has become a staple in fitness facilities across the country and, indeed, around the world. In fact, teachers of different disciplines, such as Pilates and yoga, frequently incorporate the use of stability balls into their exercise programming. A variety of different resources, including books, videos, and fitness professional training programs and seminars, have been developed. Since that time, many other fitness professionals have been instrumental in bringing stability ball exercise into the traditional fitness and performance-training arenas.

Benefits

The stability ball is perhaps the most versatile piece of equipment currently available, as it utilizes the neuromuscular system in a way that most other exercise equipment does not, requiring the integrated involvement of strength, flexibility, and balance. Ball exercises are designed primarily to enhance the exerciser's ability to move the body without restrictions and to perform functional movements necessary to meet the needs and challenges of daily life. Regular use of the stability ball can give users an improved quality of life as they develop the strength, flexibility, and balance to work and play without movement limitations.

One of the greatest benefits of stability ball usage is improved balance. The ball challenges the individual to develop the ability to continually balance and focuses effort on the core stabilizer muscles (the abdominals, low back, and hips/pelvis), regardless of the movement being performed. To train on the ball requires balance and motor control, both of which will improve through regular use of the ball. Exercises can be designed to work solely on balance, while other exercises can work on strengthening and/or stretching practically any muscle group in the body. The best feature of the ball is that while strength or flexibility work is being performed, balance work is taking place simultaneously. No muscle or muscle group can be targeted in isolation to the exclusion of the stabilizing muscles that balance the body. This time-efficient training feature makes stability ball exercises challenging and beneficial to users of all skill and ability levels.

Probably the most publicized and well-known benefit of stability ball training is that the balls allow exercisers to train and develop strength and tone of the trunk musculature, particularly the abdominals. A study conducted by researchers at San Diego State University used electromyography (EMG) equipment to examine muscle activity in 13 common abdominal exercises. Crunches on the stability ball ranked third overall in abdominal muscle activity. However, there was less activity in the hip flexor muscles during ball crunches than the bicycle maneuver and the Captain's Chair exercise, which were ranked number one

and two in the study, respectively. As hip flexion during abdominal work indicates that the exercise does not isolate the abdominals preferentially, researchers concluded that crunches on the stability ball arguably are the most effective abdominal exercise overall (American Council on Exercise, 2001). It is no wonder then that stability balls are a top pick for home exercise equipment, due to their low cost, high level of effectiveness, and versatility.

Another benefit of the ball is its demand for any movement to be performed with correct posture. Proper posture with neutral spinal alignment is a necessity as the stabilizer muscles of the core work to balance the body on the ball. Regular use of the stability ball improves spinal stability as the core stabilizer muscles become stronger at adapting to an unstable base of support. Chronically bad posture is one of the main causes of muscle imbalance that leads to low-back pain, which is statistically likely to be experienced by more than three-quarters of the adult population at some point in their lives (Darragh, 1999). Improved posture through stability ball training can be a very effective way of preventing or relieving low-back pain.

One of the greatest benefits of regular stability ball training is its effect on everyday life, yielding improved quality of life with better functioning, decreased risk of injury, and improved posture and balance. Much of traditional fitness training, while certainly effective at improving cardiorespiratory function, muscle strength, and flexibility, involves movement in a stable environment. Stability balls challenge the body to react and learn to move efficiently in an unstable environment. As so much of real-life motion involves adapting to changing conditions, such as when playing soccer, gardening, or

Group Fitness Specialities

carrying groceries upstairs, ball work is exceptional for improving functional abilities.

Participant Suitability

Because stability balls have been shown to have positive results with people with a wide variety of diagnosed medical conditions, there are very few special populations for which the ball is inappropriate. Use of the ball for strength or stretch work can be safe and effective for just about any condition, provided the exercises are chosen well. It is critical that you are familiar with the variety of common conditions and injuries and know what types of movements are most suitable to each population.

From the exerciser's perspective, the ball is lightweight, fun, and low-tech. The stability ball is large and colorful and has a comforting shape, which promotes a sense of play that makes exercise fun and interesting. Laughter is often one of the first responses from novice stability ball users, before they realize how challenging exercise on the ball can be. The endless variety of exercises possible on the ball also helps counteract boredom. Many fitness enthusiasts find themselves intimidated by complex exercises and awkward equipment. The ball is extremely user-friendly, as it supports and eases the body into proper posture and exercise positions. It is also simple to vary the resistive and/or balance challenge within each exercise by simply changing body position on the ball. Stability balls also are extremely durable and adaptable for use with just about any population.

References

American Council on Exercise (2001). Strong abs, strong core. *ACE Certified News*, 7, 4, 7–9.

Darragh, A. (1999). Training clients in back and spinal post-rehab. *IDEA Personal Trainer*, May, 43–51.

For more information on Stability Ball Training:

Stability Ball Training: A Guide for Fitness Professionals from the American Council on Exercise

ACE's Stability Ball Training Correspondence Course

Group Strength Training

The development of group strength training has undergone four distinct phases. Group strength training initially began as group calisthenics. Exercises were simple and equipment was scarce. Classes were offered as part of sports team training or physical education. A typical class included sit-ups, push-ups, and squats. Exercises were selected with little attention to safety, and modifications were rarely offered. During the next phase, group strength training developed in health clubs as group exercise classes. The emphasis of the classes was on high repetitions and "feeling the burn." Participants were attracted to the misconception that high-repetition exercises burned fat, spot reduced, or somehow slimmed the body. Exercise selection was diverse and, although attention was paid to form, safety and effectiveness were lacking.

During the third phase of group strength training, more attention was paid to safety and effectiveness. Traditional exercises (e.g., full sit-ups) were excluded and limits were placed on controversial movements such as forward flexion and deep knee flexion. A greater variety of exercise equipment became available, creating program diversity. The number of repetitions was reduced as the emphasis shifted from endurance training to strength training.

In the most recent phase, classes emphasize functional strength training along with a greater diversity of exercises, formats, and equipment. Also, classes have begun to shift from muscle-isolation exercises to functional exercises that are sport-specific and may improve participants' ability to perform activities of daily living.

Benefits

Some potential participants may avoid group strength training due to misconceptions about the effects of regular strength training. They may not understand the important role strength training plays in losing or maintaining body weight. Also, in some cases, women may believe that strength training will create bulky muscles. To keep exercise motivation high, communicate the benefits with participants before, during, and after class. For example, explain that strength training improves physical working capacity and appearance, metabolic function, and injury risk. Use positive statements to sell the benefits of strength training.

An effective strength-training program will provide the following physiological improvements:

- Increased muscle fiber size
- Increased muscle contractile strength
- Increased tendon tensile strength
- Increased bone strength
- Increased ligament tensile strength

Participant Suitability

Group strength classes are ideal for participants who enjoy exercising to music and following a structured set of exercises emphasizing muscular fitness. Typically, a variety of resistance-training equipment (e.g., hand weights, barbells, resistance tubing, medicine balls) is utilized, allowing an efficient whole-body workout during class

time. Individuals interested in increasing muscular strength, endurance, and functionality may be well-suited for participation in a group strength class.

Because group strength classes typically call for multiple repetitions of various exercises with added load or resistance, instructors should carefully screen participants prior to class. Musculoskeletal conditions, such as low-back pain, tendinitis, and arthritis, may be aggravated by certain resistance-training exercises. Instructors should be knowledgeable and experienced in providing modifications to all the exercises presented in class to accommodate all participants.

For more information on Group Strength Training:

Group Strength Training: A Guide for Fitness Professionals from the American Council on Exercise (Second Edition)

ACE's Group Strength Training Correspondence Course

For additional instructor resources and educational opportunities related to these and other group fitness specialties, visit the education center of the ACE Web site at www.acefitness.org.

Appendix E

ACE Position Statement on Nutritional Supplements

I t is the position of the American Council on Exercise (ACE) that it is outside the defined scope of practice of a fitness professional to recommend, prescribe, sell, or supply nutritional supplements to clients. Recommending supplements without possessing the requisite qualifications (e.g., R.D.) can place the client's health at risk and possibly expose the fitness professional to disciplinary action and litigation If a client wants to take supplements, a fitness professional should work in conjunction with a qualified registered dietitian or medical doctor to provide safe and effective nutritional education and recommendations.

ACE recognizes that some fitness and health clubs encourage or require their employees to sell nutritional supplements. If this is a condition of employment, fitness professionals should protect themselves by ensuring their employers possess adequate insurance coverage for them should a problem arise. Furthermore, ACE strongly encourages continuing education on diet and nutrition for all fitness professionals.

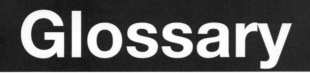

Glossary

Abduction Movement away from the midline of the body.

Accent Emphasis on a given beat.

Acromioclavicular (A/C) joint The junction of the acromion process of the scapula with the distal clavicle.

Actin One of the contractile protein filaments in muscles.

Acute injury An injury having a sudden onset, characterized by specific pain and swelling and the inability to use the injured area normally.

Addiction The devotion or surrendering of oneself to something habitually or obsessively.

Adduction Movement toward the midline of the body.

Adenosine diphosphate (ADP) One of the chemical by-products of the breakdown of ATP during muscle contraction.

Adenosine triphosphate (ATP) The immediately usable form of chemical energy needed for all cellular function, including muscular contractions.

Adherence The amount of programmed exercise someone engages in during a specified time period compared to the amount of exercise recommended for that time period.

Adipose tissue *See* Body fat.

Adult-onset diabetes *See* Diabetes *and* Type 2 diabetes.

Aerobic In the presence of oxygen.

Aerobic fitness *See* Cardiovascular fitness.

Aerobic glycolysis A metabolic pathway that requires oxygen to facilitate the use of glycogen for energy (ATP).

Aerobic power *See* Cardiovascular fitness.

Affective domain One of the three domains of learning; involves the learning of emotional behaviors.

Agility The ability to accelerate, decelerate, and quickly change direction or the position of the body in space, with speed and accuracy.

Agonist The muscle directly responsible for observed movement; also called the prime mover.

Aldosterone One of two main hormones released by the adrenal cortex; plays a role in limiting sodium excretion in the urine.

Alpha cells Endocrine cells in the islets of Langerhans of the pancreas responsible for synthesizing and secreting the hormone glucagon, which elevates the glucose levels in the blood.

Alveoli The small membranous air sacs located at the terminal ends of bronchioles where oxygen and carbon dioxide are exchanged between the blood and air in the lungs.

Amenorrhea The absence of menstruation.

American Society of Composers, Authors, and Publishers One of two performing rights societies in the United States that represent music publishers in negotiating and collecting fees for the nondramatic performance of music.

Americans with Disabilities Act Civil rights legislation designed to improve access to jobs, work places, and commercial spaces for people with disabilities.

Amino acid The simplest component of dietary protein.

Anabolic Muscle-building effects.

Anaerobic Without the presence of oxygen.

Anaerobic glycolysis A metabolic pathway that does not require oxygen, the purpose of which is to transfer the bond energy contained in glucose (or glycogen) to the formation of ATP.

Anaerobic threshold (AT) The point at which exercise intensity can no longer meet the metabolic demands of the muscles aerobically and the muscles have to rely on anaerobic metabolism for ATP.

Anatomical position Standing erect with the feet and palms facing forward.

Androgenic Effects related to masculine characteristics associated with manhood.

Anemia   A disorder caused by a low hemoglobin content in the blood, which reduces the amount of oxygen available to the body's tissues; symptoms include fatigue, breathlessness after exercise, giddiness, and loss of appetite.

Anorexia nervosa   An eating disorder characterized by self-starvation, distorted body image, and an intense fear of becoming obese.

Antagonist   The muscle that acts in opposition to the action of the agonist muscle.

Anthropometric assessment   The measurement of the human body and its parts most commonly measured using skinfolds, girth measurements, and body weight.

Antidiuretic hormone (ADH)   A hormone released by the posterior pituitary gland during exercise; reduces urinary excretion of water and prevents dehydration.

Antioxidants   Chemicals that protect membranes, lipid rich organelles, and lipoproteins (like HDL cholesterol) from being attacked by destructive agents knows as free radicals; include vitamins C and E, beta carotene, and selenium.

Aorta   The main artery exiting the left ventricle of the heart.

Apical pulse   A pulse point located at the apex of the heart.

Apparently healthy   A term to describe participants who have no known diseases, no disease symptoms, and two or fewer cardiovascular disease risk factors.

Appendicular skeleton   The 126 bones that form the extremities.

Applied force   An external force acting on a system (body or body segment).

Arrythmias   Abnormal heart rhythms.

Arteries   Blood vessels that carry oxygenated blood away from the heart to vital organs and the extremities.

Arterioles   Smaller divisions of arteries.

Arthritis   Inflammatory condition involving a joint. *See also* Osteoarthritis *and* Rheumatoid arthritis.

Articulation   The point of contact or connection between bones or between bones and cartilage; also called a joint.

Associative stage of learning   The second stage of learning a motor skill when performers have mastered the fundamentals and can concentrate on skill refinement.

Assumption of risk   A defense used to show that a person has voluntarily accepted known dangers by participating in a specific activity.

Asthma   An obstructive pulmonary disease caused by constriction of the breathing passages.

Atria   The two upper chambers of the heart (right and left atrium).

Atrophy   A reduction in muscle size (muscle wasting) due to inactivity or immobilization.

Autonomous stage of learning   The third stage of learning a motor skill when the skill has become habitual or automatic for the performer.

Axial skeleton   The bones of the head, neck, and trunk.

Balance   The ability to maintain equilibrium or a desired posture for a set amount of time while stationary or moving

Ballistic stretching   Dynamic stretching characterized by rhythmic bobbing or bouncing motions representing relatively high-force, short-duration movements.

Basal metabolic rate (BMR)   The energy required to complete the sum total of life-sustaining processes, including ion transport (40% BMR), protein synthesis (20% BMR), and daily functioning such as breathing, circulation, and nutrient processing (40% BMR).

Beats   Regular pulsations that have an even rhythm and occur in a continuous pattern of strong and weak pulsations.

Beta-adrenergic blocking agents   Medications used for cardiovascular and other medical conditions that block or limit sympathetic nervous system stimulation; commonly called "beta blockers."

Beta-adrenergic stimulating agents
Medications used for treating asthma and other pulmonary disorders that stimulate the sympathetic nervous system to cause relaxation of bronchial smooth muscles; sometimes referred to as "beta agonists."

Beta cells   Endocrine cells in the islets of Langerhans of the pancreas responsible for synthesizing and secreting the hormone insulin, which lowers the glucose levels in the blood.

Beta oxidation   *See* Fatty acid oxidation.

Binge eating disorder   Characterized by frequent binge eating (without purging) and feelings of being out of control when eating.

Bioelectrical impedance   A noninvasive body-composition assessment method measuring electrical current flow through the body.

Biomechanical balance   Balancing the musculoskeletal stress of various movements.

Blanket license   A certificate or document granting permission that varies and applies to a number of situations.

Blood pressure   The driving force that pushes blood through the circulatory system; the pressure exerted by the blood on the walls of the arteries, measured in millimeters of mercury.

Body composition   The makeup of the body considered as a two-component model: lean body mass and fat mass.

Body fat   A component of the body, the primary role of which is to store energy for later use.

Body mass index (BMI)   A relative measure of body height to body weight to determine degree of obesity.

Broad ligament   The ligament that extends from the lateral side of the uterus to the pelvic wall; keeps the uterus centrally placed while providing stability within the pelvic cavity.

Broadcast Music, Inc.   One of two performing rights societies in the U.S. that represent music publishers in negotiating and collecting fees for the nondramatic performance of music.

Bronchial tree   Name given to describe the continuous branching of the trachea into the bronchi and bronchioles of the lungs.

Bronchioles   The smallest tubes that supply air to the alveoli in the lungs.

Bronchitis   An obstructive pulmonary disease caused by inflammation of the mucus membranes and bronchial tubes in the lungs.

Bulimia nervosa   An eating disorder characterized by binge eating followed by self-induced vomiting, fasting, or the use of diuretics or laxatives.

Burnout   A state of emotional exhaustion caused by stress from work or responsibilities.

Caffeine   A relatively harmless and naturally occurring central nervous system stimulant that can be found in about 63 different species of plants (notably coffee and cocoa beans, cola nuts, and tea leaves) and any products made from those plants.

Calcium   The most abundant mineral in the body; involved in the conduction of nerve impulses, heart function, muscle contraction, and the operation of certain enzymes; an inadequate supply of calcium contributes to osteoporosis.

Calorie (note capital C)   *See* Kilocalorie.

calorie (note lowercase c)   The amount of heat necessary to raise the temperature of 1 gram of water 1 degree Celsius; often used incorrectly in place of kilocalorie (1 kilocalorie = 1000 calories).

Cancer   Uncontrolled multiplication of certain cells of the body, which can lead to death in the host.

Capacity   The total amount of energy produced.

Capillaries   The smallest divisions from arterioles and leading to venules; site of exchange of nutrients and metabolic waste products.

Carbohydrate   A primary foodstuff used for energy; dietary sources include sugars (simple) and grains, rice, potatoes, and beans

399

(complex). Carbohydrate is stored as glycogen in the muscles and liver and is transported in the blood as glucose.

Cardiac output   The amount (quantity) of blood pumped from the heart per minute.

Cardiac reserve   The work that the heart is able to perform beyond that required of it under ordinary circumstances.

Cardiorespiratory endurance   *See* Cardiovascular fitness.

Cardiorespiratory fitness (CRF)   The ability to perform large muscle movement over a sustained period; related to the capacity of the heart-lung system to deliver oxygen for sustained energy production. Also called cardiorespiratory endurance or aerobic fitness.

Cardiorespiratory segment   The portion of a group exercise class designed for improving cardiorespiratory fitness and body composition and keeping the heart rate elevated for a sustained time period.

Cardiovascular disease (CVD)   General term for any disease of the heart.

Cardiovascular endurance   The capacity of the heart, blood vessels, and lungs to deliver oxygen and nutrients to the working muscles and tissues during sustained exercise and to remove metabolic waste products that would result in fatigue.

Carotid pulse   A pulse point located on the carotid artery in the neck about 1 inch below the jaw line, next to the esophagus.

Cartilage   A smooth, semi-opaque material that absorbs shock and reduces friction between the bones of a joint.

Catecholamines   Hormones (e.g., epinephrine and norepinephrine) released as part of the sympathetic response to exercise.

Central nervous system (CNS)   The brain and spinal cord.

Cervical vertebrae   The seven vertebral bones of the neck.

Cholesterol   A fatty substance found in blood and body tissues and in certain foods (it is absorbed relatively intact in the diet). In the body it is produced by the liver and is a basic unit for many cells and hormones in the body.

Chondromalacia   A gradual softening and degeneration of the articular cartilage, usually involving the back surface of the patella (kneecap). This condition may produce pain and swelling or a grinding sound or sensation when the knee is flexed and extended.

Chronic bronchitis   Characterized by increased mucus secretion and a productive cough lasting several months to several years.

Chronic obstructive pulmonary diseases (COPD)   Term for a spectrum of airway disorders including asthma, bronchitis, and emphysema.

Circumduction   A biplanar movement involving the sequential combination of flexion, abduction, extension, and adduction.

Class objectives   Specific objectives for each class meeting, clarifying what the instructor expects the participants to accomplish during each exercise session; objectives help instructors focus on the purpose of each selected exercise and activity.

Closed-chain exercise (CCE)   Exercises that use the body muscles in a weightbearing position; co-contractors, postural stabilizers, and the neuromuscular system are all trained at the same time (e.g., squats and lunges).

Coccyx   The four small vertebral bones making up the "tailbone."

Cognitive domain   One of the three domains of learning; describes intellectual activities and involves the learning of knowledge.

Cognitive stage of learning   The first stage of learning a motor skill when performers make many gross errors and have extremely variable performances.

Collagen   The main constituent of connective tissue, such as ligaments, tendons, and muscles.

Combinations   Two or more movement patterns combined and repeated in sequence several times in a row.

Command style of teaching   A teaching

style in which the instructor makes all decisions about rhythm, posture, and duration while participants follow the instructor's directions and movements.

Compilations Original, copyrightable sequences or a program of dance steps or exercise routines that may or may not be copyrightable in themselves.

Complex carbohydrates Starch and dietary fibers made up of longer chains of carbohydrate molecules.

Concentric A type of isotonic muscle contraction where the muscle develops tension and shortens when stimulated.

Congenital Born with (i.e., a condition).

Connective tissue The tissue that binds together and supports various structures of the body. Ligaments and tendons are connective tissues.

Contract An agreement or promise between two or more parties that creates a legal obligation to do or not to do something.

Contractile proteins The protein myofilaments that are essential for muscle contraction.

Contraindication Any condition that renders some particular movement, activity, or treatment improper or undesirable.

Coordination The ability to perform multiple movements simultaneously; The ability to use the senses (e.g., sight and hearing) together with body parts to perform motor tasks or movements smoothly and accurately.

Copyright The exclusive right, for a certain number of years, to perform, make, and distribute copies and otherwise use an artistic, musical, or literary work.

Core stability When the muscles of the trunk function in harmony to stabilize the spine and pelvis to provide a solid foundation for movement in the extremities. It's a key component necessary for successful performance of most gross motor activities.

Cortisol One of two main hormones released by the adrenal cortex; plays a major role in maintaining blood glucose during prolonged exercise by promoting protein and triglyceride breakdown.

Creatine phosphate (CP) A high-energy phosphate compound found within muscle cells, used to resynthesize ATP for immediate muscle contraction.

Cueing Visual or verbal techniques, using hand signals or minimal words, to inform participants of upcoming movements.

Defendant The party in a lawsuit who is being sued or accused.

Dehydration The condition resulting from excessive loss of body fluids.

Delayed onset muscle soreness (DOMS) Soreness that occurs 24 to 48 hours after strenuous exercise, the exact cause of which is unknown.

Dependence The condition of being influenced or controlled by something else.

Depression The action of lowering a muscle or bone.

Diabetes A disease of carbohydrate metabolism in which an absolute or relative deficiency of insulin results in an inability to metabolize carbohydrates normally; also known as diabetes mellitus. *See* Type 1 diabetes *and* Type 2 diabetes.

Diaphragmatic breathing A deep, relaxing breathing technique that helps COPD patients improve their breathing capacity.

Diaphysis The shaft of a long bone.

Diastasis recti The separation of the recti abdominal muscles along the midline of the body.

Diastolic blood pressure The pressure in the arteries during the relaxation phase (diastole) of the cardiac cycle.

Dietary fiber *See* Fiber.

Dietary-induced thermogenesis The thermic (heat-producing) effect of food; energy spent on digesting and absorbing food, approximately 10% of all energy expenditure.

Disability insurance Insurance that provides

income protection in the event of an injury to the instructor.

Disaccharides   Double sugar units called sucrose, lactose, and maltose.

Distal   Farthest from the midline of the body, or from the point of attachment of a body part.

DNA adducts   A cancer-promoting condition that occurs when a molecule bonds to DNA, which can cause a cellular mutation.

Dorsiflexion   Movement of the foot up toward the shin.

Dowager's hump   An exaggerated outward curve of the thoracic spine, often associated with vertebral fractures and osteoporosis.

Downbeat   The regular strong pulsation in music occurring in a continuous pattern at an even rhythm.

Duration   The length of time of an exercise session.

Dynamic stabilizers   Muscles that contribute to core stability.

Dynamic stretching   *See* Ballistic stretching.

Dyspnea   Difficult or labored breathing.

Eating disorders   Disturbed eating behaviors that jeopardize a person's physical or psychological health.

Eccentric   A type of isotonic muscle contraction where the muscle lengthens against a resistance when it is stimulated; sometimes called "negative work."

Echocardiography   A sensitive test to identify heart defects.

Electrocardiogram (EKG or ECG)   A recording of the electrical activity of the heart.

Elevation   The action of raising a muscle or bone.

Emphysema   An obstructive pulmonary disease characterized by the gradual destruction of lung alveoli and the surrounding connective tissue, in addition to airway inflammation, leading to reduced ability to inhale and exhale.

Employee   A person who works for another

person in exchange for financial compensation. An employee complies with the instructions and directions of their employer and reports to them on a regular basis.

Endomysium   The thin layer of connective tissue covering each individual muscle fiber in skeletal muscle.

Endosteum   A soft tissue lining the internal surface of the diaphysis on a long bone.

Energy   The potential to perform work or activity.

Energy deficit   Burning more calories than one is consuming, which promotes weight loss.

Epimysium   The layer of connective tissue that entirely surrounds skeletal muscles and thickens into tendons at either end of the muscle.

Epinephrine   A hormone released as part of the sympathetic response to exercise.

Epiphysis   The end of a long bone, usually wider than the shaft (plural: Epiphyses).

Ergogenic aid   An energy-enhancing substance thought to improve athletic performance.

Essential body fat   Fat thought to be necessary for maintenance of life and reproductive function.

Essential fatty acids   Fat that cannot be produced by the body and must be supplied by the diet. Linoleic acid is the only essential fatty acid.

Estrogen   Hormones produced by the ovary.

Eversion   Rotation of the foot to direct the plantar surface outward.

Excess postexercise oxygen consumption (EPOC)   A measurably increased rate of oxygen uptake following strenuous activity. The extra oxygen is used in the processes (hormone balancing, replenishment of fuel stores, cellular repair, innervation, and anabolism) that restore the body to a resting state and adapt it to the exercise just performed. Formerly referred to as oxygen debt.

Exercise evaluation A process of evaluating an exercise based on its effectiveness and safety.

Exercise-induced asthma (EIA) More than 80% of all asthmatics experience asthma during exercise. EIA is probably caused by the cooling and then drying of the respiratory tract that accompanies the inspiration of large volumes of dry air during exercise.

Exercise intensity The specific level of physical activity at which a person exercises that can be quantified (e.g., heart rate, work, RPE); usually reflected as a percentage of one's maximal capacity to do work.

Exercise physiology The study of how the body functions during physical activity and exercise.

Exercise specificity *See* Specificity.

Extension An increase in the angle between the anterior surfaces of articulating bones.

External rotation Outward turning about the vertical axis of bone.

Fast-twitch (FT) fiber A muscle fiber type specialized for anaerobic metabolism; recruited for rapid, powerful movements such as jumping, throwing, and sprinting.

Fat An essential nutrient that provides energy, energy storage, insulation, and contour to the body. 1 gram = 9 kcal.

Fat-soluble vitamins Vitamins that, when consumed, are stored in the body (particularly the liver and fat tissues); includes vitamins A, D, E, and K.

Fatty acid The simplest component of dietary fat; important for the production of energy during low-intensity exercise.

Fatty acid oxidation A metabolic pathway involving the breakdown of fatty acids (digested dietary fat) for the production of ATP.

Feedback An internal response within a learner; during information processing, it is the correctness or incorrectness of a response that is stored in memory to be used for future reference. Also, verbal or nonverbal information about current behavior that can be used to improve future performance.

Fetus The developed embryo and growing human in the uterus, from usually three months after conception to birth.

Fiber Carbohydrate chains the body cannot break down for use and which pass through the body undigested.

Field tests Fitness tests that can be used in mass testing situations.

Flexibility The ability to move joints through their normal full range of motion.

Flexion A decrease in the angle between the anterior surfaces of articulating bones.

Food Guide Pyramid A guide to assist the public with daily food choices that will accomplish dietary goals. Published in 1992 by the U.S. Department of Agriculture and the U.S. Department of Health & Human Services.

Force A push or a pull that causes or tends to cause a change in a body's motion or shape.

Fracture Any break in the continuity of a bone, ranging from a simple crack to a severe shatter of the bone with multiple fracture fragments.

Freestyle choreography A way of designing the cardiovascular segment of a class that uses movements randomly chosen by the instructor.

Frequency The number of exercise sessions per week resulting in a training effect.

Frontal plane A plane that divides the body into front (anterior) and back (posterior) halves.

Functional capacity The maximum physical performance represented by maximal oxygen consumption.

General liability insurance Insurance for bodily injury or property damage resulting from general negligence such as wet flooring, an icy sidewalk, or poorly maintained equipment.

Glenohumeral (G/H) joint The ball and socket joint composed of the glenoid fossa of the scapula and the humeral head.

403

Glucagon A hormone released when blood glucose levels are low; stimulates glucose release from the liver to increase blood glucose. Also releases free fatty acids from adipose tissue to be used as fuel.

Glucometer A devise used by diabetics to check blood sugar.

Glucose A simple sugar; the simplest form of carbohydrate used by the body to produce energy (ATP).

Glycemic index A measurement of the impact on blood glucose levels after ingestion of carbohydrates.

Glycogen The storage form of glucose found in the liver and muscles.

Glycogenolysis Glycogen breakdown.

Glycolysis Breakdown of glucose, or its storage form glycogen.

Golgi tendon organ (GTO) A sensory organ within a tendon that, when stimulated, causes an inhibition of the entire muscle group to protect against too much force.

Graded exercise test A physician-supervised diagnostic examination to assess a participant's physiological response to exercise in a controlled environment.

Growth hormone (GH) A hormone secreted by the pituitary gland that facilitates protein synthesis in the body.

Health Belief Model suggests that individuals adopt (or do not adopt) healthy behaviors based largely on their appraisal of their susceptibility to an illness combined with their perception of the probable severity of the consequences of having the illness. An additional aspect of this model is the person's view of the benefits of the behavior change as contrasted with the difficulty of changing.

Health screening A vital process that identifies individuals at high risk for exercise-induced heart problems that need to be referred to appropriate medical care as needed.

Heart rate (HR) The number of heart beats per minute.

Heart-rate reserve The result of subtracting the resting heart rate from the maximal heart rate; represents the working heart-rate range between rest and maximal heart rate within which all activity occurs.

Heat index Guidelines regarding when exercise can be safely undertaken or when it should be avoided based on measures of heat and humidity.

Hematocrit A measure of the number of red cells found in the blood, stated as a percentage of the total blood volume. The normal range is 43–49% in men and 37–43% in women.

Hemoglobin (Hb) A protein molecule in red blood cells specifically adapted to carry oxygen molecules.

Hemorrhagic stroke Disruption of blood flow to the brain caused by the presence of a blood clot or hematoma.

Heterocyclic amines Compounds that increase cancer risk, created by charbroiling and grilling foods.

High-density lipoprotein (HDL cholesterol) Cholesterol that helps move body lipids from places of storage to places of use; referred to as "good" cholesterol.

Homocysteine A normal by-product of metabolism that can promote development of heart disease.

Hydration The process of providing an adequate amount of liquid to bodily tissues.

Hydrogenation A process by which liquid fats are turned into solids.

Hydrostatic weighing An underwater test that measures the percentage of lean body weight and body fat, based on the principle that fat floats and muscle and bone sink; considered the gold standard of body composition assessment due to its accuracy.

Hyperextension Extension of an articulation beyond anatomical position.

Hyperglycemia An abnormally high content of sugar in the blood.

Hypertension High blood pressure.

Hyperthermia A life-threatening increase in core body temperature.

Hypertrophic cardiomyopathy A congenital heart defect involving a thickening of the heart muscle.

Hypertrophy An increase in the size of individual muscle cells.

Hypoglycemia A blood sugar deficiency caused by too little glucose, too much insulin, or too much exercise in the insulin-dependent diabetic.

Hyponatremia Low blood sodium levels as a result of overconsumption of water.

Hypoxia Decrease in the amount of oxygen in inspired air that usually occurs at high altitudes.

Iliotibial band A band of connective tissue that extends from the iliac crest to the knee and links the gluteus maximus to the tibia.

Inclusion style of teaching A teaching style that enables multiple levels of performance to be taught within the same activity.

Incompletely fermented fibers Fibers that do not bind with water, fluids, or cholesterol; serve the function of "scraping" the sides of the bowel.

Incontinence The loss of sphincter control that results in the inability to retain urine, semen, or feces.

Independent contractors People who conduct business on their own on a contract basis and are not employees of an organization.

Individual medical insurance Insurance that provides hospitalization and major medical coverage.

Inferior Located below.

Informed consent A written statement signed by a client prior to testing that informs him or her of testing purposes, processes, and all potential risks and discomforts.

Inguinal ligament The ligament that extends from the anterior, superior iliac spine to the pubic tubercle.

Insoluble fiber Fiber that does not bind with water, fluids, or cholesterol, accelerating the passage of foods through the body while slowing the digestive processes (includes cellulose, hemicellulose, and lignins found in wheat bran, vegetables, and whole-grain breads/cereals).

Insulin A hormone secreted into the bloodstream by the pancreas that regulates carbohydrate metabolism.

Insulin-like growth factors Polypeptides structurally similar to insulin that are secreted either during fetal development or during childhood and that mediate growth hormone activity.

Insulin reaction The result of hypoglycemia, not enough sugar in the blood, in which diabetics experience symptoms such as anxiety, confusion, headache, and irritability; if unchecked may lead to insulin shock.

Insulin shock The condition produced when there is excessive insulin present in the bloodstream, causing rapid pulse, dizziness or headache, disorientation, and fainting with possible unconsciousness.

Intensity Physiological stress on the body during exercise; indicates how hard the body should work to achieve a training effect.

Internal fat Fat stored deep inside the body.

Internal rotation Inward turning about the vertical axis of bone.

Interval training Exercising at high-intensity levels for brief periods (10 seconds to 5 minutes) with intervening rest or relief periods at a lower intensity to allow heart rate to decline.

Inversion Rotation of the foot to direct the plantar surface inward.

Iron-deficiency anemia A nutritional deficiency characterized by a lack of hemoglobin or poorly formed red blood cells.

Ischemia Lack of blood flow to the heart muscle.

Ischemic stroke A sudden disruption of cerebral circulation in which blood supply to the brain is either interrupted or diminished.

Islets of Langerhans Irregular clusters of endocrine cells scattered throughout the tissue of the pancreas that secrete insulin and glucagon.

Isokinetic A type of muscular contraction where tension developed within the muscle changes throughout the range of motion; performed with the use of special equipment; also referred to as "variable resistance" exercise.

Isometric A type of muscular contraction where the muscle is stimulated to generate tension but no joint movement occurs.

Isotonic A type of muscular contraction where the muscle is stimulated to develop tension and joint movement occurs.

kcal *See* Kilocalorie.

Kegel exercises Controlled isometric contraction and relaxation of the muscles surrounding the vagina to strengthen and gain control of the pelvic floor muscles.

Kilocalorie (kcal) The term to express energy intake and expenditure in nutrition and exercise. A calorie is a unit of energy, specifically the amount of heat needed to increase the temperature of 1 kg of water 1°C; one kcal equals 1,000 calories.

Kinematics The study of the form, pattern, or sequence of movement without regard for the forces that may produce that motion.

Kinesiology The study of the principles of mechanics and anatomy in relation to human movement.

Kinesthetic awareness (kinethesis) The perception of body position and movement in space.

Kinetics The branch of mechanics that describes the effects of forces on the body.

Kyphosis Excessive posterior curvature of the spine, typically seen in the thoracic region.

Kyphotic A type of curve of the spine; concave anteriorly and convex posteriorly.

Lactate *See* Lactic acid (LA).

Lactic acid (LA) A by-product of anaerobic glycolysis thought to cause localized muscle fatigue associated with very high-intensity exercise.

Lateral Away from the midline of the body, or the outside.

Lateral flexion Bending of the vertebral column to the side.

Law of acceleration Newton's second law of motion stating that the force acting on a body in a given direction is equal to the body's mass times its acceleration in that direction.

Law of gravity Newton's theory stating that every object in the universe attracts every other object with a force that is proportional to the product of the masses of the two objects and inversely proportional to the square of the distance between them.

Law of inertia Newton's first law of motion stating that a body at rest will stay at rest and a body in motion will stay in motion unless acted upon by an external force.

Law of reaction Newton's third law of motion stating that for every applied force there is an equal and opposite reactive force.

Lean body mass The components of the body including muscles, bones, nervous tissue, skin, blood, and organs.

Lecithin A type of fat called phospholipid manufactured by the body and having both a water-soluble and fat-soluble portion.

Lever A rigid bar that rotates around a fixed support (fulcrum) in response to an applied force.

Liability Legal responsibility.

Ligament Strong, fibrous tissue that connects one bone to another.

Linear progression Consists of one movement that transitions into another without cycling sequences.

Linoleic acid The only essential fatty acid. *See also* Essential fatty acids.

Lipids The name for fats used in the body and bloodstream.

Lipoproteins A complex of lipid and protein

molecules, which transport cholesterol and other lipids throughout the body.

Lordosis   Excessive anterior curvature of the spine that typically occurs at the low back (may also occur at the neck).

Low-back pain (LBP)   A general term to describe a multitude of back conditions, including muscular and ligament strains, sprains, and injuries. The cause of LBP is often elusive; most LBP is probably caused by muscle weakness and imbalance.

Low-density lipoprotein (LDL) cholesterol   Cholesterol involved in the artery-blocking process; referred to as "bad" cholesterol.

Lumbar vertebrae   The five vertebrae in the low back, just below the thoracic vertebrae and just above the sacrum.

Macronutrients   The main contributors to energy intake in the diet; carbohydrate, protein, and fat.

Maximal heart rate   The highest heart rate a person can attain.

Maximal heart rate formula   A formula for determining target heart rate based on a percentage of the maximal heart rate.

Maximal oxygen uptake ($\dot{V}O_2$max)   The point at which the body's ability to take in oxygen from the atmosphere via the pulmonary system, transport it via the cardiovascular system, and utilize it via the muscular system reaches a point of little or no change with an additional workload; a direct measure of cardiorespiratory fitness.

Measure   One group of beats in a musical composition marked by the regular occurrence of the heavy accent.

Medial   Toward the midline of the body, or the inside.

Megadoses   Large intake levels of vitamins and minerals, possibly dangerous to health.

Meter   The organization of beats into musical patterns or measures.

Micronutrients   Special chemicals needed in minute amounts; found widely in foods; vitamins and minerals.

Minerals   Inorganic (non-carbon-containing) compounds the body requires that must be provided in the diet.

Mitochondria   A highly specialized structure within cells where aerobic glycolysis takes place for energy production; sometimes called the "powerhouse" of the cell.

Mobility   The degree to which an articulation is allowed to move before being restricted by surrounding tissues.

Mode   Type of exercise.

Monosaccharides   Single sugar units called glucose, fructose, and galactose.

Monounsaturated fat   A type of unsaturated fat (liquid at room temperature) that has one open spot on the fatty acid for the addition of a hydrogen atom (e.g., oleic acid in olive oil).

Motor domain   One of the three domains of learning; involves the learning of motor skills.

Motor end plate   The location of the synapse of a motor neuron and muscle cell; also called the neuromuscular junction.

Motor neurons   Nerve cells that conduct impulses from the CNS to the periphery signaling muscles to contract or relax, regulating muscular movement.

Motor skill   The degree to which movements using agility, balance, and coordination are executed.

Motor unit   A motor nerve and all of the muscle fibers it stimulates.

Multiple sclerosis   A common neuromuscular disorder involving the progressive degeneration of muscle function, including increased muscle spasticity.

Muscle spindle   The sensory organ within a muscle that is sensitive to stretch and thus protects the muscle against too much stretch.

Muscle stiffness   The capacity of muscle tissues to resist internal and external loads.

Muscular balance   The symmetry of the interconnected components of muscle and connective tissue.

Muscular endurance The ability of a muscle or muscle group to exert force against a resistance over a sustained period of time.

Muscular strength The maximal force a muscle or muscle group can exert during contraction.

Myofibrils Thread-like protein strands composing individual muscle cells.

Myofilaments Collective term for the contractile proteins of a muscle fiber; actin and myosin.

Myosin Contractile protein in a myofibril.

MyPyramid Food Guidance System An educational tool designed to help consumers make healthier food and physical-activity choices for a healthy lifestyle that are consistent with the 2005 USDA dietary guidelines.

Near-infrared (NIR) light interactance A body-composition assessment technique that analyzes the amount of near-infrared light reflected from the biceps based on the principle that body fat absorbs light while lean body mass reflects light.

Negligence Failure of a person to perform as a reasonable and prudent professional would perform under similar circumstances.

Neuron The basic anatomical unit of the nervous system; the nerve cell.

Neuropathy A chronic disease linked to diabetes involving diminished sensations in distal extremities (peripheral neuropathy) or altered heart rate (autonomic neuropathy).

Neutral spine position The balance of vertebrae in the three naturally occurring curves: two slight anterior curves at the neck and low back and one slight posterior curve in the thoracic region.

Nitrates/nitrites Preservatives used in certain foods (hot dogs, lunch meats) that are converted to carcinogenic nitrosamines, which may increase risk for stomach cancers.

Nitrosamines Carcinogenic compounds converted from nitrate/nitrite preservatives in the stomach.

Norepinephrine A hormone released as part of the sympathetic response to exercise.

Nutrients Components of food needed by the body. There are six classes of nutrients: water, minerals, vitamins, protein, carbohydrates, and fats.

Nutrition The study of nutrients in foods and of their digestion, absorption, metabolism, interaction, storage, and excretion.

Obesity An excessive accumulation of body fat. Usually defined as more than 20% above ideal weight, or over 25% body fat for men and over 32% body fat for women; also can be defined as a Body Mass Index of >30 kg/m^2, or a waist girth of >40 inches (102 cm) in men and >35 inches (89 cm) in women.

Omega-3 fatty acids Fats (found in cold-water fish) that can lower blood cholesterol, help prevent blood clots, and may lower high blood pressure.

Open-chain exercise (OCE) Exercise in which a muscle or muscle group is isolated to function alone (e.g., seated leg extension).

Osteoarthritis A degenerative bone disease involving a wearing away of joint cartilage.

Osteoporosis A condition in which bones weaken and soften due to progressive loss of calcium.

Overload The principle that a physiological system subjected to above-normal stress will respond by increasing in strength or function accordingly.

Overweight A term to describe an excessive amount of weight for a given height, using height-to-weight ratios.

Oxidative enzymes Enzymes that initiate fat metabolism by breaking down free fatty acids into aceytl CoA.

Oxidative glycolysis *See* Aerobic glycolysis.

Oxygen consumption ($\dot{V}O_2$) The process by which oxygen is used to produce energy for cellular work; also called oxygen uptake.

Oxygen deficit A situation created at exercise onset when actual oxygen consumption does not immediately meet the physiological requirement for oxygen.

Oxygen uptake *See* Oxygen consumption.

Oxylates Substances that bind and decrease calcium absorption in the body.

Part-to-whole teaching strategy A teaching strategy involving breaking a skill down into its component parts and practicing each skill in its simplest form before placing several skills in a sequence.

Partial pressure The pressure of each gas in a multiple gas system, such as air, which is composed of nitrogen, oxygen, and CO_2.

Peak flow meter A device used to measure the flow of air through the lungs; useful for COPD patients to aid in activity selection.

Pelvic floor The muscles and tissues that act as a support or reinforcement to the lower border of the pelvis.

Performing rights society An organization to which the copyright or publisher assigns the nondramatic performing rights in a musical composition.

Perineal The fibromuscular tissue located between the lower part of the vagina and the anal canal.

Periosteum A connective tissue sheath surrounding the outer surface of the diaphysis of a long bone.

Phosphocreatine *See* Creatine phosphate.

Phosphagens Adenosine triphosphate (ATP) and creatine phosphate (CP), two high-energy phosphate molecules that can be broken down for immediate use by the cells.

Phospholipid A fatty substance that has a fat-soluble end and a water-soluble end; an essential part of cell membranes that does not supply calories.

Photosynthesis Process by which plants turn radiant energy (sunlight) into chemical energy.

Phrase Two or more measures of music.

Physical activity Daily movement through either planned activity (exercise) or daily living activities; the most variable component of total energy expenditure at 10–30%.

Physical Activity Readiness Questionnaire (PAR-Q) A brief, self-administered medical questionnaire recognized as a safe pre-exercise screening measure for low-to-moderate (but not vigorous) exercise training.

Physical fitness The physical components of well-being that enable a person to function at an optimal level.

Physiological balance The balance of movement intensity (when sequencing moves) combined with movement selection based on the duration of the class.

Phytate A non-nutrient component of plant seeds that binds with minerals, forming insoluble complexes that the body excretes unused.

Phytochemicals Biologically active compounds in plants thought to have anti-cancer and anti-heart disease properties when consumed as part of a healthy diet.

Placenta The vascular organ in mammals that unites the fetus to the maternal uterus and mediates its metabolic exchanges.

Plaintiff A party who brings a suit against another party in a court of law.

Plantar fasciitis Inflammation of the plantar fascia, a broad band of connective tissue running along the sole of the foot; caused by stretching or tearing the tissue, usually near the attachment at the heel.

Plantarflexion Distal movement of the plantar surface of the foot; opposite of dorsiflexion.

Plasma The liquid portion of the blood.

Plyometrics High-intensity movements, such as jumping, involving high-force loading of body weight on the landing phase of the movement.

Polycyclic aromatic hydrocarbons Compounds that increase cancer risk, created by charbroiling and grilling foods.

Polyunsaturated fat A type of unsaturated fat (liquid at room temperature) that has two or more spots on the fatty acid available for hydrogen (e.g., corn, safflower, soybean oils).

Posterior Toward the back or dorsal side.

Postpartum The period of time after childbirth.

Power The rate at which work is performed strength over time expressed as [force x distance]/time); The ability to perform explosive work

Practice style of teaching A teaching style that provides opportunities for individualization and includes practice time and individualized instructor feedback.

Preclass preparation Methods or principles for successful group exercise instruction, including professional attributes such as knowing participants' health histories, being available to orient new participants before class, and having music/equipment cued and ready to go before class begins.

Preparticipation (pre-exercise) screening The process of determining someone's health and fitness status before beginning an exercise program.

Primary bronchi The two main branches of the trachea or windpipe.

Prime mover A muscle responsible for a specific movement.

Professional liability insurance Insurance to protect an instructor against professional negligence or failure to perform as a competent and prudent professional would under similar circumstances.

Progesterone Hormone produced by the corpus luteum, adrenal cortex, and placenta, the function of which is to facilitate growth of the embryo.

Prognosis Assessment of progress toward recovery from an accident or condition.

Program goals Goals established by the instructor to aid participants in developing personal fitness goals, reflecting what the instructor expects students to gain from participation in the group exercise program.

Pronation Internal rotation of the forearm causing the radius to cross diagonally over the ulna and the palm to face posteriorly.

Proprioception The reception of stimuli produced within the body.

Proprioceptive neuromuscular facilitation (PNF) A stretching technique involving statically stretching a muscle immediately after maximally contracting it against resistance.

Proprioceptors Somatic sensory receptors in muscles, tendons, ligaments, joint capsules, and skin that gather information about body position and the direction and velocity of movement.

Protein Compound composed of amino acids that is the major structural component of all body tissue; a complete protein is protein containing all nine amino acids essential to health.

Proximal Nearest to the midline of the body or point of attachment of a body part.

Psychological balance Balancing movement complexity with simplicity to avoid compromising form, technique, and safety, and to limit participant frustration.

Public performance Playing a recording of a copyrighted musical composition at a place where a substantial number of persons outside of a normal circle of a family and its social acquaintances are gathered.

Publisher The entity to which the owner of a copyrighted artistic, musical, or literary work assigns such copyright for licensing and income-collection purposes.

Pulmonary ventilation The total volume of gas inspired or expired per minute.

Pulse rate The wave of pressure in the arteries that occurs each time the heart beats.

Radial pulse A pulse point located on the thumb side of the wrist.

Range of motion (ROM) The number of degrees that an articulation will allow one of its segments to move.

Rating of perceived exertion (RPE) A scale that correlates the participants' perceptions of exercise effort with actual intensity level.

Receptor Nerve tissue that is sensitive to changes in its environment.

Reciprocal style of teaching Teaching style that involves using an observer or partner to provide feedback to the performer.

Recommended daily allowances (RDA) The amounts of selected nutrients that adequately meet the known nutrient needs of most healthy Americans.

Recovery heart rate The number of heartbeats per minute following the cessation of vigorous physical activity. As cardiorespiratory fitness improves, the heart rate returns to resting levels more quickly.

Relaxin A hormone of pregnancy that softens connective tissue.

Repetition reduction teaching strategy Teaching strategy involving reducing the number of repetitions that make up a movement sequence.

Repetitions The number of successive contractions performed during each weight-training exercise.

Respiration The exchange of oxygen and carbon dioxide between the cells and the atmosphere.

Respiratory ventilation The movement of air into and out of the lungs.

Resting heart rate The number of heartbeats per minute when the body is at complete rest; usually counted first thing in the morning before any physical activity.

Reversibility principle The training principle explaining that training adaptations will gradually decline if not reinforced by a "maintenance" program.

Rheumatoid arthritis A chronic disease caused by an immune response leading to inflammation of the joint membrane.

Rhythm A regular pattern of movement or sound that can be felt, heard, or seen.

RICE An immediate treatment for injury: rest, ice, compression, and elevation.

Risk factor A characteristic, inherited trait, or behavior related to the presence or development of a condition or disease.

Risk management Minimizing the risks of potential legal liability.

Risk stratification The classification of participants into risk strata to identify the need for referral to a healthcare provider, to ensure safety of exercise testing and participation, and to determine the appropriate type of exercise test or program.

Rotation Movement in the transverse plane about a longitudinal axis; can be "internal" or "external."

Rotator cuff A group of four relatively small muscles (supraspinatus, infraspinatus, teres minor, and subscapularis) that acts to oppose the constant force of gravity to dislocate the joint and stabilize the humeral head by pulling it inward and slightly downward in the glenohumeral joint.

Round ligament Ligament found on the side of the uterus near the fallopian tube insertion to help the broad ligament keep the uterus in place.

Sacral vertebrae Part of the axial skeleton; fused together into one bone as the sacrum.

Sagittal plane A plane that divides the body into right and left halves.

Sarcomere The basic functional unit of the myofibril containing the contractile proteins that generate skeletal muscle movements.

Saturated fats Fatty acids carrying the maximum number of hydrogen atoms; these fats are solid at room temperature and are usually of animal origin.

Scapulohumeral rhythm Combined action of scapular and humeral movement.

Scapulothoracic (S/T) articulation The articulation of the scapula with the thorax beneath it.

Sciatica Severe pain in the leg, running from the back of the thigh down the inside of the leg as a result of the compression of, or trauma to, the sciatic nerve.

Scoliosis Excessive lateral curvature of the spine.

Scope of practice The range and limit of

responsibilities normally associated with a specific job or position.

Screw-home mechanism A phenomenon that increases knee joint stability by locking the femur on the tibia (or vice-versa) when the knee is fully extended.

Self-check style of teaching A teaching style that relies on individual performers to provide their own feedback.

Sensory neurons Nerve cells that convey electrical impulses from sensory organs in the periphery (such as the skin) to the spinal cord and brain (CNS).

Serum lipids Lipids found circulating in the blood.

Shin splints A general term for any pain or discomfort on the front or side of the lower leg in the region of the shin bone (tibia); a common, chronic aerobics injury with several causes.

Shoulder girdle *See* Scapulothoracic (S/T) articulation.

Shoulder joint complex The three segments of the shoulder: the scapula, clavicle, and humerus.

Simple carbohydrates Single sugars (monosaccharides) and double sugars (disaccharides).

Simple-to-complex teaching strategy Advanced teaching strategy that treats a sequence of movement patterns as a whole, teaching small changes (adding small amounts of complexity) to progressively challenge the exercise participant.

Sliding filament theory Explanation for how muscle contraction occurs via the interaction of actin and myosin myofilament proteins and ATP.

Slow-to-fast teaching strategy Teaching strategy used to allow participants to learn complex movement at a slower pace, emphasizing proper placement or configuration of a movement pattern (e.g., teaching a movement at half-tempo).

Slow-twitch (ST) fiber A muscle fiber type designed for use of aerobic glycolysis and fatty acid oxidation, recruited for low-intensity, longer-duration activities such as walking and swimming.

Soluble fiber Fiber that binds fluid to delay stomach emptying and glucose absorption, lower blood cholesterol, and aid against constipation.

Spatial teaching strategy Teaching strategy used when introducing participants to a new body position, involving describing the position of different portions of the body.

Specificity Exercise training principle explaining that specific exercise demands made on the body produce specific responses by the body; also called exercise specificity.

Speed The ability to perform a movement within a short period of time or move quickly from one point to another

Sphincter A circular muscle, the function of which is constricting an opening.

Sprain Overstretching or tearing of a ligament and/or joint capsule, resulting in discoloration, swelling, and pain.

Stages-of-Change Model is a lifestyle-modification model that suggests that people go through distinct, predictable stages when making lifestyle changes; precontemplation, contemplation, preparation, action, and maintenance. The process is not always linear; individuals may move back and forth between stages. During precontemplation the individual is not intending to change soon (i.e., within six months). In the contemplation stage the client weighs the costs (effort, treatment effectiveness, finances, time) and benefits of lifestyle modification. Individuals who have decided to initiate an effort to change within a month's time are in the preparation stage. Individuals in the action stage are in the process of changing their behavior (Individuals are at the greatest risk for relapse in this stage). Maintenance is the stage of successful, sustained lifestyle modification.

Standard of care Appropriateness of an exercise professional's actions in light of current professional standards and based on the age, condition, and knowledge of the participant.

Static stabilizers The bony configuration of joints, fibrocartilages, and ligaments that contribute to core stability.

Static stretching Holding a nonmoving (static) position to immobilize a joint in a position that places the desired muscles and connective tissues passively at their greatest possible length.

Statute of limitations A formal regulation limiting the period within which a specific legal action may be taken.

Steady state The term that describes the point at which the energy needs of the body during exercise are being met aerobically.

Step test (submaximal) A test for cardiovascular fitness that requires the subject to step up and down from a bench at a prescribed rate for a given period.

Sternoclavicular (S/C) joint The junction of the sternum and the proximal clavicle.

Strain Overstretching or tearing of a muscle or tendon.

Stress fracture An incomplete fracture caused by excessive stress (overuse) to a bone. Most common in the foot (metatarsal bones) and lower leg (tibia).

Stretch reflex An involuntary motor response that, when stimulated, causes a suddenly stretched muscle to respond with a corresponding contraction.

Stroke volume (SV) The amount (quantity) of blood pumped per heart beat.

Structured choreography A way of designing the cardiovascular segment of a class that uses formally arranged movement patterns repeated in a predetermined order.

Subcutaneous fat Fatty deposits or fat pads of storage fat found under the skin.

Superior Located above.

Supination External rotation of the forearm (radioulnar joint) that causes the palm to face anteriorly.

Supine Face up.

Supine hypotension An abnormal reduction in blood pressure related to position (lying on the back).

Symphysis pubis The fibrocartilaginous joint between the pelvic bones in the midline of the body.

Symphysitis Irritation of the pubic symphysis caused by increased motion at the joint.

Systemic lupus erythematosus (SLE) An autoimmune disease that affects connective tissues and results in painful joints and arthritis.

Syncopation A rhythmic device that temporarily shifts the normal pattern of stresses to unstressed beats or parts of beats.

Synergist A muscle that aids another muscle in its action.

Systolic blood pressure The force generated by the heart during its ventricular contractile phase (systole).

Tachycardia Elevated heart rate over 100 beats per minute.

Talk test A method for measuring exercise intensity using observation of respiration effort and the ability to talk while exercising.

Target heart rate (THR) Number of heartbeats per minute that indicate appropriate exercise intensity levels for each individual; also called training heart rate.

Target heart-rate range Exercise intensity that represents the minimum and maximum intensity for safe and effective exercise; also referred to as training zone.

Tempo The rate of speed of music, usually expressed in beats per minute.

Temporal pulse Pulse point located on either temple.

Tendinitis Inflammatory response to microtrauma from overuse of a tendon.

Tendon Thickened connective tissue at the ends of skeletal muscle that connects muscle to bone.

Tennis elbow Pain on the outside of the

elbow at the attachment of the forearm muscles.

Teratogenic Nongenetic factors that can cause birth defects in the fetus.

Testosterone The primary male sex hormone; often abused in supplement form because of its potent anabolic properties.

Thermoregulation Regulation of the body's temperature.

Thoracic vertebrae The 12 vertebrae to which the ribs are attached.

Tibial stress syndrome *See* Shin splints.

Tidal volume Depth of breathing.

Total energy expenditure Amount of energy expended in a 24-hour period, which includes basal metabolism, physical activity, and dietary-induced thermogenesis.

Trace minerals Minerals required in very minute amounts for health.

Trans fatty acids Fatty acids created during hydrogenation that provoke heart disease.

Transient osteoporosis The temporary increase in the porosity of the bone as a result of dietary calcium deficiency.

Transverse plane Plane that divides the body into upper (superior) and lower (inferior) parts.

Triglycerides The form of 95% of dietary fats and stored fats in adipose tissue, consisting of a glycerol backbone and three fatty acids.

Type 1 diabetes Form of diabetes caused by the destruction of the insulin-producing beta cells in the pancreas, which leads to little or no insulin secretion; generally develops in childhood and requires regular insulin injections; formerly known as insulin-dependent diabetes mellitus (IDDM) and childhood-onset diabetes.

Type 2 diabetes Most common form of diabetes; typically develops in adulthood and is characterized by a reduced sensitivity of the insulin target cells to available insulin; usually associated with obesity; formerly known as

non-insulin-dependent diabetes mellitus (NIDDM) and adult-onset diabetes

Unsaturated fats Fatty acids that contain double bonds between carbon atoms and thus are capable of absorbing more hydrogen; liquid at room temperature and usually of vegetable origin.

Upbeat The regular, weak pulsation in music occurring in a continuous pattern at an even rhythm.

Valsalva maneuver Holding the breath when a great deal of force is exerted (such as when lifting a very heavy weight), increasing thoracic pressure and possibly impeding venous blood return.

Value statement Feedback that projects a feeling about a performance, using words such as "good," "well done," or "poor job."

Vascular disturbances A disruption of circulation.

Vascularity An increase in the number and size of blood vessels enhancing blood supply and oxygen delivery to muscle cells.

Vasoconstriction Narrowing of the opening of blood vessels (notably the smaller arterioles) caused by contraction of the smooth muscle lining the vessels.

Vasodilation Widening of the openings of blood vessels caused by relaxation of the smooth muscle lining the vessels.

Vasopressin *See* Antidiuretic hormone (ADH).

Veins Blood vessels that carry deoxygenated blood toward the heart from vital organs and the extremities.

Ventilation Rate and depth of breathing.

Ventricles The two lower chambers of the heart (right and left ventricles).

Venules Smaller divisions of veins.

Vertebrae Bones that form the spinal column.

Viscous fibers A type of dietary fiber that helps lower serum cholesterol.

Vital signs Measurable bodily functions,

including pulse rate, respiratory rate, blood pressure, skin color, and temperature.

Vitamins Organic (carbon-containing) compounds required for optimal health that the body cannot manufacture on its own and must therefore be consumed.

V̇O₂max *See* Maximal oxygen uptake.

Waiver Voluntary abandonment of a right to file suit.

Water The most important nutrient in the body, responsible for all energy production, temperature control (especially during vigorous exercise), transportation of all nutrients and waste products in and out of the body, and lubrication of joints and other structures.

Water-soluble vitamins Vitamins that must be supplied daily, as the body excretes excess amounts (rather than stores them); includes vitamin C and the B-complex vitamins.

Wolff's law Principle stating that bone is capable of adjusting its strength in proportion to the amount of stress placed on it.

Index

ACE GROUP FITNESS INSTRUCTOR MANUAL

placenta, 278, 283
plaintiff, 332
plantar fasciitis, 292, 313, 318–19
plantarflexion, 53, 56, 58, 60, 292, 299
plantarflexors, 88, 89
plantaris muscle, 58, 59, 60, 88
plasma, 36
plasma proteins, 36
platelets, 36, 45
plyometric exercises, 79, 261–62, 317, 318
polycyclic aromatic hydrocarbons, 131, 132
polypropylene, 29
polysacchrides, 116
polyunsaturated fats, 119, 129
popliteal artery, 37
popliteal space, 62
popliteal vein, 38
popliteus muscle, 58, 59, 60, 87
positive feedback, 241
positive reinforcement, 223
posterior, 39
posterior compartment (sciatic nerve), 61
posterior cruciate ligament, 321
posterior deltoid, 105, 106
posterior deltoid fibers, 71
posterior hip muscles, 82–83
posterior intermuscular septum, 61
posterior knee muscles, 87–88
posterior leg muscles, 88
posterior pelvic tilt, 97, 297
posterior shin splints, common site of, 323
posterior shoulder girdle muscles, 100, 102–4
posterior tibial artery, 37
posterior tibial compartment muscles, 60
posterior tibialis muscle, 57, 58, 59, 60, 88
posterior tibial vein, 38
postpartum depression, 278, 304
postpartum exercise, 302–5
postpartum musculoskeletal conditions, 304–5
postpartum period, prenatal exercise benefits during, 277
postural alignment, during pregnancy, 282
postural deviations, 92
postural realignments, during pregnancy, 285–86
posture, 89–91
    abnormal and fatigue-related, 91–93
    and low-back strains and sprains, 325
    perception of, 44
posture/alignment cues, 91, 220–22, 325
posture imbalance, 315
potassium, 45, 47, 121, 124, 130
power step training, 378
power walking, 83
practice style of teaching, 208–9
Pre- and Post-Natal Fitness (ACE), 295, 306
pre-class evaluation, 315

pre-class preparation, 172, 193
pre-exercise health appraisal question-naire, 145–49
pregnancy
    absolute and relative contraindications to aerobic exercise during, 279
    back alignment for exercise, 295
    back pain and changes in posture, 91, 285–86
    birth weight among exercising mothers, 283–84
    cardiovascular system and, 280–81
    concern for fetal hyperthermia, 284–85
    concern of carbohydrate utilization, 283
    contraindications and risk factors of exercise during, 278–79
    contraindications to yoga, 387
    diastasis recti, 286–87
    dysfunctions and irritations, 285–92
    effect of exercise on mood states, 277
    energy needs, 137
    exercise benefits and risks, 137, 276–80
    exercise benefits during labor and delivery, 277–78
    exercise benefits during recovery, 278
    and fasting blood glucose levels, 284
    fetal risks associated with exercise, 282–85
    high-risk exercise and, 279–80
    and hypoglycemia, 137, 284
    increase in the oxygen cost of breathing, 281
    metabolic needs, 284
    muscle cramps, 292
    musculoskeletal system imbalances and dysfunctions, 281–82, 285–92
    nerve compression syndromes, 291
    normal weight gain, 282
    overuse syndromes, 291–92
    pelvic floor weakness, 286
    physiological adaptations, 280–85
    potential conflict between the circulatory demands of exercise and those of pregnancy, 283
    proper body mechanics for getting up from the floor, 289
    proper body mechanics for rising from the side-lying position to the sitting position, 288
    pubic pain, 289–90
    reasons to discontinue exercise and seek medical advice, 280
    respiratory system and, 281
    round, inguinal, and broad ligament irritations, 287–89
    sacroiliac joint dysfunction, 290
    sciatica, 290–91

    and venous return, 282
pregnancy-induced hypertension, 277
pregnant women, exercise programming for
    cardiovascular exercise, 292–94
    conditioning exercises, 294–300
    exercise classes and programs for, 292–302
    heart-rate response to exercise, 292
    hip flexor exercises, 296–97
    programming suggestions and modifications, 301–2
    specialized classes for, 293
    standing hip exercises, 297
prenatal class format, 303
President's Council on Physical Fitness, 164
previews, 218
primary bronchi, 40
prime movers, 80
principle of specificity of training, 176
privacy policy, 355–56
professional boundaries, 357
professionalism, 232–33, 354
progesterone, 281, 287
prognosis, 317
program design and implementation, 333, 352–53
    class activities and time allocations, 203, 205
    class goals, 202–3
    class objectives, 203
    facility and equipment considerations, 205–6
    lesson planning, 203
    patterns of class organization, 205
    risk-management criteria, 337
    selecting appropriate exercises, 206–8
progressions, 202, 314
progressive relaxation, 301
prolapse, of the bladder, uterus, and rectum, 286
promptness, 231
pronation, 52, 54, 56
    of the forearm, 67, 68, 70
    of the radioulnar joint, 55
pronator quadratus, 67, 68
pronator teres, 57, 67, 68, 70
prone hyperextension, 97
prone leg lift, 83
prone plank, with forearms on mat, 96
proprioception, 318
proprioceptive neuromuscular facilitation (PNF), 15
proprioceptors, 43, 44
protein, 3, 115, 117–18
    recommended healthy intakes/day for, 117
protein synthesis, 25

433